The Failed Spine

The Failed Spine

Editors

Marek Szpalski, M.D.
Chairman
Department of Orthopedics
Associate Professor
IRIS South Teaching Hospitals
Brussels, Belgium

Robert Gunzburg, M.D., Ph.D.
Senior Consultant
Department of Orthopedics
Centenary Clinic
Antwerp, Belgium

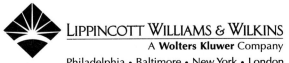
LIPPINCOTT WILLIAMS & WILKINS
A **Wolters Kluwer** Company
Philadelphia • Baltimore • New York • London
Buenos Aires • Hong Kong • Sydney • Tokyo

Acquisitions Editor: Robert Hurley
Developmental Editor: Jenny Kim
Project Manager: Bridgett Dougherty
Senior Manufacturing Manager: Benjamin Rivera
Marketing Director: Sharon Zinner
Production Service: Nesbitt Graphics, Inc.
Printer: Maple-Press

© 2005 by LIPPINCOTT WILLIAMS & WILKINS
530 Walnut Street
Philadelphia, PA 19106 USA
LWW.com

Printed in the USA

Library of Congress Cataloging-in-Publication Data
The failed spine / [edited by] Marek Szpalski, Robert Gunzburg.
    p. ; cm.
Includes index.
ISBN 0-7817-9613-X
    1. Spine—Surgery. 2. Spine—Reoperation. 3. Spine—Surgery—Complications.
4. Spine—Diseases—Physical therapy. 5. Spine—Diseases—Chiropractic treatment.
I. Szpalski, Marek. II. Gunzburg, Robert.
    [DNLM: 1. Spine—surgery. 2. Orthopedic Procedures—adverse effects.
3. Reoperation. 4. Spinal Diseases—surgery. WE 725 F1613 2005]
RD768.F33 2005
617.5'6059—dc22

          2004021702

Care has been taken to confirm the accuracy of the information presented and to describe
generally accepted practices. However, the authors, editors, and publisher are not responsible for errors or omissions or for any consequences from application of the information
in this book and make no warranty, expressed or implied, with respect to the currency,
completeness, or accuracy of the contents of the publication. Application of the information in a particular situation remains the professional responsibility of the practitioner.

The authors, editors, and publisher have exerted every effort to ensure that drug selection and dosage set forth in this text are in accordance with current recommendations and
practice at the time of publication. However, in view of ongoing research, changes in government regulations, and the constant flow of information relating to drug therapy and
drug reactions, the reader is urged to check the package insert for each drug for any change
in indications and dosage and for added warnings and precautions. This is particularly important when the recommended agent is a new or infrequently employed drug.

Some drugs and medical devices presented in the publication have Food and Drug Administration (FDA) clearance for limited use in restricted research settings. It is the responsibility of the health care provider to ascertain the FDA status of each drug or device
planned for use in their clinical practice.

10 9 8 7 6 5 4 3 2 1

Contents

Contributing Authors

Max Aebi *Professor and Chair, Institute for Evaluative Research in Orthopaedics, University of Bern, Bern, Switzerland; Chief of Staff, Orthopaedic Department, Salem Hospital, Bern, Switzerland*

Christophe Audic, M.D. *Service d'orthopédie traumatologie, CHU La Milétrie, 86021 Poitiers Cedex, France*

S. Aunoble *Spine Unit, CHU Pellegrin, Bordeaux, France*

Michel Benoist, M.D. *Consultant Rheumatologist of Paris Hospitals, University of Paris VII, Paris, France; Consultant in Rheumatology, Department of Orthopaedic Surgery, Hopital Beaujon, Clichy, France*

Alan Breen, D.C., Ph.D. *Professor of Musculoskeletal Health Care, Institute for Musculoskeletal Research and Clinical Implementation, AECC, Dorset, United Kingdom*

Dominique Brossard, CCAH *Chef de Clinique, Faculty of Medicine, Nantes University, Nantes, France; Chef de Clinique Assistant Hospitalier, Clinique Chirurgicale Orthopedique Centre Hospitalier, Regional Universitaire de Nantes, Nantes, France*

Florian Brunner, M.D. *Department of Physical Medicine and Rheumatology, Balgrist University Hospital, Zurich, Switzerland*

Frederic Camu, M.D. *Department of Anesthesiology and Pain Therapy, University of Brussels V.U.B. Medical Center, Brussels, Belgium*

Christine Cedraschi, Ph.D. *Research and Clinical Psychologist, Service of Internal Medicine for Rehabilitation and Multidisciplinary Pain Center Geneva, Service of Clinical Pharmacology and Toxicology, Geneva University Hospital, Geneva, Switzerland*

Erdal Coskun, M.D. *Associate Professor, Department of Neurosurgery, Department of Emergency Medicine, Pamukkale University, Denizli, Turkey; Chief of Emergency Medicine, Department of Neurosurgery, Department of Emergency Medicine, Pamukkale University Hospital, Denizli, Turkey*

Aina J. Danielsson, M.D., Ph.D. *Department of Orthopaedics, Sahlgrenska University Hospital, Göteborg University, Göteborg, Sweden*

Alain Deburge, M.D. *Department of Orthopedic Surgery, Beaujon Hospital, Clichy, France*

Joel Delécrin, M.D. *Associate Professor, Department of Orthopedic Surgery, Nantes University, Nantes, France; Associate Professor, Department of Orthopedic Surgery Hôtel Dieu Place Ricordeau, Nantes, France*

Stephen Eisenstein Ph.D., F.R.C.S. (Edin) *Director, Centre for Spinal Studies, Orthopaedic Institute, Keele University, Oswestry, Shropshire, United Kingdom;*

Consultant Orthopaedic Surgeon, Department for Spinal Disorders, The Robert Jones and Agnes Hunt Orthopaedic Hospital, Oswestry, Shropshire, United Kingdom

Amer Ibrahim EL-Kerdi, Ph.D., MoT (Exec) *Group Head, Faculty of Medicine, Institute for Evaluative Research in Orthopaedic Surgery, University of Bern, Bern, Switzerland*

Louis-Etienne Gayet, M.D. *Polyclinique du Maine, Laval, France*

Joseph W.M. Geurts, M.D., Ph.D. *Chief, Department of Anesthesiology Rijnstate Hospital, Arnhem, The Netherlands*

Dieter Grob *Kliniek Wilhelm Schulthess, Zurich, Switzerland*

Gerbrand J. Groen, M.D., Ph.D. *Associate Professor, Division of Perioperative Medicine, Anesthesiology & Pain Management, University Medical Center Utrecht, Utrecht, The Netherlands*

Alexander G. Hadjipavlou *Department of Orthopaedic Surgery and Traumatology, University of Crete at Heraklion*

Hamid Hamcha, M.D. *Service d'orthopédie traumatologie, CHU La Milétrie, France*

Tommy Hansson, M.D., Ph.D. *Professor, Department of Orthopaedics, Sahlgrenska Academy Göteborg University, Göteborg, Sweden*

J. Randy Jinkins, M.D., FACR, FEC *Department of Radiology, Downstate Medical Center, State University of New York, Brooklyn, New York*

Pavlos G. Katonis, M.D. *Assistant Professor of Orthopaedics, Department of Orthopaedics and Traumatology, University Hospital of Heraklion, Crete, Greece*

George M. Kontakis, M.D. *Assistant Professor, Department of Orthopaedics-Traumatology, University Hospital of Crete, Heraklion, Greece*

Jean Charles Le Huec *Spine Unit, CHU Pellegrin, Bordeaux, France*

Richel Lousberg, Ph.D. *Department of Anesthesiology Rijnstate Hospital, Arnhem, The Netherlands*

Lance M. McCracken, Ph.D. *Consultant Clinical Psychologist and Clinical Lead, Pain Management Unit, Royal National Hospital for Rheumatic Diseases, University of Bath, Bath, United Kingdom; Visiting Senior Fellow, Department of Psychology, University of Bath, Bath, United Kingdom*

A. Mehbod *Spine Unit, CHU Pellegrin, Bordeaux, France*

Maes Menno, M.D. *Staff Physician, Department of Radiology, University Hospital Antwerp, Edegem, Belgium*

Robert C. Mulholland, M.D. F.R.C.S. *Center for Spinal Studies and Surgery, Queen's Medical Center, University Hospital Nottingham, Nottingham, United Kingdom*

Alf L. Nachemson, M.D., Ph.D. *Professor Emeritus, Department of Orthopaedics, University of Göteborg, Göteborg, Sweden*

Margareta Nordin, P.T., Dr.Sci *Research Professor, Department of Orthopaedics and Environmental Health Sciences, Graduate School of Arts and Science and School of Medicine, New York University, New York, New York; Director, Occupational and*

Industrial Orthopaedic Center (OIOC), Hospital for Joint Diseases, New York University Medical Center, New York, New York

Richard B. North, M.D.   *Professor of Neurosurgery, Anesthesiology and Critical Care Medicine, John Hopkins Hospital, Baltimore, Maryland*

Özkan Özsarlak   *Department of Radiology, University of Antwerp, Belgium; Staff Member, Department of Radiology, Universitair Ziekenhuis Antwerpen, Antwerp, Edegem, Belgium*

Paul M. Parizel, M.D., Ph.D.   *Professor and Chair, Department of Radiology, University Hospital Antwerp, Belgium*

Norbert Passuti, M.D., Ph.D.   *Professor, Department of Orthopedic Surgery, Nantes University, Nantes, France; Chief, Department of Orthopedic Surgery, Hôtel Dieu Place Ricordeau, Nantes, France*

Pierre Pries, M.D.   *Service d'orthopédie traumatologie, CHU La Milétrie, 86021 POITIERS CEDEX*

Christoph P. Röder, M.D.   *Research Associate, Institute for Evaluative Research in Orthopedic Surgery, MEM Research Center for Orthopedic Surgery, University of Bern, Bern, Switzerland*

M. Romih   *Department of Orthopedic Surgery, Nantes, France*

Jacques Sénégas, M.D.   *Clinique St. Martin, Pessac, France*

Michael N. Tzermiadianos   *Department of Orthopaedic Surgery and Traumatology, University of Crete at Heraklion*

Luc Vanden Berghe, M.D.   *Orthopaedic Spine Surgeon, Department of Orthopaedic Surgery, Sint Lucas Hospitaal, Sint Lucas Laam, Brugge, Belgium*

Johan W. M. Van Goethem, M.D., Ph.D.   *Vice-Head Neuroradiology, Department of Radiology, University Hospital Antwerp, Edegem, Belgium*

Caroline Van Lersberghe, M.D.   *Department of Anesthesiology and Pain Therapy, University of Brussels V.U.B. Medical Center, Brussels, Belgium*

Roelof M.A.W. van Wijk, M.D., Ph.D.   *Clinical Senior Lecturer, Department of Anaesthesia and Intensive Care, Royal Adelaide Hospital/The University of Adelaide; Consultant, Department of Anaesthesia, The Queen Elizabeth Hospital, Adelaide SA, Australia*

Jan Van Zundert, M.D.   *Department of Anesthesiology and Multidisciplinary Pain Centre, Ziekenhuis Oost-Limburg, Genk, Belgium*

Gordon Waddell, M.D., D.Sc., F.R.C.S.   *Honorary Professor, Centre for Psychosocial and Disability Research, University of Cardiff, Cardiff, United Kingdom*

Sherri Weiser, Ph.D.   *Senior Manager, Psychological Services, Occupational and Industrial Orthopaedic Center (OIOC), Hospital for Joint Diseases, New York University Medical Center, New York, NY; Research Assistant Professor, Program of Ergonomics and Biomechanics, Environmental Health Sciences, Graduate School of Arts and Science, New York University, New York, NY*

Dr. H. (Herman) J. Wynne, Ph.D.   *WynneConsult E-learning, Amsterdam, The Netherlands*

Preface

There is no such thing as "just a little operation" and indeed, every operation has its complications. Sometimes these complications can prevent the reaching of the goal set before the intervention. Although, the operation has then actually failed, this is seldom said in so many words. In spine pathology, however, the goal to be reached is often unclear or interpreted differently by the medical team, the patient, or his/her environment. Only in spine surgery does one refer to "failed surgery." At times it is even put forward as diagnosis or even an indication for further surgery. In this book we have tried to bring together a group of experts in their respective fields with the purpose to address this delicate topic of "failed spine surgery."

Pain is often a deciding factor leading to surgery on the spine. It is therefore important to understand and evaluate this pain perception. The origin of nociception and psychosocial determinants of pain are analysed and central modulation of pain are discussed. Multifactorial and demographic aspects of pain perception are presented.

The definition of the concept of "failed spine" varies for different parts of the spine. These aspects are discussed in depth and the failures of medical treatment are taken on as a separate entity.

Specific operations each can lead to an array of "failed spine" concepts. Some of the important entities are discussed individually: fusion surgery, discectomy surgery, postoperative scoliosis, iatrogenic "flat back."

From this overview it appears imperative to improve patient selection and to be aware of the "alarm flags" before embarking on surgery. These factors are analysed and discussed. A treatment algorithm is proposed.

A "failed spine" does not necessarily require further surgery. Medications as well as physical therapy have a place in the management. Often, however, more invasive specific pain therapy is proposed. Neurostimulation and radiofrequency procedures are updated and epiduroscopy presented. When iterative surgery is proposed, however, there is always the choice between repeat surgery or the utilization of a different surgical technique or approach...

All these considerations lead us to wonder if it is not the surgeon who at times fails...

Finally some economic aspects of "failed spine" are touched on. The cost-efficacy of different procedures is analyzed and the need for central registration stressed.

Marek Szpalski, M.D.
Robert Gunzburg, M.D., Ph.D.

1

Psychosocial Factors and Surgical Outcomes

Christine Cedraschi

INTRODUCTION

The research on the determinants of pain in chronic low back problems or in the development of chronicity has moved from the search for a linear model of causality to taking into consideration the interplay among predisposing, precipitating, and perpetuating factors. Among these factors, psychosocial aspects have received considerable attention. This is not surprising because chronic pain is part of a dynamic process that results from a continual interaction among somatic, psychological, and social factors. Thus, in a multicausal perspective, identifying a factor as a predictor at one stage does not preclude the possibility that this factor may also be a consequence of pain and suffering (34). To tackle the psychosocial dimensions in no way implies the denial of somatic aspects. Indeed, studies on back pain often refer to a multicausal model, that is, a number of psychological, social, demographic, and physical aspects are considered simultaneously, whether regarding surgical or nonsurgical treatment outcomes. Such a model acknowledges the multifaceted nature of the back pain problem as well as the considerable overlap that exists among psychological variables (e.g., coping and depression).

The importance of psychosocial processes in chronic pain and the causal role of chronic pain in the development of psychosocial dysfunction have been repeatedly acknowledged over the years (12,30,48,58). Data also point to psychological factors in acute and subacute pain (6,28,59), and Linton's systematic review (28) underlines that these factors are related to pain from its inception to the chronic stage. As Main and Williams (31) have stressed, "for the vast majority of patients, the identification of contributory psychological and social factors should be seen as an investigation of the normal range of reactions to pain rather than the seeking of psychopathology."

Various studies have investigated psychological factors as outcome predictors of surgical interventions and/or assessed the consequences of surgery on psychological variables. These studies have examined these questions in the context of diverse surgical procedures: for example, they have underlined the need to address scarcity in the knowledge of outcome predictors or in the information about the psychosocial profile of the candidates for fusion surgery (17,18); they have also raised the question of the influence of these factors in the explanation of failures of lumbar discectomy even when morphological problems have been adequately managed by surgery (45).

This chapter presents an overview of the following psychosocial categories: anxiety, distress, and depression; representations, expectations, and satisfaction; pain behaviors and coping strategies; and social factors. It focuses on the role of these aspects in the outcomes of surgery.

ANXIETY, DISTRESS, AND DEPRESSION

Anxiety, distress, and depression have been reported in various studies. Exploring the association between distress (as assessed by anxiety and depression scales) and surgical outcome, Trief et al. (53) showed that subjects who were working 1 year after surgery had reported lower levels of distress before surgery than those who were disabled. The same was true for those who reported improved back and leg pain and those who reported functional gains in activities of daily living at the time of follow-up. Similarly, Schade et al. (45) have demonstrated that depression, but not anxiety, remained a significant predictor of surgical outcome in terms of pain relief and in terms of return to work after controlling for preoperative pain and disability. Various other studies have pointed to the association between depression and poorer outcomes of spine surgery (23,41,55).

In contrast with these findings, the report from the Swedish Lumbar Spine Study comparing the importance of predictors of functional and work status outcome in surgical and nonsurgical treatment (18) did not evidence any significant association between depressive symptoms and surgical outcome. The results showed, however, that pretreatment depressive symptoms predicted improvement in the nonsurgical group. Besides, self-rated improvement was associated with a decrease of depressive symptoms in both groups. Similarly, preoperative psychological distress was not a predictor of the functional status after surgical treatment in Tandon et al.'s study (50), but it was associated with a trend toward more important self-reported disability at baseline. In contrast, changes in distress were significantly associated with changes in disability, with patients reporting improvement also showing reduced distress. In light of these results and because decreased depression is linked with successful treatment, it has been concluded that depressive symptoms (18) or distress (15,50) are not an obvious contraindication to surgery.

Divergences in the results regarding the role of anxiety, distress, and depression may be related to various factors such as the diagnosis, the time frame (acute or chronic pain), and also the duration of pain before the intervention with treatment delays, which increases the likelihood of poor functional outcome (53). The preoperative work status as well as psychological aspects of work may be involved. Indeed, Schade et al. (45) have evidenced that return to work after surgery was best predicted by depression and occupational mental stress. Furthermore, preoperative selection process may also play a role: Hägg et al. (17,18) have stressed that, most probably due to their preoperative selection, the chronic low back pain surgical candidates included in their study displayed lower rates of major depression than patients in rehabilitation programs.

The association between depression or distress and surgical outcome is still an area open for debate, regarding its nature but also with respect to the possible role of other intervening variables. Rush et al. (44) have pointed out that when depression is present, it influences the pain and may, in turn, be influenced by the level of pain. However, not all chronic back pain patients suffer from clinical depression. It is thus of major importance to be clear about the distinction between clinical depression, on the one hand, and depressed mood that may not fit into a psychopathological model, on the other hand. It has been pointed out that whereas chronic pain patients may experience various levels of distress because of pain and its consequences in everyday life, they may not display the self-denigratory views and feelings that characterize clinical depression (35); this would argue for the need of a new model to account for the interaction between depression and chronic pain (42).

REPRESENTATIONS, EXPECTATIONS, AND SATISFACTION

Patients' views and patient-oriented outcomes are increasingly acknowledged, including representations or beliefs about illness, expectations of treatment, and satisfaction with treatment. Representations have been defined as "that knowledge which is formed from our experience, but also by information, learning, models of thought which we receive and transmit by tradition, education, social communication. Thus it is . . . a socially elaborated and shared knowledge" (22). It is practical knowledge to help us master our environment, to understand and explain our universe (36). Representations about health and illness—as well as expectations—exist before pain begins, but they are developed at the onset of back pain and are important determinants of affect and behavior. These representations are of particular importance when discussing the various aspects of treatment as they influence the way patients organize the information they receive, and thus patient expectations and behaviors. In clinical terms, this implies that according to the patients' prior representations, new information may be integrated, modified, or even discarded (37).

Patients' expectations about treatment have been shown to influence the outcomes; that is, functional improvement, for example, can be linked not only to the intrinsic value of treatment but also to the patients' expectations of its possible benefits. Kalauokalani et al. (24) conducted a study with chronic low back pain patients randomized in two treatment groups: either acupuncture or massage. Patients' expectations about these treatments had been investigated beforehand. The results displayed a statistically and clinically more important improvement in those patients who had received the treatment they believed in. Similarly, Lutz et al. (29) showed that patients with higher expectations of surgery had better outcomes than those with lower expectations. Iversen et al. (21) found that patients with many preoperative expectations tended to improve more than those with fewer expectations. More ambitious expectations for physical function were also associated with improved function and satisfaction with physical function; however, high expectations for pain relief were associated with greater report of pain and decreased satisfaction with pain relief, thus suggesting that these types of expectations should be addressed differently in preoperative discussions.

Investigating the relationship between expected results and actual outcomes, McGregor & Hughes (33) assessed patient expectations of surgery, and satisfaction with outcome in terms of pain, function, disability, and general health at 6 weeks, 6 months, and 1 year. The results showed that patients had high expectations of recovery and were confident of achieving this recovery. As for satisfaction, however, patients' reports at all review stages indicate that surgery had achieved only part of what they had expected, suggesting patients had unrealistic expectations leading to lower satisfaction levels.

Unrealistic expectations may influence patient outcome, whatever the type of treatment. Szpalski and Gunzburg (49) have stressed that unrealistic expectations not only in the patient but also in the surgeon may lead to poor outcomes. They may also add to abnormal pain behavior as well as hinder coping and function (46). When unrealistic expectations are set, they might prove difficult to change. Furthermore, delusion may result from failure to meet these expectations and thus lead to disruptions in the patient-therapist relationship and doctor-shopping behavior in the patient. The classical biomedical model sets the premise for a view of the body as a repairable machine whose damaged parts can be replaced or at least fixed (20). This machine model of the body may create unrealistic expectations in the mind of therapists and patients as well, without satisfactory results either for the patient or for the therapist.

Results from other studies further stress the multidimensional aspects of patient satisfaction. Patients' opinion regarding the success of surgery may yield better results than functional scores (14,41) or return to work rates (47). Atlas et al. (2) showed that surgical treatment for sciatica was associated with better results than nonsurgical treatment in terms of symptoms, functional status, and satisfaction. However, this had no significant impact either on disability or work outcomes at 5 years. The authors note that disability and work status are not related to treatment only, whereas symptoms and daily functioning may be more directly influenced by treatment, thus suggesting that patient-oriented outcomes be assessed in addition to work and disability and reported separately.

Measuring patients' satisfaction is a complex issue. As Atlas (3) summarized,

> Satisfaction is a simple concept for patients to understand, but it is a complex, multidimensional outcome measure for interested researchers. It incorporates a broad range of distinct concepts, including patient beliefs about what a treatment can provide, expectations about what the patient wants from treatment, the absolute level of symptoms and disability at baseline and follow-up, a self-rating of the relative change in outcome, and a rating of the process associated with the treatment itself.

Capturing the patient's view of change is a critical issue whenever the results of a study are likely to be applied in clinical practice (11). Comparing two methods in measurement of changes in pain and disability, that is, serial (two points in time) versus retrospective (one point in time), Fischer et al. (11) demonstrated poor agreement between both methods, with retrospective assessments displaying higher correlations with patient satisfaction. Their comments emphasize that retrospective measurements detect a particular perception of outcome insofar as serial measures are focused on a specific variable at a distinctive point in time, whereas retrospective measures capture to some extent the patient's general experience of a change over time. Retrospective measurements would thus shift the assessment toward a more composite appraisal, of greater potential relevance to the patient. As the authors stress, these results do not argue for replacing serial measures but for complementing them with the patients' retrospective evaluation of the change. Similarly, Zanoli et al. (60) demonstrated that a direct question on change in pain and the absolute visual analogue scale correlated better with patient satisfaction than calculated scores. These studies raise very interesting issues and point to the multidimensional nature of the processes involved in the patients' appraisal. They may partly account for the fact that, in spite of low levels of satisfaction, the majority of the patients may still say they had made the right decision to have surgery (33).

Patient representations of beliefs, expectations, and satisfaction are very problematic. How far patient expectations predict or influence outcomes is not yet clear. Furthermore, the nature of the relationship between expectation fulfillment and patient satisfaction is still confused (43). Clinically, when it comes to allowing patients to develop realistic expectations, it is important to provide them with information about the possibilities but also the limits of the investigation, the treatment and the course of treatment, what can reasonably be expected in the case as well as advice and reassurance about resuming daily activities (38).

PAIN BEHAVIORS AND COPING STRATEGIES

Pain behaviors refer to any physical or verbal attempt on the part of the patient to communicate suffering and disability. They include grimacing, bracing, guarding, groaning, limping, overreacting and duration of inactivity (25,57). Pain behaviors in the acute stage can be seen as appropriate and adaptive in order to avoid further injury, whereas they have no therapeutic value in the chronic stage. Instead, they perpetuate the patient's adoption of the sick role and are therefore maladaptive. Pain behaviors are therefore often targeted as intervention outcomes in chronic pain patients. Coping refers to "constantly changing cognitive and behavioural efforts to manage external and/or internal demands that are appraised as taxing or exceeding the resources of the person" (27). Coping, in this context, refers to cognitive and/or behavioral attempts to manage pain, that is, to render it more tolerable, to reduce its interferences in everyday life.

Whether pain behaviors and coping strategies are associated with outcomes of surgery is unclear. Hasenbring et al. (19) and Junge et al. (23) reported contradictory findings regarding the predictive value of coping strategies such as "general avoidance," "non-verbal pain behavior," and "search for social support" on the functional status after surgery. The Swedish Lumbar Spine Study showed no association between pain behaviors and patient global assessment of treatment effects or work status at follow-up (18).

Because functional outcomes may partly rely on patient self-management and active participation in the recovery process, the identification of cognitive and behavioral factors amenable to change and of treatment strategies favoring these changes is of considerable interest. A recent randomized trial compared the effectiveness of behavioral graded activity versus usual care provided by physiotherapists following first-time lumbar disc surgery in mostly chronic low back pain patients (39). It was expected that behavioral graded activity would alter fear of movement and pain catastrophizing and thus lead to improved functional status and higher rates of recovery. However, the results did not meet these expectations. Neither fear of movement nor pain catastrophizing seemed to be affected by the treatment program, be it behavioral graded activity or usual care. Furthermore, no between-group differences were observed regarding functional status, pain, general health, social functioning, and return to work, leading Ostelo et al. (39) to conclude that treatment principles derived from theories within the field of chronic low back pain might not apply to these patients. Another trial comparing the effectiveness of lumbar fusion surgery associated with postoperative physiotherapy versus a cognitive intervention associated with exercises in patients with chronic low back pain showed a decrease of fear-avoidance beliefs in the cognitive intervention group and equal improvements in both groups regarding back pain, use of analgesics, emotional distress, life satisfaction, and return to work at 1-year follow-up (5).

Studies assessing the effectiveness of active postsurgery rehabilitation hardly address pain-related fear aspects (39,40). Yet the body of evidence regarding pain-related fear and its mediating role in the initiation and maintenance of chronic disability in musculoskeletal pain emphasizes the importance of fear avoidance and its consequences (56) as well as that of coping and catastrophizing (54). Addressing the role of these aspects in surgical candidates as well as in postoperative interventions warrants further investigation. Indeed, as Hägg et al. (18) have noted, "An expectation of improvement after surgery alone relies on a hypothesis that surgery eliminates a sole or dominating reason for pain. Knowing that many patients develop various dysfunctional strategies as a response to chronic pain, e.g., catastrophizing and fear of movements, it may well be that successful long-term treatment also requires specific post-operative measures to overcome those."

SOCIAL FACTORS

The evaluation of social factors include variables that originate outside the individual. The measure of these factors may rely on patient self-reports and be colored by subjective perception, thus blurring the distinction between psychological and social variables.

Much research has been done in the area of chronic pain and families, but there is less ample evidence regarding the role of social support in the outcome of surgery. Reinforcement of pain behavior by the spouse has been found to reduce spine surgery benefits (10). Commenting on similar results, Schade et al. (45) nevertheless underline the multifactorial dimension of social support that may contain a tendency of the spouse to be overprotective and to encourage passivity and social companionship associated with recreational activities that may contribute to help reducing disability.

The most important bulk of research pertains to work-related aspects. Job satisfaction has been associated with low back pain disability. Similarly, psychological aspects of work, that is, occupational mental stress, general job satisfaction, and job-related resignation, were shown to be related to postoperative pain relief and disability (45).

Compensation status has often been implicated in the development of chronic low back pain. A number of studies have evaluated the role of compensation status on various outcomes of surgery, displaying contradictory results (1,32). Taylor et al. (51) examined the differences in the surgical treatment of patients covered by workers' compensation and those with other sources of payment; they showed that workers' compensation coverage was associated with a higher likelihood of receiving a fusion procedure and an increased risk of reoperation. Commenting on their results, the authors note that patients receiving compensation may be less likely to return to work, which may lead to more aggressive investigations to identify the causes of pain and reoperation attempts; they also suggest that surgeons may have a lower threshold for performing spinal fusion and reoperation in manual workers. In a community-based study, preoperative compensation payments and consultation with an attorney were shown to be negatively associated with pain relief and physical activity 1 year after surgery (52). Similarly, the presence of a compensation claim was found to be a significant prognostic factor with respect to clinical results such as satisfaction and disability scores (14).

Yet a 10-year follow-up study indicated that the negative effects of compensation on satisfaction and disability scores results seem to dissipate with time (41). Mayer et al. (32) contend that surgical interventions in disabled workers' compensation patients may have successful objective outcomes if accompanied by effective rehabilitation. Likewise, an intervention study conducted in a social security sickness fund on mandatorily insured patients emphasizes the importance of postoperative rehabilitation. This study was conducted in Belgium where medical advisers of sickness funds play an important legal role in the evaluation of working capacity and rehabilitation measures (9). This study evidenced increased return to work rates after lumbar disc surgery when medical advisers applied a rehabilitation program focused on early mobilization and return to work rather than the usual claim-based practice. Paralleling the results of other studies (e.g., 18,23,53), this study found the duration of preoperative work incapacity to be a negative predictor of outcome. In a prospective 4-year follow-up study, Atlas et al. (1) assessed the influence of workers' compensation status in operatively and nonoperatively managed patients with sciatica. The results showed that patients who had been receiving workers' compensation at baseline were more likely to be receiving disability benefits and to report less relief from symptoms and improvement in quality of life at the time of follow-up. However, they were only slightly less likely to be working at the time of follow-up. As for surgical versus nonsurgical management groups, the outcomes were comparable with respect to disability and work status, but operative management decreased symptoms and improved functional status, whether or not patients had been receiving workers' compensation at baseline.

The results also showed that patients who had been receiving workers' compensation at baseline were more likely to be young, male, less educated, and involved in physically demanding jobs. These findings parallel those of other studies regarding the association among formal education, back-related disability level, and back-related continued disability. Various factors may account for this association, including job characteristics (e.g., occupational category and strength requirement of the job, lack of job autonomy or of decision latitude, or difficulty in obtaining lighter duties during a back pain episode) but also patients' expectations. Patients' expectation of continued pain was found to be significantly associated with education on the one hand and with continued disability on the other (8). Similarly, it has been shown that manual workers, especially when unskilled, are less likely to remain in work than those in nonmanual occupations if they have a limiting illness. This is all the more so when unemployment rates are high (4).

Hence work status may be related to factors originating outside the patient or the treatment, such as job characteristics or physical accommodations in the workplace, but also local socioeconomic context or sickness and invalidity legislation. Compensation is highly dependent on the specifics of each country's health care system (13,16). These specifics may account for part of divergences in the results, along with different outcome measures, type of patients or of surgery, as well as differences in follow-up durations.

CONCLUSION

Although the complexity of the dynamic processes involved in pain makes the distinction between various psychological and social variables to some extent artificial, this division pointed to the contribution of these factors in the course of pain and in the outcomes of treatment. This overview hinted at contradictory findings but it also raised comparability issues in terms of type of patients, surgery, time frame, duration of follow-up, or outcome measures. Besides, because it is likely that many of these psychological and social variables share predictive variance, their impact can only be determined in multicausal models.

When it comes to clinical considerations, the importance of the patient-physician relationship needs to be emphasized. Various studies have shown that reassurance provided by the physician, personal interest, providing medical information, and careful listening are important components of patient satisfaction insofar as they go a long way toward meeting the patients' perceived needs. These needs include the reduction of both the cognitive and the emotional uncertainty in a situation of stress and vulnerability, which may in turn be associated with distress. In such situations, it is crucial to investigate what patients think is wrong, what their representations are of what is happening, as well as their reactions to pain and its consequences (7,26). Indeed, symptoms affect patients' perceptions of what might be wrong (cognitive states) and reactions to pain and illness (emotional states) so that perception and interpretation of symptoms influence expectations—realistic or unrealistic—and satisfaction and may thus contribute to defining what a meaningful or acceptable outcome might be. The patient-physician encounter is a cornerstone because it allows for the discussion and the negotiation of the patient's expectations so that congruent decisions can be made, taking into account medical evidence and patient values and health preferences. However, this shared decision-making approach does not involve only the patient and his or her therapist(s), but also family members, employers, and insurance providers. Meaningful goals may be different for each stakeholder. Incongruity among surgeon, employer, insurance representative, spouse, and patient expectations may have a negative impact on outcome, even if the patient achieves his or her goals. Thus goals should be clearly stated from all viewpoints at the onset of treatment, and mutually acceptable outcomes should be negotiated with the patient for the best results. This is all the more crucial for spinal surgery when the matter at stake may be the risk of failed spine.

REFERENCES

1. Atlas SJ, Chang Y, Kamman E, Keller RB, Deyo RA, Singer DE. Long-term disability and return to work among patients who have a herniated lumbar disc: the effect of disability compensation. J Bone Joint Surg 2000; 82:4-15.
2. Atlas SJ, Keller RB, Chang Y, Deyo RA, Singer DE. Surgical and nonsurgical management of sciatica secondary to a lumbar disc herniation. Five-years outcomes from the Maine Lumbar Spine Study. Spine 2001; 26:1179-87.
3. Atlas SJ. Point of view. Spine 2002; 27:1476-7.
4. Bartley M, Owen C. Relation between socioeconomic status, employment, and health during economic change, 1973-93. BMJ 1996; 313: 445-9.
5. Brox JI, Sorensen R, Friis A, Nygaard O, Indahl A, Keller A, et al. Randomized clinical trial of lumbar instrumented fusion and congitive intervention and exercises in patients with chronic low back pain and disc degeneration. Spine 2003; 28:1913-21.
6. Burton AK, Tillotson KM, Main CJ, Hollis S. Psychosocial predictors of outcome in acute and subchronic low back trouble. Spine 1995; 20:722-8.
7. Charles C, Gafni A, Whelan T. Shared-decision making in the medical encounter: what does it mean? (or it takes at least two to tango). Soc Sci Med 1997; 44:681-92.
8. Dionne C, Koepsell TD, Von Korff M, Deyo RA, Barlow WE, Checkoway H. Formal education and back-related disability. In search of an explanation. Spine 1995; 20:2721-30.
9. Donceel P, Du Bois M, Lahaye D. Return to work after surgery for lumbar disc herniation. Spine 1999; 24:872-6.
10. Epker J, Block AR. Presurgical psychological screening in back pain patients: a review. Clin J Pain 2001; 17:200-5.
11. Fischer D, Stewart AL, Bloch DA, Lorig K, Laurent D, Holman H. Capturing the patients' view of change as a clinical outcome measure. JAMA 1999; 282:1157-62.
12. Fordyce W. Psychological factors in the failed back. Int Disab Studies 1988; 10:29-31.
13. Fordyce WE, ed. Back pain in the workplace. management of disability in nonspecific conditions. Seattle: International Association of the Study of Pain (IASP) Press, 1995.
14. Greenough CG, Peterson MD, Fraser RD. Instrumented posterolateral lumbar fusion. Results and comparison with anterior interbody fusion. Spine 1998; 23:479-86.
15. Greenough CG. Point of view. Spine 1999; 24:1838.
16. Hadler NM. Disabling backache in France, Switzerland, and the Netherlands: Contrasting sociopolitical constraints on clinical judgment. J Occup Med 1989; 31:823-31.
17. Hägg O, Fritzell P, Nordwall A, and the Swedish Lumbar Spine Study Group. Characteristics of patients with chronic low back pain selected for surgery. Spine 2002, 27:1223-31.
18. Hägg O, Fritzell P, Ekselius L, Nordwall A. Predictors of outcome in fusion surgery for chronic low back pain. Eur Spine J 2003; 12:22-33.
19. Hasenbring M, Marienfeld G, Kuhlendahl D, Soyka D. Risk factors of chronicity in lumbar disc patients. Spine 1994; 19:2759-65.
20. Helman CG. The body image in health and disease: exploring patients' maps of body and self. In: Assal JP, Golay A, Visser AP (eds.), New trends in patient education: a trans-cultural and inter-disease approach. Amsterdam: Elsevier, 1995; 169-75.
21. Iversen MD, Daltroy LH, Fossel AH, Katz JN. The prognostic importance of patient pre-operative expectations of surgery for lumbar spinal stenosis. Patient Educ Counsel 1998; 34:169-78.
22. Jodelet D: Représentation sociale: phénomènes, concept et théorie. In Moscovici S (ed.), Psychologie Sociale. Paris: Presses Universitaires de France, 1984.
23. Junge A, Fröhlich M, Ahrens S, Hasenbring M, Sandler AJ, Grob D, Dvorak J. Predictors of bad and good outcome of lumbar spine surgery. Spine 1996; 21:1056-64.
24. Kalauokalani D, Cherkin DC, Sherman KJ, Koepsell TD, Deyo RA. Lessons from a trial of acupuncture and massage for low back pain. Patient expectations and treatment effects. Spine 2001; 26:1418-24.
25. Keefe FJ, Block, AR. Development of an observation method for assessing pain behavior in chronic low back pain patients. Behav Ther 1992; 13:363-75.
26. Kravitz RL. Measuring patients' expectations and requests. Ann Intern Med 2001; 134:881-8.
27. Lazarus RS, Folkman S. Stress, appraisal, and coping. New-York: Springer, 1984.
28. Linton SJ. A review of psychological risk factors in back and neck pain. Spine 2000; 25:1148-56.
29. Lutz GK, Butzlaff ME, Atlas SJ, Keller RB, Singer DE, Deyo RA. The relationship between expectations and outcomes in surgery for sciatica. J Gen Intern Med 1999; 14:740-4.
30. Main CJ, Spanswick CC. Pain management: an interdisciplinary approach. Edinburgh: Churchill Livingstone, 2000.
31. Main CJ, Williams A. Musculoskeletal pain. BMJ 2002; 325:534-7.
32. Mayer T, McMahon MJ, Gatchel RJ, Sparks B, Wright A, Pegues P. Socio-economic outcomes of combined spine surgery and functional restoration in worker's compensation spinal disorders with matched controls. Spine 1998; 23:598-605.
33. McGregor AH, Hughes SPF. The evaluation of the surgical management of nerve root compression in patients with low back pain. Part 2: Patient expectations and satisfaction. Spine 2002; 27:1471-7.

34. Melzack R, Wall PD. The challenge of pain. New York: Penguin, 1982.
35. Morley S, Williams A, Black S. A confirmatory factor analysis of the Beck Depression Inventory in chronic pain. Pain 2002; 99:289-98.
36. Moscovici S: The phenomenon of social representations. In: Farr RM, Moscovici S (eds.), Social representations. Oxford, Paris: Cambridge University Press, 1984.
37. Moscovici S, Hewstone M: De la science au sens commun. In: Moscovici S (ed.), Psychologie Sociale. Paris: Presses Universitaires de France, 1984.
38. Nordin M, Cedraschi C, Skovron ML. Patient-health care provider relationship in patients with non-specific low back pain: a review of some problem situations. In: Nordin M, Cedraschi C, Vischer TL (eds.), New approaches to the low back pain patient. Bailliere's Clin Rheumatol 1998; 12:1:75-92.
39. Ostelo RWJG, de Vet HCW, Vlaeyen JWS, Kerkhoffs MR, Berfelo WM, Wolters PMJC, van den Brandt PA. Behavioral graded activity following first-time lumbar disc surgery. 1-year results of a randomized clinical trial. Spine 2003a; 28:1757-65.
40. Ostelo RWJG, de Vet HCV, Waddell G, Kerkhoffs MR, Leffers P, van Tulder M. Rehabilitation following first-time lumbar disc surgery. A systematic review within the framework of the Cochrane Collaboration. Spine 2003b; 28:209-18.
41. Penta M, Fraser RD. Anterior lumbar interbody fusion. A minimum 10-year follow-up. Spine 1997; 22:2429-34.
42. Pincus T, Williams A. Models and measurements of depression in chronic pain. J Psychosom Res 1999; 47:211-9.
43. Rao JK, Weinberger M, Kroenke K. Visit-specific expectations and patient-centered outcomes. Arch Fam Med 2000; 9:1148-55.
44. Rush AJ, Polatin P, Gatchel RJ. Depression and chronic low back pain. Establishing priorities in treatment. Spine 2000; 25:2566-71.
45. Schade V, Semmer N, Main CJ, Hora J, Boos N. The impact of clinical, morphological, psychosocial and work-related factors on the outcome of lumbar discectomy. Pain 1999; 80:239-49.
46. Schofferman J, Reynolds J, Herzog R, Covington E, Dreyfuss P, O'Neill C. Failed back surgery: etiology and diagnostic evaluation. Spine J 2003; 3:400-3.
47. Slosar PJ, Reynolds JB, Schofferman J, Goldtwaite N, White AH, Keaney D. Patient satisfaction after circumferential lumbar fusion. Spine 2000; 25:722-6.
48. Sternbach R. The psychology of pain. New York: Raven Press, 1978.
49. Szpalsky M, Gunzburg R. The role of surgery in the management of low back pain. In: Nordin M, Cedraschi C, Vischer TL (eds.), New approaches to the low back pain patient. Bailliere's Clin Rheumatol 1998; 12-1:141-59.
50. Tandon V, Campbell F, Ross ERS. Posterior lumbar interbody fusion. Association between disability and psychological disturbance in noncompensation patients. Spine 1999; 24:1833-38.
51. Taylor VM, Deyo RA, Ciol M, Kreuter W. Surgical treatment of patients with back problems covered by workers compensation versus those with other sources of payment. Spine 1996; 21:2255-9.
52. Taylor VM, Deyo RA, Ciol M, Farrar EL, Lawrence MS, Shonnard NH, Leek KM, McNeney B, Goldberg HI. Patient-oriented outcomes from low back surgery. A community-based study. Spine 2000; 25:2445-52.
53. Trief PM, Grant W, Frederickson B. A prospective study of psychological predictors of lumbar surgery outcome. Spine 2000: 25:2616-21.
54. Turner JA, Jensen MP, Romano JM. Do beliefs, coping, and catastrophizing independently predict functioning in patients with chronic pain? Pain 2000; 85:115-25.
55. Van Susante J, Van de Schaaf D, Pavlov P. Psychological distress deteriorates the subjective outcome of lumbosacral fusion. A prospective study. Acta Orthop Belg 1998; 64:371-7.
56. Vlaeyen JWS, Linton SL. Fear-avoidance and its consequences in chronic musculoskeletal pain: a state of the art. Pain 2000; 85:317-22.
57. Waddell G. Understanding the patient with back pain. In: Jayson M (ed.), The lumbar spine and back pain (3rd ed.). Edinburgh: Churchill Livingstone, 1987.
58. Waddell G. A new clinical model for the treatment of low back pain. Spine 1987; 12:632-44.
59. Weiser S, Cedraschi C. Psychosocial issues in the prevention of low back pain—a literature review. In: Nordin M, Vischer TL (eds.), Common low back pain: prevention of chronicity. Baillieres' Clin Rheumtol 1992; 6-3:657-84.
60. Zanoli G, Strömqvist B, Jönsson B. Visual Analog Scales for interpretation of back and leg pain intensity in patients operated for degenerative lumbar spine disorders. Spine 2001; 26:2375-80.

3

In Vivo Effects of Iatrogenic Injuries of the Spine on Intervertebral Motion and Biomechanics

Tommy Hansson

Several potential iatrogenic injury mechanisms are related to surgical treatment of spinal disorders. The mechanisms range from those unavoidable injuries to the fascias, muscles, and ligaments that even the most skilled and careful surgeon has to excise (e.g., the painful disc herniation or freeing the compressed nerve roots in the cauda equina in spinal stenosis) to unnecessary or damaging dissection or removal of active or passive stabilizing structures. Whether the injuries are premeditated or not, some will heal without any significant sequelae, whereas others may generate detectable profound pathological changes, however hard or impossible it is to relate them correctly to a certain injury.

This chapter evaluates the immediate, acute, and late chronic effects of different iatrogenic injuries to the intervertebral joint in vivo and in vitro. At least hypothetically, an iatrogenic injury can involve all the different tissues in and around the spine. If such an injury changes the biomechanics of the spine, its consequences most probably will materialize at or around the intervertebral joint. The most likely consequence of a direct or indirect injury is that it causes or accelerates a degenerative process of the intervertebral joint and especially the disc. Other injuries to passive or active structures around the spine might alter the motion, kinematics, between the vertebrae in such a way to cause acute as well as chronic changes also to the intervertebral joint.

This chapter presents results from studies of static and dynamic properties of the intervertebral disc at different grades of degeneration but also the acute and long-standing effects in vivo, with and without muscular activity on the spinal kinematics of sequential experimental injuries to different structures of the intervertebral joint.

THE INTERVERTEBRAL JOINT

Determinations of the mechanical properties of the human spinal column are of significance for understanding the biomechanical and thus the clinical behavior of the spine under both normal and pathological conditions. In its normal role, the spine is a complex structure capable of motion in three planes: to transfer loads between adjacent vertebrae, to stabilize the spine, and to protect the spinal cord and the nerve roots in the cauda equina.

The motion segment consisting of two vertebrae and the intervening intervertebral joint (disc and facets) is the basic functional unit of the spine. During normal motions and daily activities, the motion segment is subjected to a combination of compression, torsional, and bending loads. The loads might be of a static or dynamic nature.

Changes within the disc because of factors like normal aging (degeneration of the disc) and injuries (iatrogenic or noniatrogenic) to different extents may compromise the mechanical resistance of the disc and consequently the other part of the intervertebral joint.

MECHANICAL PROPERTIES OF NORMAL AND DEGENERATED DISCS

Many studies have demonstrated that the mechanical properties of the spine are influenced by both the duration and the frequency of the applied load (12,17–20). The effect of duration is indicated when the spine is subjected to a static load. Here it behaves in a viscoelastic manner; that is, it deforms (strains) with time or undergoes creep when subjected to a static load. Dynamic loads produce deformations (strains) as well but now depend on the rate and frequency of the applied loads. Both static and dynamic biomechanical experiments can provide valuable information on the structural stability and competence of the intervertebral joint, irrespective of the injury mechanisms to the joint. To determine the effects of degeneration on compressive mechanical behavior, normal and degenerated human lumbar motion spine segments can be tested in a static or dynamic way.

Static in Vitro Testing

A static test model subjects intact human motion segments to a constant load corresponding to the estimated body weight above each segment (15). In this experiment, a total of 18 segments were tested from levels ranging between T11 and L5. The load was kept constant for 30 minutes while the compressive load and axial displacement were recorded simultaneously. Following testing, the degree of disc degeneration was visually graded (grades I to IV, where grade I meant no macroscopic degeneration and grade IV, severe degeneration). Many studies have shown that an intervertebral disc exhibits both viscous and elastic behavior (1,11–13,16). When subjected to a compressive force, for example, that means the disc will undergo creep or plastic flow with time. It also means that on removal of the applied load, the disc recovers to almost its initial state if the applied load has not exceeded the disc's elastic limit (15). Rheological laws provide a mathematical solution to the deformation and flow of different materials. The different "components" are often represented graphically by mechanical models, including the Hooke body, or "spring," and the Newton body, or "dashpot." The former represents pure elastic, whereas the latter represents pure viscous behavior. The Hooke body acts to store mechanical energy; the Newton body absorbs or dissipates energy. In this way, the intervertebral joint can be modeled as series or parallel combinations of springs or dashpots, the simplest combination of which is called a Kelvin body.

When the strain-time behavior (where strain is the deformation divided by the average disc height) of motion segments in the present experiment was determined, it was evident that degeneration typically was characterized by a larger initial strain and equilibrium was approached at a higher rate than nondegenerated segments. Degeneration also meant a decreased stiffness coefficient, something shown in several other studies. At large it was evident that the viscous modulus, the elastic modulus and viscosity of the segments with grade III disc degeneration, were lower than the discs with grades I or II degeneration.

Disc Degeneration and Static Properties of the Disc

Static tests of intervertebral discs suggested that disc degeneration must be relatively advanced (>grade II) to influence significantly the mechanical behavior of the human lumbar disc. That might be one reasonable explanation for the fact that light or moderate disc degeneration has questionable clinical significance.

Dynamic in Vitro Testing

When the segments were tested dynamically, they were first subjected to a compressive load corresponding to the load of the trunk above each segment (4) (Fig. 3.1). The static load was maintained for 30 minutes after which time each segment was subjected to a cyclic compressive load ranging between the load of the trunk above the segment and a percentage (60% to 100%) of each segment's ultimate compressive strength. The initial maintaining of the compressive loads functioned to "condition" the segments to the "normal" in vivo stresses. After the "conditioning," a sinusoidal loading regimen with a frequency of .5 Hz was superimposed on the segments. Dynamic testing of the segments continued until fracture or 1,000 load cycles, whichever occurred first. Fatigue fracture criteria were an audible cracking sound or a sudden increase in axial deformation.

Irrespective of the grade of macroscopic disc degeneration, the relation was characterized by an initial rapid increase in stiffness (decreased deformation) followed by an approach to an equilibrium state in which the segment stiffness became stable and almost constant. Disc degeneration grades II and III tended to stabilize much earlier than the segments with no visible disc degeneration (grade I). Segments with most degeneration tended to be less fatigue resistant, although no statistically significant differences were found.

When acute injuries have been inflicted on the intervertebral disc, for example through puncture of the annulus fibrosus with a scalpel, that has resulted in an immediate decrease of the disc's stiffness after the disc was loaded (17). When a repeat loading was superimposed on the injured disc, however, an equivalent or even greater stiffness was noted after just a few loading cycles.

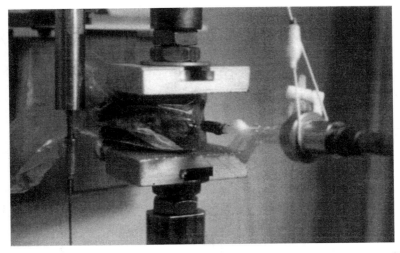

FIG. 3.1. A human motion segment during repeat loading. Disc pressure was monitored continuously.

Disc Degeneration and Dynamic Properties of the Disc

Degeneration of the disc influenced the stiffness of the disc. Irrespective of grade of degeneration, the stiffness stabilized after a few loading cycles to become relatively constant. A tendency toward a reduced fatigue resistance was noted with more pronounced degeneration; however, it was not significant. Those results indicated that the immediate effect of disc degeneration on the dynamic properties was quite restricted (4). The effects of prolonged repeated loading have not been studied.

In Vivo and in Vitro Testing

More or less immediately, significant changes of the intervertebral disc's viscoelastic properties have been found in animals first tested in vivo and then in vitro (14). Although concentrating on properties strongly dependent on normal rheological conditions, the relatively profound differences found in this study between in vivo and in vitro testing situations suggested that the design of a biomechanical experiment and how that influences the results must be kept in mind when interpreted.

Dynamic Loading of the Intervertebral Joint in Vivo

It is reasonable to assume that the testing conditions (i.e., in vivo or in vitro) might be of even greater importance when dynamic loads are applied as compared with static loading. For that reason, the in vivo dynamic stiffness was studied in intact and injured intervertebral discs of lumbar motion segments subjected to vibratory loading (2,3,6). A porcine model was used that allowed application of a miniaturized servo-hydraulic testing apparatus designed for applying controlled force or displacement in the spine of the anesthetized animal (6). The design of the device is based on two shanks, a mobile and a stationary one, located on the thrust bar (Fig. 3.2) (5). The compression induced by this device is an arch-type movement rather than a pure axial compression movement. The difference between those two movements is negligible when small movements (<5mm), as in this experiment, were used. No other coupled forces are induced by the device, leaving the vertebrae free to rotate axially, bend laterally, and shear anteroposteriorly and laterally. Force or displacement is applied via the actuator and can be computed at the geometric center of the disc (5).

Animals weighing between 80 and 95 kg were used, and the testing occurred at the L2-L3 level. The animals were grouped into three groups: (a) 12 animals with intact (uninjured) discs, (b) 6 animals with an acutely injured disc, and (c) 6 animals with a degenerated (chronic lesion) disc. During testing, each animal was placed prone on the operating table. All animals were operated on at the decided level. The testing device was rigidly fixed to the spine through intrapedicular screws inserted bilaterally at the L2 and L3 vertebrae.

Group a was sinusoidal compressed from 0.05 to 25 Hz and at a peak load of either 100 or 200 N. Group b with the acutely injured disc (injured through a 15 mm deep anterolateral scalpel stab injury in the annulus parallel to the endplates of the adjacent vertebrae) was subjected to a peak load set of 200 N. For group c, with a degenerated disc at L2-L3, the same loading protocol as in group b was used. The disc degeneration was created with a similar injury as in group b. In this experiment, the animals recuperated after the surgical procedures and were monitored daily for 3 months.

The results showed no significant differences in dynamic stiffness between the intact and acutely injured discs. For the degenerated disc group, a significant increase in stiffness was found when compared with the intact disc group. Qualitatively there were no distinct alterations in the shape of the frequency response compared with the intact disc.

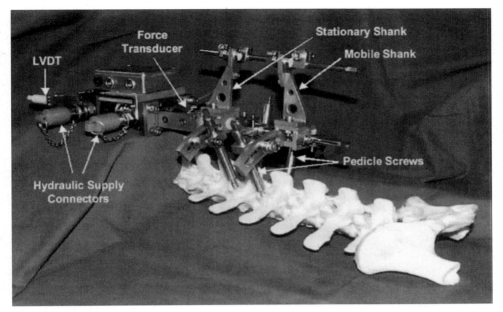

FIG. 3.2. The miniaturized servo-hydraulic testing machine used for in vivo loading of the porcine spine. It is designed to allow controlled force or displacement and can be used for static or repeat loading (>30 Hz).

It was concluded that the in vivo dynamic axial stiffness of the intervertebral joint depends on excitation frequency, load magnitude, and load history and the biomechanical properties of the disc were significantly affected by the degenerative changes of the disc but not by the acute injury (10).

Kinematics after Iatrogenic Injuries to the Lumbar Spine

Unavoidable injuries to the posterior ligaments/musculature and/or bony elements of the spine are accepted consequences of most spine surgical procedures. Those injuries are now and then accompanied by likewise unavoidable and sometimes accidental injuries also to the facet joint capsule or the joint proper, for example. As mentioned earlier, the intervertebral joint allows mobility while providing stability of the spine. Surgical alterations of those structures might change both load-bearing and kinematic characteristics of the spine and by that initiate pathological processes (e.g., accelerated degeneration of the intervertebral joint). In vitro studies have shown that partial or complete violation of the facet joints can affect the biomechanical relationship of the entire intervertebral joint significantly. Because iatrogenic injuries can alter not only passive stabilizing structures like ligaments and bony elements but the actively stabilizing muscles as well, it is necessary to perform in vivo experiments to include both those aspects. To investigate systematically the acute effects of iatrogenic injuries to both active and passive stabilizers of the spine, the study described next was performed.

The Kinematics after Acute Intervertebral Joint Injuries

A porcine animal (33 domestic pigs, 55 to 65 kg weight) model was used (7). With the animal prone on the operating table and through a midline incision, the tip of the spinous

TABLE 3.1. *Injuries Created in Different Sequences in the Four Animal Groups*

1. The sham injury: nothing but insertion of k-wires in the spinous processes of L3 and L4.
2. Transverse process injury: L4 transverse process was excised close to the pedicle.
3. Minor disc and anterior ligament injury: a scalpel incision (20 mm width) through the central part of the anterior longitudinal ligament, the annulus fibrosus, and into the nucleus pulposus.
4. Severe disc and anterior ligament injury: an incision through the central part of the anterior longitudinal ligament and the disc, leaving intact the superficial layer of the posterior aspect of annulus facing the posterior longitudinal ligament and the spinal canal venous complex.
5. Interspinous ligament injury: the entire ligament was transacted in the A-P direction.
6. Facet joint capsular opening: central incisions through the collagen capsule, into the synovial joint, bilaterally.
7. Facet joint slit: bilateral 2-mm slits in the facet joints, removing the cartilage on both joint surfaces.
8. Facetectomy: a total bilateral facetectomy.

processes of L3 and L4 were identified and freed. A k-wire was inserted in each process to a depth of around 20 mm to obtain rigid fixation. An intervertebral motion device (IMD), which allows for measurement of the dynamic intervertebral motion, was then fixed to the k-wires (9). The placement of the animal on the operating table was adjusted so the L3-L4 level could be moved through movements of the hinged table. The animals were divided into four groups. In each group, a different type and/or sequence of injuries was created (Table 3.1).

Kinematics

After each sequential injury, kinematic testing took place. With the animal securely fixed and with the L3-L4 level placed directly over the hinge of the operating table and beginning and ending in a neutral position, the spine was flexed and extended through lowering and raising the caudal end of the table. During the flexion-extension maneuvers, the motions between L3 and L4 were continuously monitored with the IMD (Fig. 3.3). The flexion-extension protocol was repeated three times.

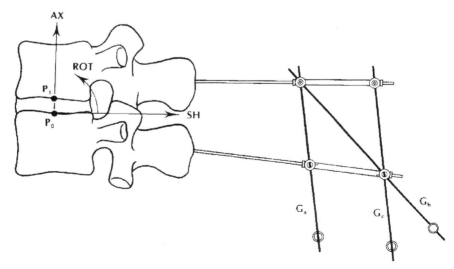

FIG. 3.3. The intervertebral motion device (IMD), which allows precise determination of the intervertebral motion in rotation (ROT), axial (AX), and shear (SH) translation in the sagittal plane.

Muscular Stimulation

The effect of muscular stimulation after each injury was also studied in two of the groups. Bipolar wire electrodes were placed bilaterally around the paraspinal muscles at the L2 and L6 levels, respectively. Stimulation with square voltage repetitive pulses caused intense contraction of the lumbar musculature.

Flexion-extension with and without stimulation was performed, with time for recovery of the musculature in between. The effect of the injuries on the dynamic motion pattern was compared with that found in the sham lesion group. In that comparison, the transverse process injury caused significantly less shear.

The minor disc injury created no significant differences, whereas the severe disc injury caused a significantly greater axial rotation. When transsection of the interspinous ligament was added to the severe disc injury lesion, significantly more rotation and shear translation was noted. The facet joint capsule opening produced significantly less shear translation than what was found in the sham group.

For the isolated facet joint slit lesion, no significant differences were found. With the excision of the transverse processes, an increased rotation and shear translation was found as well as less axial translation and that in both the joint opening and the joint slit groups.

Facetectomy caused more rotation along with less shear translation when compared to the behavior after capsular injury. The complete removal of the facets produced a paradoxical kinematic behavior that enhanced the unstable condition of the motion segment. Muscular stimulation, although increasing the range of motion, also had a stabilizing effect and especially in reducing abrupt kinematic behavior, particularly in the so-called neutral zone (8,10). From these acute in vivo experiments, we learned there are passive and active stabilizing structures of the spine that interact, sometimes in an unexpected way.

The Kinematics in the Chronically Injured Intervertebral Joint

A similar model was used to study the influence of the kinematics of the intervertebral joint after a "chronic" iatrogenic injury (8). Almost identical injuries were created as in the "acute" experiments. In the chronic experiments, however, the animals recuperated after the surgical procedures and were monitored daily for 3 months.

Three months after injury, the animals once again were anesthetized and their spines opened through a posterior midline approach. The injured intervertebral joint, L3-L4, as in the acute experiment, was positioned directly over the hinged operating table, allowing for flexion-extension motions in the 3 months earlier injured joint. The kinematics of the joint during flexion-extension motions of the table was then continuously monitored with the IMD device (Fig. 3.3). The range of motion occurring at the end points (END ROM) of full flexion-extension was calculated for each kinematic variable (ROT = rotation, AX = axial, and SH = shear). In the case of what we called paradoxical motion, the END ROM did not necessarily coincide with the maximum range of motion (MAX ROM) occurring during full flexion-extension, nor was it necessary that the MAX ROMs for ROT, AX, or SH occur simultaneously—that is, at the same global flexion-extension angle (Fig. 3.4).

Morphological Findings

Three months after the initial injury, the sham motion segments revealed normal morphology. The discs injured through a stab incision in the annulus healed in the outermost

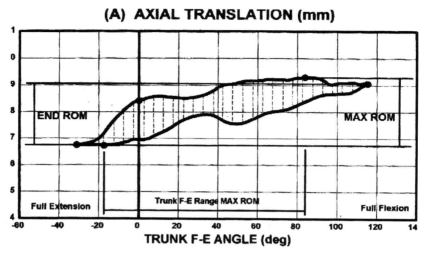

FIG. 3.4. The marked area within the figure marks the difference (hysteresis) in motion pattern between flexion and extension in the axial direction.

annulus but not in the inner. Nucleus pulposus maintained its normal appearance. Adjacent discs were completely normal.

Discs with injuries of the nucleus showed pronounced degenerative changes in the annulus as well as in the nucleus. Healing occurred in the outermost annulus, but there was considerable disruption of the inner annulus. The nucleus was fibrous and discolored. The disc height was reduced, and there were visible osteophytes in most specimens. With the exception of one animal, there was no visible change of any adjacent discs. The exception was a caudal disc with a disc herniation. Facet joint injuries caused scaring and discoloration of the cartilage, and in those where the cartilage had been removed, ossification and formation of nonmature cartilage were noted.

HYSTERESIS

The kinematic behavior of the lumbar motion segment can be different in loading and unloading phases. This can be manifested by an opening in the kinematic curve, an opening we named *hysteresis* (Fig. 3.4).

Iatrogenic Patterns of Motion

Comparisons between hysteresis lines, with and without muscle stimulation (see the section on acute injury), were made within each group of chronic injury (8). The muscle stimulation influenced the kinematic in different ways. In the disc annulus injury group, muscle stimulation of the paraspinal muscles tended to increase the hysteresis in the flexion phase for all three kinematic variables, whereas in the disc nucleus group, axial hysteresis decreased with muscle stimulation. The greatest hysteresis changes in comparison to the sham lesion group were noted in AX and especially for the disc annulus, the disc nucleus, the facet joint wedge, and the facet capsule lesion groups.

After 3 months, the different iatrogenic injuries to the motion segment had caused degenerative changes of the discs and the facet joints, seemingly very similar to those seen in the human spine. The different injuries caused various disturbances of the normal intervertebral kinematics. Some characteristics could be determined through these in vivo experiments:

1. It was obvious that the maximum range of motion, MAX ROM, measured dynamically, is the most sensitive kinematic parameter in detecting the effect of a chronic injury to the intervertebral joint.
2. Axial translation, AX, is the kinematic variable that shows the most change in these chronic lesions.
3. In comparison to the acute injury model, the lumbar paraspinal musculature overall was less potent in providing stability during flexion-extension in the chronic lesion groups. Possible reasons for that could be altered mechanisms in the neuromuscular feedback system or a fatiguing of the stabilizing muscles in the chronic injury groups.

SUMMARY

Injuries to the spine can affect different structures and in that way influence the biomechanical properties and kinematics of the intervertebral joint in different ways. Some injuries can, at least early on, be detected in vivo only, whereas others are time dependent and reveal themselves long after the initial injury. To be able to detect and possibly correct iatrogenic injuries in the human spine of a kind similar to those injuries created experimentally in this presentation, better and more sensitive methods must be invented.

REFERENCES

1. Burns ML, Kaleps I, Kazarian LE. 1984. Analysis of compressive creep behavior of the vertebral unit subjected to a uniform axial loading using exact parametric solution equations of Kelvin-solid models—Part I. Human intervertebral joints. J Biomech 17: 113-30.
2. Ekstrom L, Kaigle A, Hult E, Holm S, Rostedt M, Hansson T. 1996. Intervertebral disc response to cyclic loading—an animal model. Proc Inst Mech Eng [H] 210: 249-58.
3. Ekström L, Holm S, Holm AK, Hansson T. 2004. In vivo porcine intradiscal pressure as a function of external loading. J Spinal Disord Tech 17: 312-316.
4. Hansson TH, Keller TS, Spengler DM. 1987. Mechanical behavior of the human lumbar spine. II. Fatigue strength during dynamic compressive loading. J Orthop Res 5: 479-87.
5. Hult E, Ekstrom L, Kaigle A, Holm S, Hansson T. 1995. In vivo measurement of spinal column viscoelasticity—an animal model. Proc Inst Mech Eng [H] 209: 105-10; discussion 35.
6. Kaigle A, Ekstrom L, Holm S, Rostedt M, Hansson T. 1998. In vivo dynamic stiffness of the porcine lumbar spine exposed to cyclic loading: influence of load and degeneration. J Spinal Disord 11: 65-70.
7. Kaigle AM, Holm SH, Hansson TH. 1995. Experimental instability in the lumbar spine. Spine 20: 421-30.
8. Kaigle AM, Holm SH, Hansson TH. 1997. 1997 Volvo Award winner in biomechanical studies. Kinematic behavior of the porcine lumbar spine: a chronic lesion model. Spine 22: 2796-806.
9. Kaigle AM, Pope MH, Fleming BC, Hansson T. 1992. A method for the intravital measurement of interspinous kinematics. J Biomech 25: 451-6.
10. Kaigle AM, Wessberg P, Hansson TH. 1998. Muscular and kinematic behavior of the lumbar spine during flexion-extension. J Spinal Disord 11: 163-74.
11. Kaleps I, Kazarian LE, Burns ML. 1984. Analysis of compressive creep behavior of the vertebral unit subjected to a uniform axial loading using exact parametric solution equations of Kelvin-solid models—Part II. Rhesus monkey intervertebral joints. J Biomech 17: 131-6.
12. Kazarian LE. 1975. Creep characteristics of the human spinal column. Orthop Clin North Am 6: 3-18.
13. Keller TS, Hansson TH, Holm SH, Pope MM, Spengler DM. 1988. In vivo creep behavior of the normal and degenerated porcine intervertebral disc: a preliminary report. J Spinal Disord 1: 267-78.
14. Keller TS, Holm SH, Hansson TH, Spengler DM. 1990. 1990 Volvo Award in experimental studies. The dependence of intervertebral disc mechanical properties on physiologic conditions. Spine 15: 751-61.
15. Keller TS, Spengler DM, Hansson TH. 1987. Mechanical behavior of the human lumbar spine. I. Creep analysis during static compressive loading. J Orthop Res 5: 467-78.

16. Kulak RF, Belytschko TB, Schultz AB. 1976. Nonlinear behavior of the human intervertebral disc under axial load. J Biomech 9: 377-86.
17. Markolf KL, Morris JM. 1974. The structural components of the intervertebral disc. A study of their contributions to the ability of the disc to withstand compressive forces. J Bone Joint Surg Am 56: 675-87.
18. Nachemson AL, Schultz AB, Berkson MH. 1979. Mechanical properties of human lumbar spine motion segments. Influence of age, sex, disc level, and degeneration. Spine 4: 1-8.
19. Tencer AF, Ahmed AM. 1981. The role of secondary variables in the measurement of the mechanical properties of the lumbar intervertebral joint. J Biomech Eng 103: 129-37.
20. Tencer AF, Ahmed AM, Burke DL. 1982. Some static mechanical properties of the lumbar intervertebral joint, intact and injured. J Biomech Eng 104: 193-201.

4

Lumbar Fusion: Looking
for Failure

Stephen Eisenstein and Alan Breen

Pseudarthrosis, perhaps the most common cause of recurrent or new low back pain after lumbar fusion surgery, is probably underdiagnosed. This is a judgment based on clinical impressions: there does not appear to be any large recent series to provide a ranking of other technical causes such as adjacent segment pain. A conscientious search for pseudarthrosis is a tedious and potentially humiliating endeavor. In one large study, pseudarthrosis was found in 8.5% of 342 patients who had posterior fusion and pedicle screw fixation, but the relationship with postoperative pain was not described (1). Plain radiographs and clinical examination were used to diagnose the pseudarthroses. Plain X-ray will reveal gross evidence of failure such as breakage and displacement of internal fixation (Figs. 4.1, 4.2) or resorption of bone graft (Fig 4.3). Such gross evidence is unusual: there are more subtle signs of pseudarthrosis and movement to be found on plain X-ray before a confident verdict of technical success can be given. Where metal fixation has been used, a dark line of demarcation between the metal implant and the surrounding bone is strongly suggestive of pseudarthrosis. This applies whether the metal implant is a pedicle screw, a cage, or a plate (Fig 4.4).

It is surprising how seldom even simple and inexpensive stress lateral views (in flexion and extension) of the fused area have been requested for patients who have been referred for assessment of their continuing or recurrent back pain after fusion surgery. These views often reveal intervertebral movement where there should be none, and no further explanation is necessary. The method of acquiring these views is of some importance: movement is most likely to be demonstrated if the patient is lateral recumbent on the X-ray table and encouraged with physical assistance to adopt maximum possible flexion and extension in the lumbar spine. Having the patient standing for these views will produce limited results because there must be some fear of losing balance before maximum postures can be reached (2). The latter quoted authors nevertheless found that flexion/extension views, assessed by the Hutter method (3) (superimposition) and the Simmons method (1) (>1° of intervertebral angle difference), were more successful than plain static radiographs in revealing a pseudarthrosis. Blount et al. (4) suggested at least 5 degrees of intervertebral angle difference as a criterion for pseudarthrosis, but this generosity would surely produce an exaggerated rate of assessed fusion and would be bound to be shown excessive on surgical exploration.

Where metal implants were used in the original surgery, they may be useful as an additional marker against which to measure movement within bone, even when there can be no certainty as to persisting intervertebral movement (Fig. 4.5). The fact

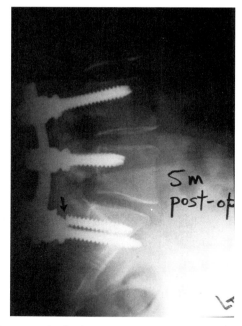

FIG. 4.1. Broken pedicle screw in S1 in patient with persistent postoperative back pain and pseudarthrosis.

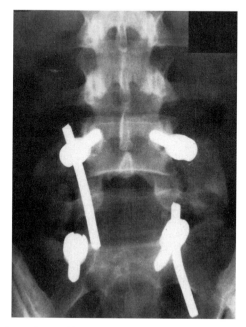

FIG. 4.2. Loose fixation in patient with persistent postoperative back pain and pseudarthrosis at L5-S1.

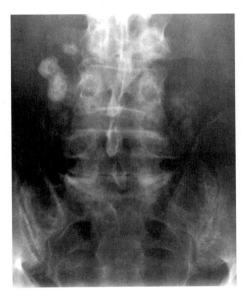

FIG. 4.3. Granular appearance of paravertebral bone graft in patient with 1-year postoperative pain and pseudarthrosis.

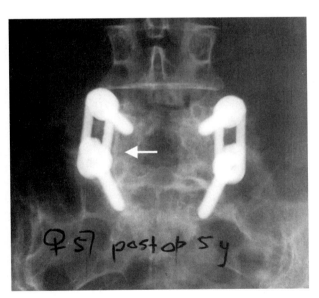

FIG. 4.4. Black demarcation of metal suggesting pseudarthrosis in patient suffering relapse of back pain 5 years postoperatively: confirmed at revision surgery.

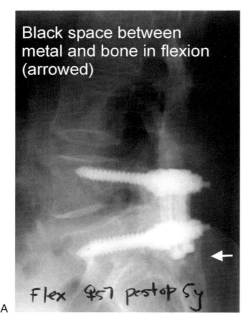
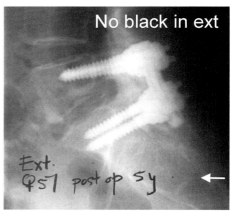

A   B

FIG. 4.5. A, B: Metal implants may be useful as markers against which to measure movement of adjacent host bone. Stress laterals here were not helpful in showing intervertebral movement.

remains that even with stress views, plain radiographs will reveal no more than 68% of pseudarthroses discovered at surgical exposure (5). Plain radiographs have been found inadequate to the task of defining pseudarthrosis in several other studies (6–10).

Plain tomography is a forgotten and prematurely abandoned imaging technique that has been successful far beyond expectation on a number of occasions (Fig. 4.6). Many departments of imaging have disposed of their tomogram machines; others require some days' notice for reinstalling the machine for just one patient.

The introduction of metal interbody cages of various designs into fusion surgery has produced further difficulty in the diagnosis of pseudarthrosis. The metal obscures all attempts to visualize the state of the bone graft within the cage. The more recent introduction of carbon fiber cages was expected to solve this problem, but plain radiographs will still not always adequately confirm a pseudarthrosis within the cage (Fig. 4.6a). The benefit of carbon fiber cages is that they will at least permit plain tomography to reveal the condition of the bone graft within (Fig. 4.6b).

It is possible that there will be nothing amiss to see on plain X-ray alone. The surgeon is then confronted with a range of more sophisticated imaging possibilities of varying complexity and expense.

The greatest obstacle to a diagnosis of fusion failure is the reluctance of the treating surgeon to search for failure. There is a very human perception by surgeons that persistent pain after fusion surgery represents some sort of personal failure of ability or even a manifestation of lack of gratitude on the part of the patient. The temptation to blame psychosocial factors in the patient as the cause of symptom failure is strong indeed. A particularly dogged persistence and a lack of pride is required of a surgeon to continue with

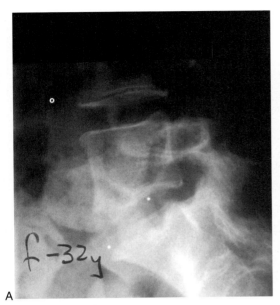
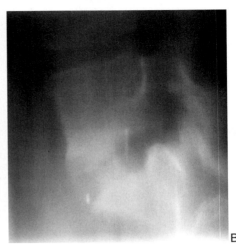

FIG. 4.6. A: Apparent solid anterior fusion L5-S1 within carbon cage on plain radiograph 18 months after fusion surgery. Recurrent back pain. **B:** Same patient as in Figure 4.6a. Plain tomography reveals pseudarthrosis at waist of interbody graft within carbon cage.

the search for pseudarthrosis in his or her own patients and then to deal with the consequences of finding the failure.

Radioisotope bone scan and MRI are both inadequate to the task of reliably exposing a pseudarthrosis. They are also relatively expensive. Isotope scanning cannot be judged conclusively inside of 2 years after surgery: even then, a pseudarthrosis will not necessarily show increased uptake. However, single photon emission CT (SPECT) with planar scintigraphy was found to be superior to plain radiography in a small series of symptomatic patients tested at surgical exploration (11). Where infection of the previous surgical area has been a feature of the suspected pseudarthrosis, any uptake on the isotope scan is likely to represent the residual inflammation rather than a pseudarthrosis alone.

Standard axial CT scanning cannot adequately reveal the hairline defect that frequently characterizes a pseudarthrosis after posterior fusion, especially in the frequent presence of metal fixation. However, there is evidence that thin-section helical CT is currently the most successful method of proving fusion or pseudarthrosis in interbody fusions with carbon cages (2). Likewise, sophisticated manipulation of CT images in various planes and formats can be useful in demonstrating pseudarthroses in posterior fusions (12,13). MRI currently does not offer the degree of resolution required for the detection of subtle pseudarthroses (Fig. 4.7). If internal fixation was used in the original surgery, MRI will in any event produce such an artifact as to render this investigation useless.

A recent development led by Professor Alan Breen holds promise of the ability to expose very small movements at intervertebral segments (1.85 degrees, root mean square). The technology represents a combination of software and hardware for the

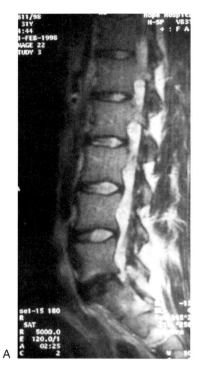
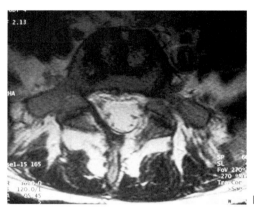

FIG. 4.7. A, B: Same patient as in Figure 4.6. MR scan less revealing than plain tomography in search for pseudarthrosis L5-S1 within carbon cage.

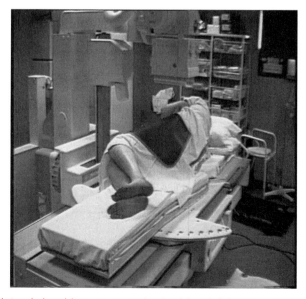

FIG. 4.8. Patient lateral decubitus on motorized table of OSMIA system for lateral digitized lumbar spine views in flexion and extension.

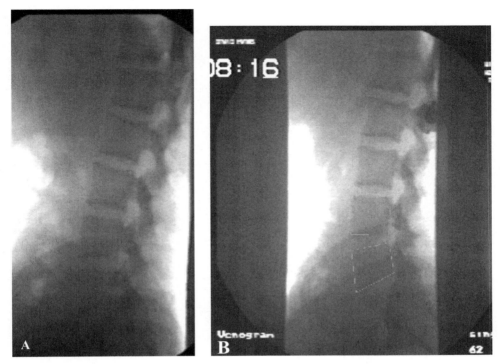

FIG. 4.9. A, B: OSMIA: after image capture (left), relevant vertebral bodies are "framed" (right). Framing applies automatically to all images. Interframe angles digitally measured and represented graphically (Figs. 4.10, 4.11, 4.12).

analysis of multiple digitized low-dose fluoroscopic images taken in flexion, extension, and lateral bending (objective spinal motion imaging assessment: OSMIA). The patient is placed supine for lateral bending or lateral decubitus for flexion/extension (Fig. 4.8) on a tabletop fixed to a conventional X-ray table. The tabletop is motorized to move its distal half at a hinge placed at the lumbar spine. The movement is continuous through an arc of 80 degrees over approximately 20 seconds. Lumbar spine low-dose radiographs are taken at a rate of 25 frames per second and digitized (Fig. 4.9). The differential intervertebral movements (if any) can be plotted on a graph representing the total collection of images. The presence of small movements suggesting the likelihood of pseudarthrosis is easily read on the graph (Figs. 4.10, 4.11, 4.12). Early testing suggests that this technique is more sensitive than any other imaging in the diagnosis of pseudarthrosis. For all its sophistication, the apparatus is robust and capable of adaptation to existing facilities in most hospital radiographical departments. The total irradiation is no more than that for lumbar spine plain films with stress views.

In the absence of this technology and without a positive finding from any other investigation, all that remains for the diligent surgeon investigating failure in his patients is exploration surgery based only on some speculation that there may be a pseudarthrosis to find and repair. An algorithm (Fig. 4.13) is appended here, intended as an aid to clinicians prepared to take the trouble to look for failure.

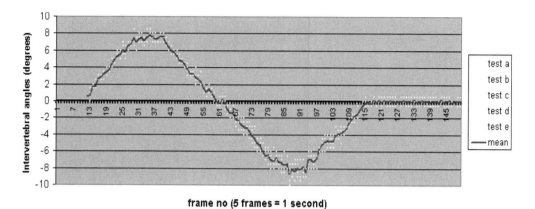

FIG. 4.10. Normal volunteer. Side bending at L4/L5.

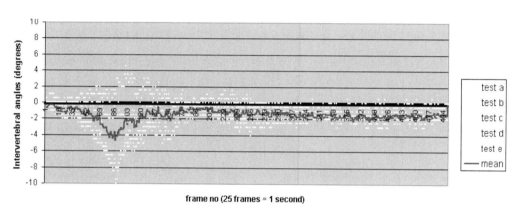

FIG. 4.11. Solid fusion on side bending.

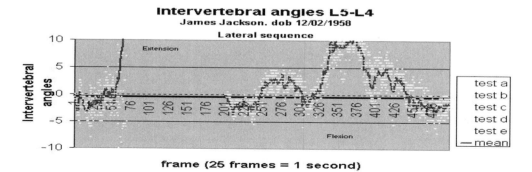

FIG. 4.12. Failed fusion L4/L5 with segmental movement on laterals in flexion/extension.

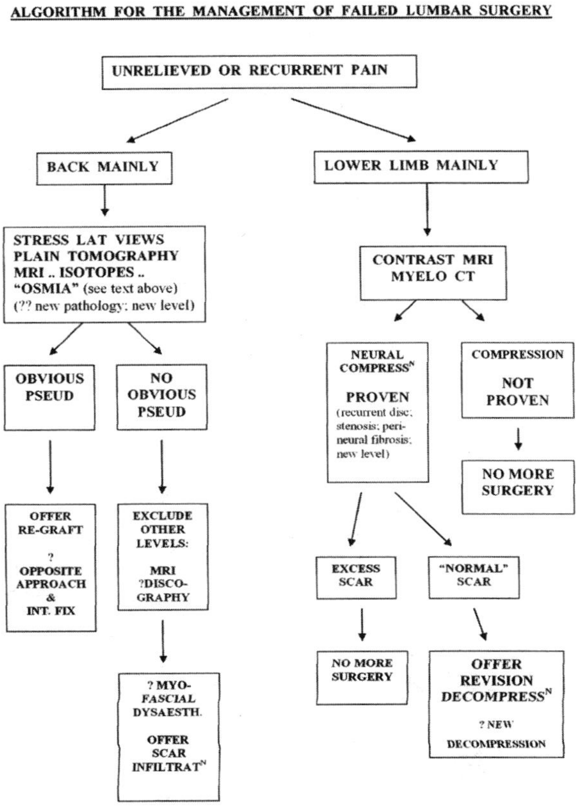

ALGORITHM FOR THE MANAGEMENT OF FAILED LUMBAR SURGERY

UNRELIEVED OR RECURRENT PAIN

BACK MAINLY — LOWER LIMB MAINLY

STRESS LAT VIEWS / PLAIN TOMOGRAPHY / MRI .. ISOTOPES .. / "OSMIA" (see text above) / (?? new pathology: new level)

CONTRAST MRI / MYELO CT

OBVIOUS PSEUD — NO OBVIOUS PSEUD

NEURAL COMPRESS^N PROVEN (recurrent disc: stenosis: perineural fibrosis: new level) — COMPRESSION NOT PROVEN

NO MORE SURGERY

OFFER RE-GRAFT / ? / OPPOSITE APPROACH & INT. FIX

EXCLUDE OTHER LEVELS: / MRI / ?DISCO-GRAPHY

EXCESS SCAR — "NORMAL" SCAR

? MYO-FASCIAL DYSAESTH. / OFFER SCAR INFILTRAT^N

NO MORE SURGERY — OFFER REVISION DECOMPRESS^N / ? NEW DECOMPRESSION

FIG. 4.13. Algorithm for the management of failed lumbar surgery.

REFERENCES

1. Simmons JW, Andersson GB, Russell GS, Hadjipavlou AG. A prospective study of 342 patients using transpedicular fixation instrumentation for lumbosacral spine arthrodesis. J Spinal Disord 1998; 11:367-74.
2. Santos ER, Goss DG, Morcom RK, Fraser RD. Radiologic assessment of interbody fusion using carbon fibre cages. Spine 2003; 28:997-1001.
3. Hutter CG. Posterior intervertebral body fusion. A 25-year study. Clin Orthop 1983; 179:86-96.
4. Blount KJ, Krompinger WJ, et al. Moving towards a standard for spinal fusion outcomes assessment. J Spinal Disord Tech 2002; 15:16-23.
5. Kant AP, Daum WJ, Dean SM, Uchida T. Evaluation of lumbar spine fusion: plain radiographs versus direct surgical exploration and observation. Spine 1995; 20:2313-7.
6. Blumenthal SL, Gill K. Can lumbar spine radiographs accurately determine fusion in postoperative patients? Correlation of routine radiographs with a second surgical look at lumbar fusions. Spine 1993; 18:1186-9.
7. Brodsky AE, Kovalsky ES, Khalil MA. Correlation of radiologic assessment of lumbar spine fusions with surgical exploration. Spine 1991; 16:S261-5.
8. Cizek GR, Boyd LM. Imaging pitfalls of interbody spinal implants. Spine 2000; 20:2633-6.
9. Herzog RJ, Marcotte PJ. Assessment of spinal fusion: critical evaluation of imaging techniques. Spine 1996; 21:1114-8.
10. Pearcy M, Burrough S. Assessment of bony union after interbody fusion of the lumbar spine using biplanar radiographic technique. J Bone Joint Surg [Br] 1982; 64:228-32.
11. Slizofski WJ, Collier BD, Flatley TJ, Carrera GF, Hellman RS, Isitman AT. Painful pseudarthrosis following lumbar spinal fusion: detection by combined SPECT and planar bone scintigraphy. Skeletal Radiol 1987; 16:136-41.
12. Laasonen EM, Soini J. Low back pain after lumbar fusion: surgical and computed tomographic analysis. Spine 1989; 14:210-3.
13. Lang P, Genant HK, Chafetz N, Steiger P, Morris JM. Three-dimensional computed tomography and multiplanar reformations in the assessment of pseudarthrosis in posterior lumbar fusion patients. Spine 1988; 13:69-75.

5

Failed Medical Spine

Michel Benoist and Alain Deburge

DEFINITION

Before discussing this important issue, a clear definition of the present topic is necessary. Webster's dictionary defines "to fail" as "to come short of a result" but also "to deteriorate, to become weaker." Obviously the aim of this presentation is not to review the numerous aspects of therapeutic negative results, but rather to examine how medicine can be a cause of deterioration. The spine deteriorated by medicine is equivalent to "iatrogenic disorders of the spine." According to the Concise Oxford Dictionary, "medical" is defined as "the art of medicine in general" or "as opposed to surgery, obstetrics etc." In this review the term "art of medicine in general" is considered.

Iatrogenic disorders of the spine imply morbidity created by a physician. These disorders must be differentiated from the unavoidable complications secondary to validated procedures performed with adequate indications and technique. For example, there is a clear difference between a thromboembolism occurring after a well-indicated and performed surgical intervention, in spite of an appropriate anticlotting treatment, and complications secondary to an inadequate, poorly performed surgical operation. Iatrogenic disorders imply a notion of guilt recognized in legal proceedings. This latter notion, on which experts are supposed to evaluate a responsibility, separates these two categories of complications. However, it must be recognized that in some instances the line of separation is then debatable and can be the source of expert dispute.

ETIOLOGY

Medical nonsurgical caregivers, including, for example, rheumatologists and specialists in physical or sports medicine, may generate iatrogenic disorders in different ways. First, with wrong or delayed diagnosis; second, with a passive or defensive attitude (or perhaps the absence of a therapeutic action due to an apprehension of taking responsibility). Third, by directing patients toward inappropriate surgical procedures or channels. Finally, with ineffective programs of conservative therapy or failure to recognize central influence on pain. For example, it is now established that passive procedures such as massage and physiotherapy are ineffective in the treatment of subacute or chronic low back pain. Their extended use leads to distress, chronicity, and pain behavior.

When the term "medical" is considered as the art of medicine in general, the area of potential iatrogenic disorders is considerably extended. These disorders may be related to various causes. First, wrong indications of validated methods; second, validated procedures but poor inadequate techniques; third, use of nonvalidated treatments, and finally, imprudent indications and misuse of risky procedures. We discuss these main topics in turn.

A wrong indication of a validated technique is probably the main cause of iatrogenicity. By definition, failure of a procedure can be expected if the use of that technique does

TABLE 5.1. *Number of operations in 40 patients (12)*

No. patients	No. operations
28	2
6	3
6	4
40	98

not correspond to the clinical and pathological problem of the patient. Abuse and misuse of discal surgery is a good example. It is universally recognized that surgery for discal herniation is an effective procedure if the spinal nerve irritation and compression has been clearly demonstrated by clinical and imaging data, following a period of an appropriate conservative treatment. Unfortunately, misuse and abuse of discal surgery can lead to disaster. This is especially true in the case of persisting or relapsing radiculopathy after a primary negative exploration. A failed first therapeutic action can be the source of a noxious escalation. For example, Revel et al. (11) studied 40 patients, recruited in a pain clinic, with a postoperative radiculopathy. Two criteria of inclusion were necessary: first, at least two operations, second, all clinical pre- and postoperative imaging data and operations reports of each operation had to be available. Patients were reviewed and evaluated using adequate outcome measures. The number and results of operations in these 40 patients are shown in Tables 5.1 and 5.2.

Ninety-eight operations were performed with catastrophic results. Review of the clinical, imaging, and operative data was particularly instructive. A real discal herniation was disclosed in the first preoperative imaging in only 15 out of the 40 cases and only mentioned in 50% of the operative reports. Review of the imaging studies performed between repeat surgery disclosed discal tissue in 22% of the patients, although discal herniation was in all cases the pretext of reoperation. Repeat surgical insults generate the so-called battered root. Structural changes of the nerve tissue, deafferentation, provoke an excess of nociception, activation of the cells of the cord and glia, and central sensitization. Perception of chronic pain in the brain and associated psychosocial factors generate positive feedback on the nociceptive system. What is the cause of the discordance between the preoperative work-up and results that are catastrophic for the patients? At best, repeat clinical and radiological diagnostic errors or an insistence on seeing on the images what the surgeon would like to see. It is recognized that in discal surgery, a first operation, based on debatable clinical symptomatology and doubtful imaging data, may generate a noxious escalation. This iatrogenic effect is worse with repeat surgery. In that case, presence of scar tissue and periradicular fibrosis complicates the nerve root liberation, and repeat surgical insult worsens the radicular lesions (1). The pathogenic role of scar tissue is not exactly known, but it has been demonstrated that excision of scar tissue yields poor results (2). Repeat surgery should only be decided if a clear relapse of discal herniation and/or an associated stenosis is clearly observed. As shown in Table 5.2, multiple

TABLE 5.2. *Results of 98 operations (12)*

- 60% have never resumed any kind of work.
- 40% had an intermittent professional activity. 22% of these had to change for a lighter sedentary job.
- Only 5 patients could resume normal activity at home and at leisure.

nonmotivated operations lead to chronic pain and invalidity. These patients fill the pain clinics and rehabilitation centers.

Iatrogenicity is not limited to discal surgery. The misuse of percutaneous methods can be iatrogenic in the absence of an appropriate indication. These techniques are often presented to the patient as noninvasive, necessitating a short hospitalization and avoiding the risks of surgery. For such reasons, mini-invasive procedures are easily accepted by the patient and indications may be abusively increased. However, even when the technique is a "minima," the risk of complications exists (11). The principal danger is the absence of positive results, which obviously is to be expected if indication of such a technique is wrong. It must be emphasized again that failure of a first therapeutic action can be the first step of a noxious escalation.

The second cause of "failed medical spine" is related to the use of a validated procedure with a good indication but with an inadequate technique. For example, in the United States, 48 severe neurological complications with serious sequelae were observed following chymopapain chemonucleolysis (9). During the same period in Europe, 15 neurological complications were disclosed, most of them reversible in a comparable number of patients (3). It has been shown that neurological complications in the United States were due to intrathecal injection of the enzyme following insufficient training of the practitioners. In spinal surgery, technical education of the surgeons is essential. The best surgical program with the best indications can be disastrous, if poorly performed.

Untimely use of a nonvalidated procedure is another cause of iatrogenicity. The widespread, commercially motivated dispersal of automated percutaneous discectomy, which proved to be ineffective, is a good example. Intradiscal injections of hexacetonide triamcinolone for treatment of discal herniation were introduced in France in 1986 (4) as a substitute to chymopapain. This technique was popularized without animal experiments, pharmacological studies, or long-term pilot trial. Although displaying short-term good results, it turned out to be an ineffective and hazardous method with time. Moreover, calcified deposits in the epidural space were frequently observed, generating low back and radicular pain. The calcified deposits were difficult to remove surgically and could reappear after surgical removal (7).

Due to its simplicity and its supposed cost effectiveness, this technique rapidly found numerous followers with the iatrogenic consequences just described. It is a striking example of a nonvalidated procedure disseminated without a precaution. As emphasized by Waddell, "New therapies and techniques cannot be promoted on the basis of personal series with sometimes commercial interest. Properly designated and conducted studies published in peer-reviewed journals are mandatory before routine use" (14). Inefficacy of a procedure is iatrogenic; it can be the first step of escalation with its own potential complications.

A final source of iatrogenic disorders of the spine is related to the abusive use of risky procedures. At the lumbar level, reduction of severe spondylolisthesis is not exempt from potential neurological complications (13). Pedicular screws are used more and more in traumatic and degenerative pathology. Anatomical studies have shown that even in the hands of the best surgeons, intracanalar penetration of the screws is possible with an evident danger of radicular lesions. In less expert hands the risk is higher (15). The same remarks can be applied to the use of cages. Moreover, the neurological complications and morbidity of surgery for scoliosis should also be noted. Before deciding to use such risky procedures, they should be classified as iatrogenic if their use is not justified by the clinical symptoms and imaging data. Benefit-risk ratio is the best criteria of iatrogenicity.

In summary, we have briefly discussed the main causes of the failed medical spine: we have seen that the distinction is sometimes difficult between iatrogenic disorders and complications following an adequate, justified, and properly performed procedure.

PREVENTION

Those potentially responsible for creating a "failed medical spine" are numerous and constitute a complex network. They include the medical caregiver, the radiologist, the patient, the media, the government, and academic institutions.

Medical caregivers, whether surgical or nonsurgical, are on the front line, responsible for both indications and technique. As emphasized by Deburge (8), the technical education of practitioners can be considered satisfactory related to the quality and duration of their fellowship, which is its essential basis. However, residents should be taught that surgery or other technical procedures are not always the best solution to all problems and natural evolution is sometimes better. Moreover, and most importantly, education must also be ethical and include the awareness of the patient's distress and suffering, the health care expenses, and the cost of ineffective care and disability. For example, in the study of Revel et al. (12), there is a clear discordance between the preoperative workup and the catastrophic results. Abusive indications are the most probable explanation. It has been established that there is a direct relation between the amount of discal surgery in a given geographical region and the number of surgeons in the area (6).

The amazing progress in the technology of imaging can paradoxically be a source of iatrogenicity. CT and MRI are noninvasive procedures without side effects. They are often performed without any motivated clinical indication. Trivial abnormalities may be disclosed leading to wrong therapeutic indications. The role of the radiologist is important. He or she is responsible for the quality of imaging and for the reading, which are often crucial in the indications. As emphasized by Nordby (10), "CT and MRI appear to take the place of a well-conducted history and physical examination. Too often we see a radiologist reading of a possible small defect which may represent a possible herniated nucleus pulposus become a definitive voluminous discal herniation in the following note forming the basis of a failed procedure."

The patient's belief and expectations can also be iatrogenic. Nowhere else in medicine are so many different treatments proposed for the same condition. This leads to confusion. Some noninformed patients may request quick, active, radical, mini-invasive therapies for moderate symptoms and become involved in disproportionate treatment programs or nonvalidated procedures. Alternatively, others fearing the classical approach are seeking help in fake alternatives. It is therefore the physician's role to analyze carefully the patient's beliefs and expectations. Educating the patient regarding natural evolution and the nature and risks of the various alternative procedures is mandatory.

The patient's confusion is often fostered by the media, always seeking new and sensational therapies without having verified their risks and effectiveness. There is an ethical responsibility of the medical profession and of the medical media to disseminate the best information available.

The legal and health insurance systems may influence health care delivery in many ways. For example, the fear of malpractice suits may encourage a defensive attitude on the part of practitioners. Alternatively, the health insurance system is able to prevent the use of validated procedures or approve only a portion of therapy. For example, the French social security system has always denied payment or reimbursement of chymopapain chemonucleolysis in private practice, refusing this treatment to a patient not able to afford the payment.

Academic institutions are also involved. It is imperative that they keep their tradition of excellence in research. Most importantly they must avoid a conflict of interest with industry, thereby producing reliable "nonfailed" trials. We have already stated that the use of ineffective procedures is iatrogenic. Repeat therapeutic failures, whether conservative or surgical, generate distress, anxiety, depression, and chronic pain. The same remarks can be applied to industry, which must keep excellence in research and development (5). Ethical considerations must be maintained in spite of the financial pressure. For example, the recent and brutal halt of the production of chymopapain is a perfect case of an unethical move.

REFERENCES

1. Benner B, Ehni G. Spinal arachnoiditis: the post-operative variety in particular. Spine 1978;3:40-4.
2. Benoist M, Ficat C, Baraf P, et al. Sciatiques post-opératoires par fibrose épidurale et arachnoidite lombaire. Rev Rhum 1979;46:593-9.
3. Bouillet R. Treatment of sciatica. A comparative survey of complications of surgical treatment, and nucleolysis with chymopapain. Clin Orthop 1990:144-52.
4. Bourgeois P, Frot B, Folinais, et al. Traitement de la lombosciatique par hernie discale par nucléorthese à l'hexacetonide de Triamcinolone. Presse Med 1986;15:2073-6.
5. Burton CV. The ethics of spine care. In: Wiesel SW, Weinstein JN, Herkowitz H, Dvorak J, Bell J (eds.), The lumbar spine (Vol. 2). Philadelphia: WB Saunders 1996; 1339-46.
6. Cherkin D, Deyo R, Loeser J, et al. An international comparison of back surgery rates. Marseille: International Society of the Study of the Lumbar Spine, 1993.
7. Debiais AF, Lambert de Dursay G, Alcalay M, et al. Complications des injections introdiscales de corticoids. In: Simon L, Revel M, Herisson CH (eds.), Pathologie iatrogene du rachis. Paris: Masson, 1993; 93-101.
8. Deburge A. De la pathologie iatrogene en général et de la pathologie iatrogene du rachis en particulier. In: Simon L, Revel M, Herisson CH (eds.), Pathologie iatrogene du rachis. Paris: Masson, 1993; 1-7.
9. McDermott HD, Agre K, Brim, et al. Chymodiactin in patients with herniated lumbar disc. An open label multicenter study. Spine 1985;10:242-9.
10. Nordby EJ. Chemonucleolysis. In: Frymoyer JW (ed.), The adult spine. New York: Raven Press, 1991; 1733-48.
11. Ratsiouras T, Bulstrode C, Cook P, et al. Percutaneous nucleotomy: an anatomic study of the risk of foot injury. Spine 1991;16:38-45.
12. Revel M, Auleley GR, Amor B. La fuite en avant thérapeutique en quête d'une hernie discale. In: Simon L, Revel M, Herisson CH (eds.), Pathologie iatrogene du rachis. Paris: Masson, 1993; 8-13.
13. Transfeldt E, Dendrinos GK, Bradford DS. Paresis of proximal lumbar roots after reduction of L5-S1 spondylolisthesis. Spine 1977;14:774-7.
14. Waddell G, Gibson A. Disc herniation: are recent surgical developments also recent advances? In: Gunzburg R, Szpalski M (eds.), Lumbar disc herniation. Philadelphia: Lippincott Williams and Wilkins, 2001; 181-4.
15. Zucherman J, Hsu K, Picetti G, et al. Clinical efficacy of spinal instrumentation in lumbar degenerative disc disease. Spine 1992;17:734-8.

6

Failed Spinal Fusion

Jean Charles Le Huec, A. Mehbod, and S. Aunoble

Failed fusion surgery of the spine occurs when poor clinical outcomes are associated with fusion procedures. In order to study failed fusion, one must fully understand the indications for performing a fusion, including (a) adjunct to decompression for patients with spinal stenosis associated with degenerative or iatrogenic spondylolisthesis, (b) adjunct to excessive decompression causing iatrogenic instability of the spine, (c) progressive degenerative lumbar scoliosis, and (d) recurrent disk herniation. Fusion for incapacitating nonradicular back pain should only be performed after all nonoperative treatments have been explored (1).

Can a pseudarthrosis in and by itself with good clinical results be considered failed fusion surgery? Scientifically, it might be deemed a failure, but the clinical outcome is the aim of the treatment. In this particular case, the deal with the patient is broken according to the X-rays, but the clinical result is good and cannot be evaluated as a failed procedure. Unfortunately, this situation is not so rare. Conversely, a solid fusion with poor clinical results should be viewed as a failed fusion. Greenenough (4) reported on 135 patients with instrumented posterolateral fusion. Out of 82% patients who were fused, only 65% had clinical improvement. Herkowitz's group (7), in contrast, reported on patients undergoing posterolateral fusion for degenerative spondylolisthesis where there were good or excellent clinical results in 85% or patients with only a 45% fusion rate. Therefore, it seems that clinical results do not always correlate with fusion status (2).

Consequently, in order to determine the reason for the failed fusion surgery, one must consider several variables. Initially, one must assess the fusion status because the pain could be due to nonunion. If a nonunion is diagnosed, one must determine the factors leading to it. If the fusion is solid, one must assess the indications for surgery. Finally, one must consider the treatment options for failed fusion surgery, which leads to a better analysis of the pain generator before the indication for fusion. When the fusion is there without good outcome or when the fusion did not occur with a good clinical result, it probably means the surgical procedure modified something: the extensile approach with damage to muscles and ligaments, the section or destruction of nerve captors, the damage of some proprioceptive elements, and so on. The surgical procedure by itself creates new biomechanical balance and modifies the anatomy with collateral damages. This has to be taken in account when evaluating the clinical outcomes.

Evaluating failed fusion surgery begins with assessing the fusion status. Although surgical exploration is the gold standard, radiographical evaluation may be a more prudent diagnostic tool. Historically, plain anteroposterior and lateral radiographs have been used to define fusions as having spanned trabecular bone between two fused levels. Further radiographical evaluation with dynamic flexion and extension films may be used to define fusion as lack of translatory or angular motion between two fused levels. Most recently, computed tomography (CT) has increased the diagnostic sensitivity of determining fusion.

In a recent study by Santos, the use of plain radiographs was compared to CT scan to determine fusion status. Using plain radiographs, 86% of surgical cases were assessed as fused, whereas using CT scan, the fusion rate of the same patient population was 65% (6). Therefore, it may be wise to use CT scans in assessing fusion status.

If a pseudarthrosis is diagnosed, one must consider the possible reasons, including both technical and biological factors. Technical factors that may decrease the fusion rate include inclusion of multiple levels in the fusion, inadequate preparation of the fusion bed, malpositioned instrumentation, malpositioned bone graft, and inadequate restoration of balance. These factors are very important and can explain the varieties of fusion rate and clinical outcome between different series. The surgical procedure and the personal experience of the surgeon is a very important factor (7). Biological factors that may decrease the fusion rate may be the type of bone graft used, smoking status of the patient, or presence of metabolic or systemic disease. Each of these possible reasons should be critically evaluated for their contribution to the pseudarthrosis (3,5). Finally, in doubtful cases, a late infection with unusual germs like corinae bacterium acnes has to be evaluated. Acute infection with staphylococcus is well known and easy to diagnose in many cases. Low-grade infection is a reason often underestimated.

If the patient is assessed as having a solid fusion with CT scan but continues to have poor clinical results, one must consider several options. If one truly believes the indications for surgery were correct and the patient has a pseudarthrosis, one can surgically explore the fusion and remove the instrumentation at the same time. In a study by Wild (8), up to 70% of patients had clinical improvement after removal of instrumentation. If after the removal of instrumentation and assessment of a solid fusion, the patient continues to have poor clinical results, one must consider the indications for surgery. The work-up should begin with a history and physical examination, followed by new radiographical and diagnostic tools to identify the source of pain. Functional and psychological evaluations of the patient before the surgery are tremendously important in diseases of the spine.

REFERENCES

1. Deyo RA, Nachemson A, et al. Spinal-fusion surgery—the case for restraint. N Engl J Med 2004; 350(7): 722-6.
2. Fischgrund JS, Mackay M, et al. 1997 Volvo Award winner in clinical studies. Degenerative lumbar spondylolisthesis with spinal stenosis: a prospective, randomized study comparing decompressive laminectomy and arthrodesis with and without spinal instrumentation. Spine 1997; 22(24): 2807-12.
3. Greenough CG. Results of treatment of lumbar spine disorders. Effects of assessment techniques and confounding factors. Acta Orthop Scand Suppl 1993; 251: 126-9.
4. Greenough CG, Peterson MD, et al. Instrumented posterolateral lumbar fusion. Results and comparison with anterior interbody fusion. Spine 1998; 23(4): 479-86.
5. Greenough CG, Taylor LJ, et al. Anterior lumbar fusion: results, assessment techniques and prognostic factors. Eur Spine J 1994; 3(4): 225-30.
6. Santos ER, Goss DG, et al. Radiologic assessment of interbody fusion using carbon fiber cages. Spine 2003; 28(10): 997-1001.
7. Sidhu KS, Herkowitz HN. Spinal instrumentation in the management of degenerative disorders of the lumbar spine. Clin Orthop 1997; 335: 39-53.
8. Wild A, Pinto MR, et al. Removal of lumbar instrumentation for the treatment of recurrent low back pain in the absence of pseudarthrosis. Arch Orthop Trauma Surg 2003; 123(8): 414-8.

7

Postoperative Scoliosis

Max Aebi

Postoperative scoliosis, or in a wider sense deformity, can be considered as (a) an iatrogenic scoliosis when it is present immediately after a surgical intervention or (b) a mid- to long-term complication of a surgical procedure that may end up in a failed implant situation inducing a frontal and possibly sagittal malalignment or a secondary scoliosis or deformity above or below a surgically treated area of the spine (Table 7.1).

Such deformities and deviations in the frontal plane can occur in more or less the whole spectrum of spinal pathology but mostly in deformities, degenerative spinal disease, trauma, or tumor surgery. Most of the so-called postoperative scoliosis are not scoliosis in the true sense of the word, since they are deviations of the spine in the frontal or sagittal plane and very rarely true three-dimensional rotational deformities. This may, however, be the case in scoliosis surgery, where a compensatory curve is induced by the correction maneuver. The literature concerning postoperative scoliosis is sparse except for scoliosis surgery itself (3,5–7,9,12). In the category of immediately postoperative iatrogenic scoliosis belong all the deviations, which occur in the context of a surgical procedure either on traumatized, degenerated, or deformed spines.

SPINAL TRAUMA

Scoliotic deformities may occur after an asymmetrical fracture, mostly in asymmetrical compressive injuries (A-type injuries) or in C-type injuries, which are characterized by a rotational dislocation in the cervical, thoracic, or lumbar spine. The scoliotic deformity may be due to insufficient correction of such an asymmetrical fracture or to an inability to correct the rotation by reduction or simply by not recognizing the lesion. An asymmetrical compression fracture differs from a rotational injury like an unilateral dislocation in that the latter is a true rotational deformity, whereas the first is a scoliotic deviation of the spine in the frontal plane. With segmental posterior instrumentation, an asymmetrical correction is rather improbable except if the type of the fracture has not been recognized properly. An asymmetrical fracture needs unequal distraction and/or segmental derotation on the shorter side in order to restore equal height. To gain such correction it may be necessary to restore the mechanical integrity of the anterior column by bone grafting or expandable cages. When using anterior plates in lumbar fractures, a frontal deviation is possible, although the surgical restoration of the anterior column seems to have succeeded (Fig. 7.1).

In the Harrington era, fractures were treated with a system originally designed for deformity surgery. This led usually to a long fixation and overdistraction of B-type injuries, ending up in a kyphosis as well as a frontal deviation. These were unfavorable mechanical conditions. A nonunion and progressing deformity was the consequence, which could become a problem for the patient even many years after the initial

TABLE 7.1. *Matrix of Possible Postoperative Deformities*

Postoperative Deformity	Fracture	Deformities	Degenerative Disease
Short term: immediately, during, or after the surgery	• insufficient correction • misinterpretation of the fracture • unstable fixation	• overcorrection of a secondary lumbar curve when the original thoracic curve is fused • overcorrection of one curve of a double major	• asymmetrical stabilization (e.g., PLIF) not balanced • instrumentation asymmetrical, compressed, or distracted
Midterm: within a year after the surgery	• implant failure • adjacent segment degeneration due to unrecognized trauma	• implant failure • overcorrection of a curve decompensation of countercurve • nonunion, pain, asymmetrical posture unbalanced curve	• implant failure • asymmetric discectomy combined with facet joint damage • decompression at the apex of a degenerated scoliosis • secondary asymmetrical degeneration of an adjacent segment
Long term	• implant failure • nonunion • adjacent segment degeneration	• implant failure • Cranckshaft phenomenon • secondary curve progression	• implant failure • status after discectomy, asymmetrical collapse • adjacent segment pathology in fusion

trauma (Fig. 7.2). Fracture patients with lateral deviation in the frontal plane usually are in as much pain as patients with sagittal malalignments.

DEFORMITIES

One of the most prevalent problems concerning postoperative scoliosis is a decompensation curve above and/or below the corrected spinal area, which may occur immediately after the surgery. This mostly became a problem with the pedicular and other segmental systems, which have a significant correction power, specifically when used according to the principles of rod rotation to achieve so-called derotation of the spine. These problems have not been seen to this extent in the Harrington rod era, although decompensation problems have been described for Harrington rods, too, up to 30% (2,3,9–11).

This obviously leads to the basic question: From where to where does a fixation need to be extended to correct and stabilize optimally a scoliotic deformity in order to avoid postoperative decompensation (3,5,11)? When using the Harrington instrumentation, the implant needed to be anchored in "the stable zone" of the lumbar spine.

Later, after introducing segmental instrumentation systems (CD-Instrumentation and next generation), Dubousset created the term "vertèbre d'élection," which is determined in the frontal as well as in the sagittal projection.

For curves that decompensate, those basic rules have not been respected. Decompensation occurs more frequently distally than proximally to the instrumented zone. The Cranckshaft phenomenon, however, is a decompensated proximal curve mostly initiated by not including growing parts of the curve into the fusion (4).

There is also the possibility that patients who have been treated for a vertebral fracture had an additional, unrecognized asymmetrical discal lesion above or below the treated fracture. Over the years this diskal lesion may progress in asymmetrical discal degeneration and finally end up as true degenerative scoliosis.

DEFORMITY

A scoliosis may increase mid to long term when a decompression is done at the level of the apex. This is specifically true in degenerative scoliosis, where it must be considered as a contraindication to do decompressive maneuvers alone at the apex, respectively above and below. Correction of this complication can be quite demanding (8) and may require a major reconstructive surgery to maintain the balance of the spine (Fig. 7.6).

If we find a broken implant, in anterior or posterior surgery, and it concerns rods and screws or disassembled hooks, usually we can assume there must be a nonunion in the fusion mass, which facilitates rod breakage or screw breakage through fatigue. There are secondary deformities in scoliosis surgery that occur slowly over time as an expression of a delayed chronic decompensation. These are reactive curves that may not occur

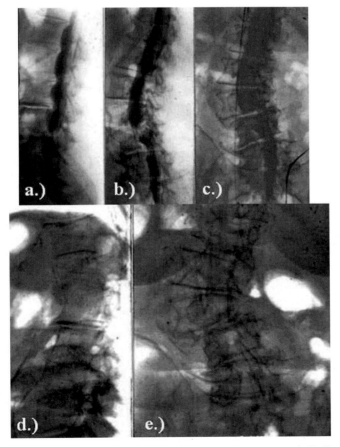

FIG. 7.6. A, B: 78-year-old patient with degenerative adult scoliosis. **C-E:** Decompressed at the apex: progression of the curve.

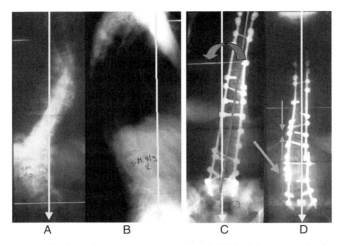

A   B   C   D

FIG. 7.7. A, B: 41-year-old female patient with a painful rigid triple curve. **C:** Correction followed by decompensation, lumbosacral nonunion. **D:** Repair with a circumferential fusion (PLIF) L5/S1 and realignment by cutting the left rod and applying tension banding forves (arrows).

immediately after correction of a scoliosis but are delayed. An unbalanced spine may induce a nonunion of the fusion mass, which may even increase the imbalance due to a localized pain reaction (Fig. 7.7).

DEGENERATIVE SPINAL DISEASE

A mid- to long-term deformity after interventions at the lumbar spine for degenerative disease—a unilateral decompression or asymmetrical decompression on several levels—is relatively rare today. Careful preservation of the joint structures and stabilizing elements while doing a decompression practically avoids the postoperative development of a scoliotic deformity due to unilateral joint damage. The treatment is again a reconstructive stabilizing procedure, which today can easily be avoided when localized stability preserving procedures are chosen. It is, however, advisable, specifically in degenerative scoliosis, to stabilize the curve apex prophylactically when a decompression is necessary, for example in a case with a complete stop in the myelogram (Fig. 7.8).

Furthermore, if decompressions are done at the adjacent segment of a lumbar instrumented fusion with a secondary collapse in this decompressed segment and a consecutive scoliosis, extension of the stabilization and fusion mass is necessary in such cases.

TREATMENT PRINCIPLES

Acute postoperative deformities can be treated usually by reversing the procedure just outlined and equilibrating the stabilized segment in trauma and degenerative reconstruction and restoring the spinal balance in decompensated spinal deformities. The principle is to disassemble the preceding construct and reassemble it in a better balanced configuration.

The mid- to long-term postoperative scoliotic complication usually requires a more complex analysis in order to address the real cause of the problem. Usually the surgical measures are different from what has been done originally, necessitating a major reconstructive salvage surgery that is clearly bigger and more extensive than the original sur-

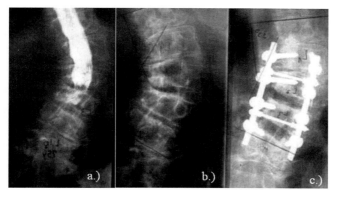

FIG. 7.8. A, B: 75-year-old female actress with paraparesis; prevention of a progressive post-operative curve after decompressive surgery for a complete block (**A**) at the level of the apical vertebra through prophylactic in situ stabilization of the apex (**C**).

gery. In rare cases of complex scoliosis where compensatory curves have been treated sequentially and getting a balanced spine has proved impossible, a complete removal may induce the spine to find its own balance unhindered by powerful, rigid instrumentation (1).

REFERENCES

1. Arlet V, Marchesi D, Papin P, Aebi M. Decompensation following scoliosis surgery: treatment by decreasing the correction of the main thoracic curve or "letting the spine go." Eur Spine J 2000; Apr 9(2): 156-60.
2. Bradford DS, Tribus CB. Vertebral column resection for the treatment of rigid coronal decompensation. Spine 1997; Jul 15;22(14): 1590-9.
3. Bridwell KH, McAllister JW, Betz RR, Huss G, Clancy M, Schoenecker PL. Coronal decompensation produced by Cotrel-Dubousset "derotation" maneuver for idiopathic right thoracic scoliosis. Spine 1991; Jul 16(7): 769-77.
4. Dubousset J, Herring JA, Shufflebarger H. The Crankshaft phenomenon. JPO 1989; 9: 541-50.
5. Edwards CC II, Bridwell KH, Patel A, Rinella AS, Kim YJ, Berra A, Della Rocca GJ, Lenke LG. Thoracolumbar deformity arthrodesis to L5 in adults: The fate of the L5-S1 disc. Spine 2003; 28(18): 2122-31.
6. Kamimura M, Ebara S, Kinoshita T, Itoh H, Nakakohji T, Takaoka K, Ohtsuka K. Anterior surgery with short fusion using the Zielke procedure for thoracic scoliosis: focus on the correction of compensatory curves. J Spinal Disord 1999; Dec 12(6): 451-60.
7. Lenke LG, Betz RR, Bridwell KH, Harms J, Clements DH, Lowe TG. Spontaneous lumbar curve coronal correction after selective anterior or posterior thoracic fusion in adolescent idiopathic scoliosis. Spine 1999; Aug 15;24(16): 1663-71.
8. Marchesi D, Aebi M. Pedicle fixation devices in the treatment of adult lumbar scoliosis. Spine 1992; 17(8 Suppl): S304-9.
9. Mason DE, Carango P. Spinal decompensation in Cotrel-Dubousset instrumentation. Spine 1991; Aug 16(8 Suppl): S394-403.
10. Muschik M, Schlenzka D, Robinson PN, Kupferschmidt C. Dorsal instrumentation for idiopathic adolescent thoracic scoliosis: rod rotation versus translation. Eur Spine J 1999; 8(2): 93-9.
11. Patwardhan A, Rimkus A, Gavin TM, Bueche M, Meade KP, Bielski R, Ibrahim K. Geometric analysis of coronal decompensation in idiopathic scoliosis. Spine 1996; May 15;21(10): 1192-1200.
12. Puno R, Johnson JR, Ostermann PAW et al. Analysis of the primary and compensatory curvatures following Zielke instrumentation for idipathic scoliosis. Spine 1989; Jul 14(7): 738-43.

8

Postoperative Flat Back

Aina J. Danielsson and Alf L. Nachemson

DEFINITION/MEASUREMENT OF LUMBAR LORDOSIS

Flat back syndrome has been defined as occurrence of lumbar pain ("fatigue") subsequent to a postoperative reduction of the lumbar lordosis and an inability to stand erect without flexing the knees; that is, the plumb line from C7 falls anterior to the sacrum (1,2). A definition of the normal range of lumbar lordosis as well as the lower normal limit is mandatory for a diagnosis. However, controversy still exist on these values. Furthermore, lordosis is measured in different ways and from different levels, partly a result from insufficient imaging techniques of the lower lumbar disc and the top of sacrum, making the lower level of lordosis difficult to define. Most authors use the upper level of L1 for the upper measurement level, but for the lower level, both lower L5 and upper S1 have been used. The segmental contribution to the lordic curve increases distally, with the greatest contribution coming from the two most caudal segments. From L1 to L5, mean segmental lordosis has been reported to be 40 to 44 degrees (3,4) and normal values between 20 to 40 degrees (1,5). When including the lower lumbar disk (i.e., measured from L1 to S1), mean segmental lordosis has been reported between 55 to 72 degrees (6–8), with a wide normal distribution between 20 to 80 degrees (9). In general, a lumbar lordosis of less than 20 degrees (L1 to S1) should be regarded as "flat back." The best overall agreement when measuring lumbar lordosis was achieved by measuring from L1 to L5 (10).

The relation between the thoracic kyphosis and the lumbar lordosis as well as the line for center of gravity are also of importance. It has been stated that the patient should have 30 degrees more lumbar lordosis than thoracic kyphosis.

It is not clear whether the reduced lumbar lordosis per se is the reason for pain. Some studies suggest that a loss of segmental lordosis in the lower lumbar area might be associated with low back pain (7,11), but many other studies have found no clear correlation (12,13), including our own series of surgically treated patients with Adolescent Idiopathic Scoliosis (AIS) (14–16).

ETIOLOGY

Postoperative flat back occurs in the following situations:

1. After fusion for scoliosis, usually in distraction of the lumbar spine below L3, if shortening of anterior column or lengthening of the posterior column (1,11,13,17,18)
2. After surgical treatment of spondylolisthesis (19)
3. "Degenerative disc disease" or after fusion for this entity (20,21)

These are the etiological factors for development of flat back syndrome (22):

1. Distraction instrumentation with the lower end at the L5 or S1 vertebra
2. Thoracolumbar junction kyphosis greater than 15 degrees, especially if associated with a hypokyphotic thoracic spine
3. Degenerative changes above and below a previous fusion

The incidence of the flat back syndrome is variable and depends on patients studied and levels and type of instrumentations used. Swank et al. (17) reported that 5% out of 222 adults treated for adult scoliosis with Harrington instrumentation had a marked loss of lordosis. Kostuik 1983 (11) found that 50% of patients fused with Harrington distraction rods had a significant loss of lordosis and half of these required surgery. Luque instrumentation was initially promising in the respect that it was supposed to decrease the rate of flat back syndrome, but reports on using it down to L5 or sacrum have shown a reduction of lordosis in 40% of patients, and 15% had significant pain or cosmetic change (11).

For multilevel hook systems, such as Cotrel-Dubousset (CD), reports have shown that sagittal curves are preserved after surgery or with a modest increase of lumbar lordosis (5,12,23). Over a 9-year follow-up period of patients treated with fusion using CD instrumentation (12), a slight but significant increase in lordosis of the unfused lumbar spine was found, but the clinical significance of this was uncertain. Out of the 30 patients, 23% developed degenerative changes and 20% had low back pain, not correlated to the degree of lumbar lordosis, however.

In our own 25-year follow-up of 156 consecutive cases of Harrington fusion for adolescent idiopathic scoliosis, of which 40 were fused below L3, 26 out of the evaluated 142 patients had a lumbar lordosis of less than 20 degrees. However, only four of those developed a flat back syndrome, of which two patients exhibited severe enough symptoms to warrant surgical correction (14). Our previously published 10-year follow-up (24) seems to indicate it is the long fusion per se that is mostly to blame for the occurrence of the flat back syndrome. More low back pain was observed with a more distal fusion, but there was no correlation to the degree of lordosis. Pain was more severe when a retrolisthesis was found.

Out of those 40 patients that had undergone a fusion down to L4, L5, or L6, respectively, which left one or two unfused disc levels below the fusion, 32 also underwent MRI of the lumbar spine (15). They had significantly ($p<0.0001$) less lumbar lordosis (mean 21.5 degrees, L1-L5) compared with matched controls (mean 43.6 degrees). No correlation was found between the lumbar lordosis and lumbar back pain (VAS) in any of the groups, but correlations between lumbar lordosis and degenerative signs could be found.

TREATMENT

The most important aspect is prevention, which includes the following:

1. Avoiding distraction fusion that extends into the lower lumbar spine
2. Maintaining normal lordosis at the time of the primary surgery
3. Considering total hip movement, extension in particular

Surgical treatment includes correction of the deformity by performing one or several closing wedge osteotomies through the fusion mass, with or without anterior release and possibly structural grafting prior to the correction (1,2,22,25). Goal for surgery is to restore a normal sagittal contour and place head over feet/C7 over sacrum in the coronal plane and head over hips/C7 over L5-S1 or just behind in the sagittal plane. Correction for this troubling sequel of spine surgery is best performed, according to our view,

management of degenerative lumbar spondylolisthesis, spinal fusion significantly improves patient satisfaction, and adjunctive spinal instrumentation enhances fusion rates."

Surgeons reported that instrumentation improved fusion rates, although we are all aware that determining if bony fusion is present, when there is a rigid fixation device in place, using, at most, flexion films but usually just viewing the X-rays, must be most imprecise. It was known that fusion improved the results of decompression in degenerative spondylolisthesis (Herkowitz) (7), but to add these two observations together as an endorsement for pedicle screws is questionable, when in the same study you have established that those with pedicle screws do less well.

The other major paper was by Yuan (8), representing a rapidly mounted "Historical Cohort Study of Pedicle Screw Fixation in Thoracic, Lumbar and Sacral Spinal Fusions." This was a collection of data on patients treated for fractures and degenerative spondylolisthesis from January 1990 to December 1991. The cohort of patients analyzed was 2,121 who had been treated with pedicle screws and 449 who were uninstrumented. There is no statistical assessment of the significance of the results, despite the widely disparate groups, which showed patients who were uninstrumented had an 84% improvement rate, as against a 91% improvement rate for those treated with pedicle fixation. Regarding leg pain, the respective figures were 88.2% as opposed to 91%. This was hardly a ringing endorsement for pedicle fixation. Complications were all self-reported by the surgeons and indeed are not dwelled on in any detail in the paper. Because a pedicle penetration rate of only 0.3% is reported, one must conclude the data is rather questionable. This paper, the Mardjetko paper, and the comments in an editorial by Garfin (9) led to a ringing endorsement of the use of the pedicle screw, ignoring the fact that the disorder treated was degenerative spondylolisthesis, not degenerative spondylosis. On the basis of these papers, showing in one paper a very marginal value of pedicle fixation in spondylolisthesis, the FDA climbed down, and the era of the pedicle screw continued.

Because those papers showing the questionable value of pedicle fixation, however, we finally had in 1998 the Volvo award-winning paper demonstrating that in treating low back pain, instrumentation leads to the same or worse clinical results (9,10). We have also had papers demonstrating the complications of pedicle screws (11,12). The development of specific steering devices to allow safe placement of the screw suggested the 0.3% misplacement result quoted in the Yuan paper was very inaccurate. The paper by Fischgrund et al. in 1997 (11) further confirmed that even in spondylolisthesis, fixation conferred no benefit. However, the most dramatic condemnation of the use of pedicle screws when doing a low lumbar fusion are the results of the prospective Swedish fusion study (13), which showed the results were uninfluenced by the surgical technique, that is, posterolateral, alone, or with fixation or a 360-degree fusion, and all had similar outcomes. Thus I believe to continue using pedicle fixation in carrying out a low lumbar fusion for back pain, where correction is not required, represents a misuse of instrumentation.

THE CAGE

Surgeons are pragmatists, and it was of course clear to many as the 1990s progressed that the pedicle screw had not been the solution to achieving better clinical results with spinal fusion. Hence the cage found a ready market, and as the sales of pedicle screws fell, so the sales of a multitude of cages went up. We started to use the BAK cage soon after it was cleared by the FDA, after the 2-year results were reported. Our results were very disappointing. What concerned us was that despite an apparently solid fusion, patients continued to have pain.

I had at that stage come to the conclusion the pain generator in low back pain was endplate and vertebrae (both very richly enervated), rather than the outer annulus, which is poorly innervated and related to load, not movement, so stopping movement and not addressing loading pattern was doomed to failure. I believe the reason for pain is excessive point loading on the endplate, due to the fact that the disc is no longer isotropic, and in certain positions very high-point loading occurs over a relatively small area of endplate. It was the same, of course, as the pain generated in hip and knee: osteoarthritis. We could in those disorders realign the load bearing and often cure patients (especially early unicompartmental knee arthritis). But the best cure was the artificial hip, which replaced the bearing surface and ensured an even pattern of weight transmission. Prior to the use of hip replacement, the literature abounds with theories as to where the pain is from, and needless to say the capsule was blamed (rather like the annulus), but we soon learned that capsulectomy played no role in hip arthroplasty; with increasing experience we even stopped spending time doing capsular releases as part of hip replacement (14–16).

We had published our work on the correlation between abnormal load patterns and positive discography in 1994 (17), and we reviewed our BAK patients a couple of years later and reported the dismal results. I suspected the problem might be that although union was achieved, the actual load bearing continued to be through the cage, and the BAK cage had a small load-bearing area. Work we did in collaboration with researchers in Aberdeen supported this view, showing, using a finite element model, the intense loads beneath the BAK cage, and this was supported by much more elegant work done by Polykeite in Berne (18).

McAfee in published an excellent review of the results of cages, commenting that the results were no better than previous techniques (19). He made the important observation that success clinically was associated with bone developing outside and around the cage. Another interesting observation he makes in an interview for *Argus Spine News* is the fact that without this surrounding bone, cages lead to associated vertebral osteoporosis, load goes through the cage, and the surrounding vertebrae becomes osteoporosis. Of course bone outside and around the cage increases the load-bearing area, leading to the better clinical result observed by McAfee in his review. It is unlikely that bone within a cage, even if integrated with the cancellous bone beneath and above it, will be load bearing. Because the cage is subjected to load, it will not deform and allow the bone to take load. As demonstrated so well in telemetric experiments some years ago, even after a solid anterior fusion, the plate and screws placed posterior continue to take maximal load, load sparing as long as they remain rigid. Cages have been made bigger—with a bigger footprint—as it was appreciated that the larger the bearing surfaces, the better.

We have just completed a prospective study comparing the Syn cage with femoral ring allografts, reviewed at 2 years (20). The results still show that for back pain, fusion is not a very good operation, but what is most dramatic is that the femoral all grafts do so much better. We cannot be certain as yet why this is the case, the union rate in both was similar, and in any event union was not a factor that affected clinical success. However we know that slowly but surely the femoral ring is replaced by normal weight-bearing bone, appropriately developed to transmit load across the segment in a normal fashion. We are reviewing what CT scans we have to see if the bone pattern below the Syn cage is less organized than that below the femoral ring.

In my view the evidence is mounting that cages are not an advance, and the recent prospective study from Sweden where it was shown that irrespective of what method of fusion was used, the results, although better than doing nothing, where all in the 60% to

70% success rate. I believe the continued use of cages, especially small cages that rest mainly on the cancellous bone, represents a misuse of the device.

DISC ARTHROPLASTY

The development of disc arthroplasty is fueled by two factors. First is our disenchantment with fusion, despite all the new advances such as cages and pedicle screws. Over the last 50 years, we had regarded fusion as the only effective treatment for low back pain due to degenerative disease. We ascribed failure to a failure to achieve fusion, and because of this many patients had further operations to refuse the spine, with dismal results. However we got steadily better in getting a fusion, and indeed with pedicle fixation we were certain that flexion and extension and translation movement was abolished (but not loading), yet still clinical success eluded us. We also felt, on rather questionable evidence it must be said, that adjacent segment disease was a clinical problem with spinal fusion. Of greater importance, especially with two or more level fusions, especially if they are in a flexed position, is the long-term effect on the ability of a patient to achieve satisfactory saggital balance when sitting or walking, without placing adjacent levels in an uncomfortable position of lordosis.

Arthroplasty certainly deals with both these concerns because it allows a degree of movement. However by serendipity it also has one other great advantage: the potential to create a normal loading pattern over the endplate and vertebrae. The failure of rigid fixation to cure back pain due to disc degeneration was because it did not unload the disc. Anterior surgery autologous bone graft could, but it was necessary that the graft be sufficiently large to transmit load over all the endplate. Cages have failed because they may transmit load in a concentrated pattern. Femoral ring allografts may succeed somewhat better because they can respond to load patterns and remodel to transmit load normally. The one obvious fact is that the success of arthroplasty rather conclusively proves that movement itself is not an important factor in back pain. Arthroplasty allows much more movement than any failed fusion could ever do, and in all planes, but it has the potential to transmit load evenly over the endplate. Over the next few years, it is incumbent on us all to look very critically at the new developments in arthroplasty and critically evaluate any publications.

NUCLEOPLASTY

The principal nucleoplasty device in clinical use is the Ray device. It was Charlie Ray's (17) intention that his device should replace the isotropic disc that would load equally over the endplate and most importantly load against the inner annulus. We are all aware that nuclear degeneration precedes annular failure because it ceases to protect the inner annulus, and enfolding and splitting occur. The Ray device does not load against the annulus; the material cage it is in prevents this. The initial design allowed it, but then there was a high rate of dislocation. It is being used most frequently as an adjunct to an operation for sciatica when there is a protruding or herniated disc. This is removed, ensuring a 90% success rate, and then the inside of the disc is meticulously cleared, so that most, if not all, of the nucleus is removed. The Ray device then replaces it. It does not replace the important function of the device in protecting the annulus. In many ways it functions like the Fermstrom balls used in the 1950s, loading the endplates alone but not tensioning the annulus. We are all aware that the majority of patients who have a disc herniation do not get a serious low back pain problem, and indeed the propensity to get a problem is not related to disc space narrowing (21). One could therefore predict that the generalized use of the Ray nucleoplasty will lead to an increase of annulus disruption and a greater propensity to a major back problem in patients who have it inserted as an add-on to having a herniated disc removed. I believe its continued use; especially in patients with sciatica and a herniated disc rather then back pain, is misuse, not based as in the two previous examples on clinical trials but on the inherent defect in the design and concept.

IDET

Intradiscal Electro Therapy (IDET) is another flawed concept. It was introduced initially with the view that it coagulated the collagen at the back of the disc and tightened it to make it more stable. A recent comprehensive study had shown it does not actually do this, and combined with a clinical study it has been shown to be ineffective. The questions are whether these results will be read critically by surgeons and will they review their use of the technique (22).

SUMMARY

With the increasing recognition that back pain can be cured, and movement maintained, and that fusion has certain other disadvantages, even if it does produce a normal loading pattern, we are now entering the era of the artificial total disc and so-called flexible stabilization. I have great hopes for both. I am not nihilistic. However, from our experience in the last 30 years, I believe surgeons have a number of responsibilities concerning the use of new devices. They must be sufficiently scientific themselves to assess the likelihood that a device will be of value. Most of us viewed with some scepticism the IDET concept that heating and possibly shrinking some collagen at the back of the disc would produce a cure, when at the same time we routinely left a gaping hole in the back of the disc and expected our patients to do well, and they usually did.

Regarding the study by Freeman et al. (19), surgeons must await the results of carefully clinically controlled trials of a new device before using it. When using a new device they must assess their own results meticulously. If reporting their results, or indeed assessing them themselves for their guidance, they ideally should have their results independently reviewed. They must read any such reports with some care, reading the whole paper, not just the abstracts, which are often rather tailored to avoid upsetting those who might be supporting the study. If reports of devices show a pattern of failure or ineffectiveness, they must react.

When I was first appointed as a consultant surgeon, I worked alongside some splendid experienced senior surgeons, who refused to do hip and knee replacements, however, and patients were denied a very valuable new advance in treatment. A certain caution is necessary in a surgeon, but it will be a sad day if such caution denies our patients of the benefits of some very important advances in surgery, especially surgery of the back. Therefore we must be innovative, but assess innovation very critically.

A second important philosophical consideration is that usually and indeed preferably a new treatment for back pain is based on an hypothesis as to its cause. The clinical use of the procedure is essentially a test of that hypothesis. If we delude ourselves and others that the treatment is successful, we validate the hypothesis and cease looking for other reasons. This is what happened with the use of fusion for back pain. A failure to recognize the very modest effect it had in many patients, and the lack of success in many was really not appreciated, and for 40 years no further research was done as to alternative methods of treatment, merely better methods of achieving a fusion. We now have moved on, recognizing that abnormal load bearing is crucial, not movement, and this opens the way to the use of devices that alter loading but do not stiffen the segment.

REFERENCES

1. Camille R, Sealant G, Maze C. Internal fixation of the lumbar spine with pedicel screw plating. Clin Orthop 1986;203:7-17.
2. Panjabi MM. The stabilizing system of the spine. Part II: Neutral and instability hypothesis. J Spinal Disord 1992 Dec 5;(4):396-406.
3. Panjabi MM et al. On the understanding of clinical instability. Spine 1994 Dec 1;19(23):2642-50.
4. Panjabi MM. Clinical spinal instability and low back pain. J Electromyogr Kinesiol 2003 Aug 13;(4):371-9.
5. Zdeblick TA. A prospective randomized study of lumbar fusion. Spine 1993 Jun 15;18(8):983-91.
6. Mardjetko SM, Connolly PJ, Shott S. Degenerative lumbar spondylolisthesis. A meta-analysis of the literature 1970–1993. Spine 1994(20):S2256-61.
7. Herkowitz HN. Degenerative lumbar spondylolisthesis with spinal stenosis. A prospective study comparing results of decompression alone, and decompression combined with posterior intertransverse fusion. J Bone Joint Surg 1991 July 7;396:802-8.
8. Yuan H, Garfin SR, Dickman CA, Mardjetko SM. A historical cohort study of pedicle screw fixation in thoracic, lumbar and sacral spinal fusions. Spine 19(20):S2279-92.
9. Steven R Garfin. Summation. Spine 19(20):S2300S-5S.
10. 1997 Volvo Award winner in Clinical Studies. The effect of pedicle screw instrumentation on functional outcome and fusion rates in posterolateral lumbar spinal fusion: a prospective randomized and clinical study. Spine 1997 Dec 15;22(24):2813-22.
11. Katonids P, Christofarakis J, Katonis G, Aligizakic AC, Papadopoulos C, Sapkas G, Hadjipavlou A. Complications and problems related to pedicle screw fixation of the spine. Clin Orthop 2003 June; (411):86-94.
12. Jutte OC, Castelain RM. Complications of pedicle screws in lumbar and lumbosacral fusions in 105 consecutive primary operations. Eur Spine J 2002 Dec 11;(6):594-8. E-pub 2002 October.
13. Fischgrund JS, Mackay M, Herkowitz HN, Brower R, et al. Prospective study comparing instrumented posterolateral fusion and uninstrumented fusion in treatment of degenerative spondylolisthesis. Spine 1997 Dec 15; 22(24)2807-12.
14. Complications in lumbar fusion surgery for chronic low back pain: comparison of three surgical techniques in a prospective randomized study. A report from the Swedish Lumbar spine Study Group. Eur Spine J 2003 Apr 12; (2): 178-89. E-pub 2003 February.
15. Kuslich K. I.D.E. study. Spine 1998 June 23;(11):1267-78.
16. Kuslich K, et al. Four-year follow up results of lumbar spine arthrodesis using the Bagby and Kuslich lumbar fusion cage. Spine 2000 Oct 15; 25(20):2656-62.
17. McNally D, Shackleford I, Mulholland RC. In vivo stress measurement can predict pain in Discography. Spine 1996 Nov 15;21(22)2580-7.
18. Polikeit A, Nolte L-P, Orr TE, Muller ME. Factors affecting the behavior of interbody cages in the lumbar spine: finite element analysis. Bern, Switzerland: Institute for Biomechanics, University of Bern.
19. McAfee PC. Current concepts review. Interbody fusion cages in reconstructive operations on the spine. J Bone Joint Surg; 81-A June 1999: 859-80.
20. Klara PM, Ray CD. Artificial nucleus replacement. Spine 2002 June 15;27(12):137-7.
21. Clarke A, Freeman BJC, Leung YL, Mehdian SH, Grevitt MP, Mulholland RC, Webb JK. The Centre for Spinal Surgery, University Hospital, Queen's Medical Centre, Nottingham, UK. Prospective randomized trial comparing femoral ring allograft versus a titanium cage for circumferential spinal fusion. Presented at EuroSpine Prague 2003.
22. Freeman B, Grevitt M, Webb JK, Mehdian H, Mulholland RC. Two year functional and radiological outcome, a randomized double-blind controlled study: IDET versus placebo for the treatment of chronic discogenic LBP. Presented at Prague EuroSpine and in print. In press, Eur Spine J.

10

Delayed Infections After Posterior Arthrodesis of the Spine for Idiopathic Scoliosis

Pierre Pries, Louis-Etienne Gayet, Christophe Audic, and Hamid Hamcha

This chapter discusses the incidence of delayed infections after posterior spinal instrumentation-arthrodesis for idiopathic scoliosis, outlines the accurate management of these delayed infections, and identifies the potential risk factors.

All the patients operated for idiopathic scoliosis by posterior spinal instrumentation-arthrodesis between 1986 and 2001 are included in this study. Delayed infections appearing more than 1 year after the first intervention were studied retrospectively. All the patients of this study were operated on by the same senior surgeon, in identical operative conditions. The following parameters were studied: clinical signs of the infection, delay of outbreak, sedimentation rate, presence of a pathogenic germ in the perioperative sample cultures, existence of a pseudarthrosis, surgical method, and the infection's treatment and antibiotherapy duration.

Between 1986 and 2001, 162 patients were operated for an idiopathic scoliosis by posterior spinal instrumentation-arthrodesis. The CD instrumentation (Medtronic-Sofamor-Danek) was used for the 148 first patients, the TTL (Scient'x) for the other 14 cases.

Among those patients, nine presented a delayed infection, at least 1 year after the initial surgery (i.e., 5.56%). The average appearance of late infection was 51 months with extremes of 22 to 89 months. Seven patients had a productive fistula; two suffered pains and local fluctuation. The sedimentation rate was increased in all cases. The identified germs were four propionibacterium acnes, one pseudomonas aeruginosa, one corynebacterium amycolatum, and one unspecified cocci Gram +. For two patients, no germ was identified. One of them had an initial coral arthrodesis; the other one was proved allergic to nickel. Among the nine infected patients, seven underwent a complete removal of the instrumentation, two a partial one. The mean delay between the initial intervention and the removal was 66 months, with extremes from 24 to 130 months. The average time between the diagnosis of the delayed infection and the removal of the instrumentation was 15 months, with extremes from 1 to 108 months. The last case is the one initially treated with coral arthrodesis. After instrumentation removal, only two patients had no antibiotics. The seven others benefited from intravenous antibiotherapy for an average of 32 days (7 to 180 days) followed by antibiotherapy by mouth for an average of 50 days (43 to 180 days). All the patients healed after a mean recoil of 28 months after antibiotherapy. No pseudarthrosis was observed when removing the instrumentation. In seven cases, the Cobb angle gain was maintained; in two cases a loss below 5 degrees was observed.

Usually, the responsible germs for the appearance of delayed infections are low-virulent ones, like propionibacterium acnes. The perioperative contamination is followed by a quiescent period. The increased number of implants and the complexity of the mountings used in idiopathic scoliosis treatment are probably the roots of local inflammatory phenomenon, contributing to the disclosure of the infection. The infection treatment has to be univocal: complete removal of the instrumentation, antibiotherapy, first parenteral, then oral, fitting the germ identified on cultures maintained for 14 days, and primary closure on drainage. This therapeutic strategy secures the proper healing of the infection.

INTRODUCTION

The modern segmental instrumentations, which appeared after 1984 from Cotrel and Dubousset's work, permitted optimum correction in idiopathic scoliosis treatment. Unfortunately, the increased complexity of the systems and the multiplicity of the implants required a longer surgery. The quantity and bulk of the devices, positioned near the skin, increased during the years of this study.

In the meantime, several studies reported late infections, with a 1% to 6.7% rate (1,2,5,9,10). Several authors concluded that those infections were the consequence of soft tissue inflammation, in reaction to the fretting corrosion of the metallic implants (2,10). Others concluded it was the consequence of perioperative contamination by low virulent bacteria, responsible for the late revelation of the infection (1,5,9).

In 1995, Stephens Richards (5) reported 10 delayed infections on 149 patients (i.e., an incidence of 6.7%). These infections were due to germs like propionibacterium acnes, staphylococcus epidermidis, and micrococcus varians. He concluded that, if the cultures of the preoperative samples were maintained for 72 hours only, the responsible germs were not identified. This was confirmed by Clark and Shufflebarger's study in 1999 (1). Among 22 infected patients in their study, the cultures were maintained 72 hours for the first 10 patients: no germ was identified for 9 cases. In contrast, when the cultures were maintained for 7 days, for the remaining 12 patients, 11 results showed pathogen germs, among which staphylococcus epidermidis was predominant.

Our study aims at the determination of the delayed infections' incidence in a population of 162 operated idiopathic scoliosis, to identify the best therapeutic management and possible risk factors.

MATERIAL AND PATIENTS (TABLE 10.1)

A group of 162 patients were operated on using posterior instrumentation-arthrodesis for idiopathic scoliosis between 1986 and 2001. All of them was operated on by the same senior surgeon, in the same operation room, in identical anesthesia conditions. The first 148 patients had Cotrel-Dubousset (Medtronic-Sofamor-Danek) instrumentation, and the 14 last ones, the TTL instrumentation (Scient'x). The arthrodesis was performed using the same technique: resection of all the articular process of the merged area, decortication of the posterior arch of the uninstrumented vertebrae, and posterior arthrodesis by autograft. Among this population, 9 patients presented a delayed infection, appearing more than a year after the initial surgery. For those 9 patients, we compiled the following parameters, retrospectively analyzed: sex, age at surgery time, initial Cobb angle in degrees, preoperative associated pathologies, height, and weight. The following surgical parameters were analyzed: duration of the operation in hours and minutes, estimated blood loss, number of vertebrae included in the arthrodesis, arthrodesis type, and instrumentation type. The postoperative parameters studied were mechanical complication seven patients who had a total removal of the osteosynthesis instrumentation, an angular loss, below 5 degrees, was observed in two cases.

Average Time since Infection Healing

The average elapsed time since the clinical, biological, and radiological healing of the infection is 28 months; extremes 8 to 48 months. It was 97 months for one of the patients who benefited only from a partial removal of the osteosynthesis instrumentation and 46 months for the second one.

DISCUSSION

Several studies about the development of late infections, beyond 1 year after arthrodesis for idiopathic scoliosis, using instrumentation with multiple hooks and two rods, were recently published (1,2,4,5,7,9).

In 1995, Richards et al. (5) found 10 cases of late infections in 149 operated cases (i.e., an occurrence of 6.71%). The average infection time of emergence was 11 to 45 months. The identified germs were staphylococcus aureus and propionibacterium acnes in 90% of the cases. After complete removal of the instrumentation, the parenteral antibiotherapy lasted for 2 to 14 days; the oral one lasted 14 to 60 days. The authors concluded, "We suspect—but cannot prove—that several of the delayed infections resulted from intraoperative seeding and remained subclinical for an extended period of time."

In 1999, Clark et al. (1) reported that in 1,247 cases operated by CD instrumentation (Medtronic-Sofamor-Danek), then Moss Miami (DePuy), 22 delayed infections occurred, showing an average of 1.7%. The mean time of appearance ranged from 14 to 101 months, identified germs being staphylococcus aureus, propionibacterium acnes, and enterococcus. The identified germs occurrence was only 10% if the cultures were maintained for 72 hours, and it was 90% when prolonged 7 to 10 days. The parenteral antibiotherapy lasted 3 days, the oral one 10 days. The authors concluded, "The treatment is implant removal and short-term antibiotics. . . . The effect of lower volume implants on the incidence of late infection is unknown."

In 2001, Gaine et al. (3) reported six cases of late infection after arthrodesis for scoliosis, happening in a mean delay of 10 to 22 months. Staphylococcus aureus and streptococcus were found in 50% of the cases. The authors conclude, "Fretting at cross connection junctions may provide the environment for the incubation of dormant or inactive microbes."

In 2001, Richards et al. (6) find 23 cases of late infections in 489 cases of operated scoliosis by means of arthrodesis instrumentation (i.e., a 4.7% occurrence) observed in a mean delay of 11 to 79 months after the initial intervention. The identified germs were staphylococcus aureus and epidermidis, propionibacterium acnes, and micrococcus varians in 90% of the cases. The parenteral antibiotherapy duration was 2 to 14 days followed by an oral one for 14 to 60 days. The authors conclude, "intraoperative seeding followed by subclinical quiescent periods appears to be the method by which infection occurs."

In 2003, Soultanis et al. (8) reported 5 late infections in 60 operated scoliosis cases (i.e., an 8.33% occurrence), developing within 12 to 60 months. In all the cases, the pathogen germs were identified: coagulase negative staphylococcus, acinetobacter baumani, and peptostreptococcus. The parenteral antibiotherapy was administered for 7 days, followed by oral antibiotherapy during 45 days, after complete removal of the osteosynthesis device. The authors conclude, "The findings suggest a correlation between instrumentation failure and loosening and late infection."

In our series, none of the pre, per, or postoperative studied parameters could be sig-nificantly pointed out as risk factors for the emergence of late infection. The occurrence of the late infection in our series, 1.7%, is consistent with the literature data. Even if no parameter was identified as a statistically consistent risk factor, we observed that in most cases it concerned extended arthrodesis on an average of 10 levels. The infected patients were always lean, with the height/weight ratio 164 cm for 49.8 kg.

Only one patient presented with a preoperative hepatitis C, potential risk factor to the breaking out of infection. The average age at intervention time was 17 years 9 months; mean Cobb angle was 55 degrees. The average duration of the initial intervention was 4 hours 30 minutes with extremes of 3 h 20 to 5 h 05, sensibly more than the average dura-tion of the interventions performed for scoliosis of patients during the same lapse of time, without any statistically significant difference found. The blood loss during the operation was also superior to the average in the series: 1,500 ml (i.e., 150 ml per arthrodesis level). Apart from the case with coral graft, which is the only one in the 162 operated patients, the nature of the arthrodesis had no influence on the late infection nature. This data is sim-ilar to the examples in the literature and confirms the necessity to abandon the coral grafts.

Three of our nine infected patients presented with a mechanical complication after the initial surgery, leading to a revision. In one case it was a lumbar pedicular screw break-age, diagnosed after a road accident, which led to a revision 15 months after the initial surgery. In another case, it was the aggravation of a curvature adjacent to the fusion site, implying an extension of the arthrodesis, 16 months after the initial operation, and in another case, it was a pseudarthrosis with distal screw breakage, needing an arthrodesis' extension at 20 months postoperatively. For us, the apparition of a mechanical complica-tion leading to a reintervention constitutes an additional risk factor to the outbreak of a late infection. Nevertheless, the bacteriological cultures of the samples systematically performed when reintervening remained negative for those three patients after 10 days.

In our series, the diagnosis of late infection occurred an average 51 months postoper-atively, in front of local signs of infection, with local productive fistula in seven cases, and pain syndrome and fluctuation in front of the material in the other two cases. The ini-tial management of the late infection varied because no consensus existed at the time of the diagnosis as to the required management of these late infections. It is why three patients only, after a short time necessary to the infection assessment, were treated by complete removal of the instrumentation and adapted antibiotherapy. They were the last three cases of the series. At the time of their undertaking, the therapeutic attitude con-sensus was known, and the treatment of their late infection was thus conforming to the consensus, meaning complete removal of the instrumentation and adapted antibiotherapy. Three other patients, whose infection was anterior to the consensus, were treated by local care and antibiotics during 1 to 3 months for two of them. Finally, two patients were treated by partial removal of the instrumentation and antibiotherapy and one by surgical debridement. Even if this attitude is no more used, we note that the two patients who underwent a distal partial removal of the osteosynthesis device can be accepted as healed of their infection, with a 46 months recoil for one and 86 months for the other. In the first of these two cases, the inflammation seemed very localized in front of the failing hook. This patient did not receive any antibiotics after surgery and healed after a simple clean-ing and drainage of the wound, performed contemporarily with the removal of the hook. He is now working as a car mechanic and is an amateur rally pilot.

The results of the bacteriological samples in our series are similar to those of the liter-ature: four propionibacterium acnes, one pseudomonas aeruginosa, one corynebacterium amycolatum, one unspecified cocci Gram+; only two patients had no identified germs, the patient with coral graft and the patient allergic to nickel. The purulent aspect of the observed liquid at the removal of the material led us to include them in the infected group.

The complete removal of the osteosynthesis instrumentation, even if technically delicate, especially with the first CD instrumentation, appears to us as the sine qua non condition for the infection healing, with a complementary parenteral then oral antibiotherapy, adapted to the identified germ. The duration of the antibiotherapy, parenteral or oral, fluctuates in the literature. We take as a base the clinical as well as biological and radiological evolution of the infection parameters. A parenteral antibiotherapy duration of 2 to 4 weeks, followed by an oral one of 3 months, seems adequate to us.

With mean recoil of 28 months since the clinical and biological healing of the infection, we did not observe any pseudarthrosis, only an angular loss of less than 5 degrees in two patients.

SUMMARY

The incidence of late infection after arthrodesis instrumentation of scoliosis is 5.6% in our series of 162 operated cases. Mostly, low-virulent germs like propionibacterium acnes are responsible for those late infections. We attribute the late infections to peroperative seeding remaining quiescent for a long time. Local mechanical complications (partial dismantling of the osteosynthesis), fretting phenomenon at anchoring site of the rods on the vertebral implants, seem to be risk factors involved in the delayed infection. The presence of membranes surrounding the osteosynthesis material (Glycocalix biofilm) is a barrier to the efficacy of simple medical treatment by antibiotherapy. Hence the univocal treatment of these delayed infections seems to us, as to most of the authors, the complete removal of the osteosynthesis material, followed by a parenteral antibiotherapy adapted to the identified germ for 2 to 4 weeks. An oral complementary antibiotherapy is usually administered for 1 to 3 months. Sticking to this therapeutic strategy leads to the healing of the late infection, with, at the worst, a small angle loss and no identified pseudarthrosis.

REFERENCES

1. Clark CE, Shufflebarger HL. Late developing infection in instrumented idiopathic scoliosis. Spine 1999; 24: 1909-12.
2. Dubousset J, Shufflebarger H, Wenger D. Late "infection" with CD instrumentation. Orthop Trans 1994; 18: 121.
3. Gaine WJ, Andrew SM, Chadwick P, Cooke E, Williamson JB. Late operative site pain with isola posterior instrumentation requiring implant removal: infection or metal reaction? Spine 2001; 26: 583-7.
4. Heggeness MH, Esses SI, Errico T, et al. Late infection of spinal instrumentation by hematogenous seeding. Spine 1993; 18: 492-6.
5. Richards BS. Delayed infections following posterior spinal instrumentation for the treatment of idiopathic scoliosis. J Bone Joint Surg Am 1995; 77: 524-9.
6. Richards BS, Emara KM. Delayed infections after posterior TSRH spinal instrumentation for idiopathic scoliosis. Spine 2001; 18: 1990-6.
7. Schofferman L, Zucherman J, Schofferman J, et al. Diphtheroids and associated infections as a cause of failed instrument stabilization procedures in the lumbar spine. Spine 1991; 16: 356-8.
8. Soultanis K, Mantelos G, Pagiatakis A, Soucacos PN. Late infection in patients with scoliosis treated with spinal instrumentation. Clin Orthop 2003; 411: 116-23.
9. Viola RW, King HA, Adler SM, et al. Delayed infection after elective spinal instrumentation and fusion. Spine 1997; 22: 2444-51.
10. Wimmer C, Cluch H. Aseptic loosening after CD instrumentation in the treatment of scoliosis: a report about eight cases. J Spinal Disord 1998; 11: 440-3.

11

How Important is Postoperative Infection in the Spine, and What are the Available Therapeutic Options?

Alexander G. Hadjipavlou, Michael N. Tzermiadianos, Pavlos G. Katonis, and George M. Kontakis

INTRODUCTION

This is an update and modified version of the original chapter on postoperative spinal infections edited by Calhoon and Mader (1). Any invasive diagnostic spinal procedure or surgery, whether noninstrumented or instrumented, can be complicated by infection. This incidence generally increases with the complexity of the procedure (2). Infections after instrumentation may be manifested as an early or late (delayed) complication. Early infections are not uncommon and, if not treated promptly and appropriately, they may have significant implications. Delayed spinal infections after elective spinal instrumentation and fusion are uncommon, and the diagnosis is frequently challenging (3).

Infections following spinal surgery can have devastating consequences, from enormous social implications to jeopardizing the patient's life. The complications can be classified into local complications, general complications, and socioeconomic problems. The best treatment for postoperative infections is prevention; therefore special attention to the so-called reversible risk factors must be paid. Successful outcomes in terms of restoring the purpose of the original surgery can be achieved by prompt diagnosis and appropriate treatment based on available medical reports and the authors' experience.

SOCIOECONOMIC PROBLEMS

The magnitude of the socioeconomic problem of spinal infections is enormous; consequently, the reduction of infection rates is of paramount importance (4). The prognosis of discitis varies markedly in different series. Clinical studies generally support the concept that when treatment is instituted early in the process of infection, the prognosis is definitely better (5,6). Available clinical studies indicate that after spondylodiscitis complicating discectomy, 50% to 87.5% of patients were unable to resume their previous occupation (7-12). The average cost per patient with infected spinal wound was $100,000, indicating the cost of postoperative infection is four times greater than in uncomplicated spine surgery (13). The socioeconomic aspect of postoperative infections after spinal instrumentation was well outlined in a prospective, multicenter study by Thalgott and associates (14). For mild infections, necessitating only one surgical debridement-irrigation treatment, the average hospital stay was 14 days (ranging from 8 to 28 days) with an average hospital cost of $42,000 (ranging from $14,000 to $87,000). In more severe infections, the patients required multiple hospital admissions and an average of three surgeries per patient (ranging from one to seven) to resolve their infections. The average hospital stay was 51.6 days (ranging from 8 to 180 days), and the average hospital cost was $128,000 (ranging from $10,500 to $778,000). Patients with extensively infected wounds, with extensive tissue damage and myonecrosis, required an average of six surgeries per patient (ranging from four to eight) and eventually needed muscle flaps for closure. The average hospital stay was 77.5 days (ranging from 65 to 90 days), and the average hospital cost was $437,000.

RISK FACTORS

Several risk factors can predispose a patient to postoperative spinal infection, particularly to early postoperative spinal infection after spinal instrumentation. To a lesser extent, however, these factors may also play a role in late infections and infections after noninstrumented spinal surgery, particularly after discectomy. On the basis of available reports (14-21), the medical conditions widely accepted as risk factors are listed in Table 11.1.

The type of surgical approach also has an important bearing on postoperative infections. The infection rate for spinal instrumentation through an anterior approach has been reported to range between 0% and 0.1% (16,21), as opposed to a relatively high infection rate when the posterior approach (Table 11.7) for instrumentation was used (16). It is postulated that the extensive surgical exposure required for posterior instrumentation, compounded by prolonged retraction of the paraspinal muscles (large retractors, etc.), devitalizes the paraspinal muscles. The ensuing liquefaction necrosis predisposes to tissue colonization

TABLE 11.1. *Risk Factors Predisposing to Spinal Surgical Wound Infections*

Preoperative factors
Concomitant infections: acute or chronic (skin, visceral, pressure sores, etc.)
Immunocompromised host (cancer, chemotherapy, HIV, etc.)[a]
Corticosteroid therapy
Rheumatoid arthritis
Advanced age
Obesity
Malnutrition
Diabetes mellitus (uncontrolled)
Smoking
Previous spinal surgery
Cardiovascular disease

Intraoperative factors
Posterior spinal instrumentation greater than anterior
Prolonged duration of surgery (more than 5-7 hours)
High-volume blood loss (average 1600 mL)
High-volume operating room personnel traffic
Violation of sterile conditions
Use of allograft
Contaminated irrigation solution

Postoperative factors
Paralysis (incontinence, genitourinary infections, etc.)
Prolonged hospital bed rest
Skin maceration (dressing, orthosis, etc.)
Contamination of wound drains

[a] HIV, human immunodeficiency virus.

by contaminated microorganisms, which eventually leads to sepsis. Postoperative wound infection has been frequently observed in paralytic patients. In two reports the incidence ranged between 20% to 32% (22,23). Long surgical time (over 5 hours) and a high volume of blood loss (mean volume 1,620 mL) (17,24) have also been implicated as risk factors for the development of postoperative infections. The presence of relatively large numbers of people in, or moving through, the operating room (OR) during surgery is also a consideration. The number of colony-forming units per cubic foot has been shown to be almost proportional to excessive traffic and number of persons in the OR (25,26).

A history of previous surgery was noted in 37% of infected cases in one report (2). Additionally, biomaterials may make the adjacent tissues susceptible to both immediate and delayed infection by impeding host defense mechanisms (27), suggesting the presence of instrumentation may be a risk factor by itself (28). This instrumentation may protect inoculated microorganisms, allowing them to form a nidus of infection, making treatment more difficult.

The length of the patient's hospital stay may also be a risk factor for infection. An extended preoperative hospital stay leads to colonization of the patient with hospital flora, which may increase the incidence of postoperative infections (29). Additionally, the patient's nutritional status may be a risk factor for postoperative infection. One study reports that the prevalence of nutritionally challenged patients undergoing elective spinal surgery was noted in 25% of cases, with a higher number (42%) encountered in the older population group (30). Preoperative nutritional status is an extremely significant independent predictor of postoperative complications in patients undergoing elective lumbar spinal fusion; 85% of postoperative infectious complications were noted in malnourished patients in one report (31). Weight loss greater than 10 pounds should be considered indicative of malnutrition. Finally, diabetes mellitus has been widely accepted as a risk factor for infection. In some studies (12,32), 19.4% to 26% of patients who developed postoperative spondylodiscitis had associated diabetes mellitus. The incidence of diabetes mellitus in all surgical patients is 6.8% (32). However, a 2000 study challenges this conclusion (33). Uncontrolled diabetes mellitus, particularly when associated with cardiovascular or renal complications, should be considered a potential risk factor. It seems that the presence of more than two or three risk factors predisposes the patient to infection (16).

LABORATORY INVESTIGATION

Conventional Inflammatory Parameters

The conventional inflammatory parameters, white blood cell, C-reactive protein, and erythrocyte sedimentation rate, although useful, lack specificity and sensitivity, particularly for low-grade infections (34-36).

Erythrocyte Sedimentation Rate

In the majority of patients, erythrocyte sedimentation rate (ESR) increases to peak levels about 4 to 5 days after surgery (37,38), followed by a slow and irregular decrease, usually with a return to normal after 2 weeks (37). However, ESR may remain elevated even *21 to 42* days after surgery (38). More specifically, the maximal mean peak values seen 4 days after disc surgery were 45 to 75 mm/h (6,37,38) and exceeded 100 mm/h after spinal fusion (37). When deep wound infection complicates spinal surgery, ESR values exceed the corresponding mean values by +2 SD. In delayed spinal infection, ESR was elevated in 87.5% of cases, averaging 57 mm/h.

C-Reactive Protein

The normal values for C-reactive protein (CRP) are usually less than 10 mg/L (µg/mL). These values can increase to certain peak levels, without reflecting infection, after different types of spine surgery, such as microdiscectomy (46 ± 21 mg/L), anterior fusion (70 ± 23 mg/L), conventional discectomy (92 ± 47 mg/L), and posterolateral inter-transverse fusion (173 ± 39 mg/L). These values reach peak levels on the second and third postoperative days and tend to normalize in 5 to 14 days. The expected rapid decline in CRP is often interrupted by a second rise, or CRP level remains persistently elevated if infection supervenes (39). CRP may be a better index than ESR for early detection of postoperative infection (3,39).

White Blood Cell Count

White blood cell count (WBC) usually is not expected to show any changes after uncomplicated spinal surgery, even in the presence of infection. Usually, this test is not a reliable index of infectious activity. Total WBC was found to be slightly elevated in only 20% of patients with acute postoperative spinal infection (37) and in 25% of patients with delayed postoperative infection after instrumentation (3).

Imaging Resources

Available imaging recourses for assessing infections are labeled leukocyte scanning, bone scanning, and fluorodeoxyglucose positron emission tomography (FDG PET). CT scan is not useful in the early diagnosis of postoperative spondylodiscitis (5). Although MRI is an excellent test for primary hematogenous spinal infection, it may not play a major diagnostic role in the presence of metallic implants but may be useful to indicate whether epidural abscess or discitis is complicating the infection (42,43).

Scintigraphy has been widely used in joint infections (44). However, more emphasis is given to the clinical diagnosis in this situation and radionuclide testing should not create unnecessary delays of treatment. Radionuclide imaging after removal of hardware is a useful tool for assessing the treatment and evaluating the infectious process (44). The high concentration of labeled leukocyte in hematopoetically active bone marrow of the vertebrae renders this test inaccurate when assessing spinal infections (45).

Sequential imaging with technetium Tc99 methylene diphosphonate and gallium citrate (Ga67) is an accurate method of disclosing musculoskeletal infections of the spine prior to definite radiographical changes. The two radiopharmaceutical modalities are synergistic—they are more specific in combination than either one alone (44,46,47). Sequential gallium citrate Ga67 scanning is a reliable and sensitive tool to evaluate not only the disease activity but also the response to antibiotic therapy (44). As an instrument for assessing the evolution of infection, subsequent gallium scans do not require combination with bone scan. This makes them a cost-effective as well as accurate method for assessing the level of the infection (44).

FDG PET images the increased utilization of activated neutrophils and macrophages in inflammatory reactions (48,49), and because it is not hindered by the presence of metallic implants, it makes this test a very valuable tool in the diagnosis of postinstrumentation spinal infections (50). In one publication, the overall accuracy was reported to be 86% with a negative predictive value of 100% (50), suggesting this test may become the standard imaging technique for suspected infections after spinal instrumentation (50).

TABLE 11.6. *Comparison of commonly used antibiotics and their antimicrobial activity*[a]

	Cephalosporin generation		Vancomycin	Clindamy	Penicillin	Ciprofloxacin	Tobramycin
	First	Second					
Staphylococcus aureus (MSSA)	S	S	S	S	S	S	S
Staphylococcus aureus (MRSA)	R	R	S	R	R	R	R
Staphylococcus epidermidis	S	S	S	S	S	S	S
Escherichia coli	S/I	S	R	R	S	S	S
Klebsiella pneumoniae	S	S	R	R	R	S	S
Proteus mirabilis	S	S	R	R	S	S	S
Proteus indole (+)	R	R	R	R	R	S	S
Pseudomonas aeruginosa	R	R	R	R	R	S	S
Beta-hemolytic *Streptococcus* spp.	S	S	S	S	S	I	R
Enterobacter spp.	R	R	R	R	R	S	S
Serratia marcescens	R	I	R	R	R	S	S
Gram-negative	R	V	S	S	R	S	S

[a] MSSA, methicillin-sensitive S. aureus; MRSA, methicillin-resistant S. aureus; S: sensitive; R: resistant; V: variable; I: intermediate.
* Cefazolin and cephalothin.
** Cefoxitin and cefamandole.

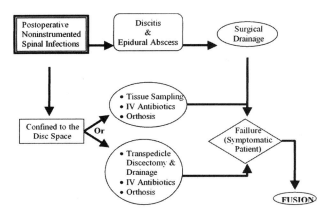

FIG. 11.1. Management of spinal infection without instrumentation.

prostatitis (Escherichia coli) and the other from infected facial acne (Staphylococcus aureus). We have been using cefuroxime (a second-generation cephalosporin), 1.5 g IV, just before induction of anesthesia, and 750 mg IV 6 hours after surgery in the recovery room as a routine prophylactic antibiotic. This antibiotic was not expected to cover the organism in the first three cases and probably was ineffective in the fourth case. The last two cases should have been treated prophylactically with more specific and culture-directed antibiotics.

According to one report, only 35.5% of cases were cured with antimicrobial treatment. The rest required a more aggressive approach (12). On the basis of available reports (38) and our experience with the management of hematogenous pyogenic spondylodiskitis (67,82,87) and postoperative infections (61), we recommend the following guidelines for the management of postdiscectomy infections (Fig. 11.1):

- If the infection is confined to the disc space, one may elect a conservative treatment with IV antibiotics (38), unless it fails (8,9,67,83).
- If the infection spreads to form a retrodiscal abscess (epidural abscess), we recommend a more aggressive approach with surgical drainage, debridement, and irrigation as the treatment of choice (38,67,84,88).
- Minimally invasive surgery, such as transpedicle discectomy and drainage of infection, has proved to be a cost-effective treatment in the management of primary hematogenous pyogenic discitis, provided it is not complicated by a serious neurological deficit or destructive bony lesions (67,88).
- Most available reports advocate some type of immobilization by means of either bed rest until the patient is comfortable (8,63,84) or orthotic devices (84). We recommend the use of rigid or semirigid orthosis until fibrous or bony ankylosis takes place.
- Finally, we recommend interbody fusion, when conservative treatment, debridement/irrigation, or transpedicle discectomy fails (88).

EARLY POSTOPERATIVE SPINAL INFECTION
AFTER INSTRUMENTATION

The most common infections encountered after spinal instrumentation are superficial and deep wound infections (64). Complications such as osteomyelitis, discitis (spondylodiscitis), epidural abscess, infected meningocele with or without cerebrospinal fluid leak, meningitis, sepsis, and even death are fortunately by far less common (24). In general, epidural abscesses

TABLE 11.7. *Reported infection rates for spinal surgery after posterior instrumentation*

Complication rate	Authors
11.0%	Tamborino et al. 1964 (163)
20%	Moe 1967 (96)
8.0%	Levine et al. 1971 (164)
4.0%	Keller and Pappas 1972 (95)
8.0%	Kostuik et al. 1973 (165)
9.3.%	Lonstein et al. 1973 (104)
13%	Swank et al. 1979 (166)
8.0%	Swank et al. 1981 (167)
9.0%	McCarthy et al. 1986 (168)
6.0%	Roy-Camille et al. 1986 (86)
6.0%	Luis et al. 1986 (169)
7.0%	Micheli et al. 1986 (170)
0%	Alien and Ferguson 1988 (171)
6.0%	Zuckerman et al. 1988 (172)
0%	Gurr and McAfee 1988 (173)
6.0%	Thalgott et al. 1989 (174)
7.5%	Whitecloud et al. 1989 (175)
4.0%	Esses and Saches 1991 (176)
11.9%	Kretzler and Banta 1992 (177)
2.6%	Davne and Myers 1992 (144)
6.0%	Massie et al. 1992 (17)
3.7%	Abbey et al. 1995 (91)
3.6%	Wimmer and Gluch 1996 (142)
9.7%	Perry et al. 1997 (18)
7.2%	Levi et al. 1997 (156)
8.7%	Szoke et al. 1998 (99)
4.6%	Aydinli et al. 1999 (178)
3.2%	Picada et al. 2000 (100)
12%	Sponseller et al. 2000 (19)
8%	Labbe et al 2003 (23)
7.24%	Average

complicating spinal surgery represent 16% of all presentations (89). With the advent of spinal implants, infection has become more prevalent, with reported rates reaching as high as 20%, but averaging 7.24% (Table 11.7).

Pathogenesis

The organism may have been inoculated during surgery, and any number of sources may be responsible. The source of gram-negative organisms is a matter of speculation (17). Polymicrobial infections are more likely to inoculate the wound either at the time of surgery or secondarily through drains and wound contamination in the presence of urinary bladder or bowel incontinence.

The most commonly isolated organisms are gram positive; Staphylococcus aureus is the most common organism, with incidence rates ranging from 17% to 63%, followed by

Staphylococcus epidermidis with incidence rates ranging from 36% to 50%. Negative culture findings are not unusual (6% to 16%), and multiple organisms are found in approximately 20% to 59% of infections (2,5,16,17) (Table 11.3).

In paraplegic patients, the flora seems to be different: gram-negative organisms (Enterobacter spp., 35%, Escherichia coli, 28%, Proteus spp., Acinetobacter spp., and Pseudomonas spp.) are seen as often as gram-positive organisms (coagulase-negative Staphylococcus spp., 50%, Enterococcus spp., Streptococcus spp., and Staphylococcus aureus) and are polymicrobial in 50% of cases (19). Arguably, the presence of enteric organisms suggests fecal contamination (19).

Clinical Manifestation

The most common clinical presentation is partial wound dehiscence associated with drainage of fluid that may or may not appear purulent, approximately 15 to 17 days after surgery (ranging from 4 to 80 days) (2,17,20,24) (see also risk factors). Other common manifestations are pain and redness around the wound. Fever is uncommon (2,15) and, at most, pyrexia at presentation was reported in 30% of cases (1). Unexplained hyperglycemia in diabetic patients, malaise, exacerbation of back pain, and sweat and chills, particularly at night, are important clues for prompt diagnosis of suspected infection (17). The mean age ranges from 44 to 57.2 years (20,24). We would like to emphasize that usually early diagnosis is established on clinical grounds.

Pseudoarthrosis and Spinal Infection

Available reports tend to indicate that, in contrast to delayed infection after spinal instrumentation in which increased rates of pseudoarthrosis are observed, early infections do not significantly alter the rate of pseudoarthrosis (2,20,24). One report, however, implicated the use of an allograft and the extension of the graft mass to the sacrum as a risk factor for pseudoarthrosis (90).

TREATMENT

The most appropriate surgical method for managing early wound infection after spinal instrumentation has been widely debated. For this reason we attempt here to analyze the different concepts and methods of treatment in an objective fashion.

The surgical management of early spinal infections after instrumentation is divided into two different camps. One group thinks that the presence of spinal instrumentation precludes successful treatment of spinal infection (28,91), and therefore all the hardware should be removed. This option, however, may result in an unstable spine. The majority of surgeons (14,16,24,92,93) try to salvage the instrumentation at least until fusion takes place.

The principle of maintaining internal fixation in the presence of infection has been well recognized in the management of long bone fracture (94) that consolidates satisfactorily despite the infection. This concept also has been applied successfully in the management of instrumented spinal infections (95,96).

The objective of treating spinal infection with instrumentation is to eradicate the infection without removing the hardware, which is required to maintain alignment of the spine, especially after extensive laminectomy, until the fusion consolidates. This precludes the need for additional surgery and even orthosis.

Three main, different, and distinct surgical techniques are available for salvaging infected spinal instrumentation until fusion takes place. In general, these surgical methods are known as surgical debridement/irrigation, constant antibiotic irrigation/suction, and muscle flaps. The surgeon may choose any combination of these techniques, depending on the local wound condition and the general physical status of the patient.

Guidelines for Surgical Treatment

For a rational method of treating postoperative infection after spinal instrumentation, Thalgott and colleagues (14) have developed a classification scheme in which the patients have been categorized according to two parameters. The first deals with the severity of infection, and the second takes into account the host response or physiological classification of the patient. This classification system is based on the clinical staging system for adult osteomyelitis developed by Cierny and coworkers (97). The severity of infection is divided into three groups: group I involves a single-organism infection, either superficial or deep; group II is a multiple-organism deep wound infection; and group III is a multiple-organism infection with myonecrosis. The host response is divided into three classes: class A requires normal systemic defenses and metabolic capabilities and vascularity; class B patients demonstrate local or multiple systemic diseases, including effects of cigarette smoking; class C is an immunocompromised or severely malnourished host.

According to Thalgott and associates (14), patients in group I can be managed by single surgical debridement/irrigation and closure over suction-drainage tubes without the use of an inflow-outflow irrigation system. The group II patients, with a multiple-organism infection, require more surgical debridement/irrigation sessions and, usually at the completion of the third debridement/irrigation treatment, the installation of a closed inflow-outflow device for constant irrigation with antibiotics. They found that patients in this group responded better with this technique when compared with surgical debridement/irrigation with a simple suction drainage system without constant inflow irrigation. The group III patients with multiple-organism infections and myonecrosis have a poor prognosis and are best managed with muscle flaps. Tissue expanders or vacuum-assisted closure are alternatives for these patients (Fig. 11.2).

Surgical Techniques

Surgical Debridement/Irrigation Method

Surgical debridement should be carried out in the operating room with general anesthesia. The surgeon should meticulously remove all the infected tissues, necrotic material, and nonviable bone grafts or substitutes by aggressive debridement and obtain tissue for immediate Gram stain and culture. Then the wound should be thoroughly irrigated by antibiotic-containing saline solution (5 to 9 L, depending on the situation), preferably by using a pulsatile lavage system. All the subfascial plains should be cultured, debrided, and irrigated separately in a systematic order. We advocate bacitracin, 50,000 units in 1,000 mL, because its soapy quality adds a detergent effect to the solution. This practice has been supported experimentally as well (98).

One report argues that a single suction irrigation treatment does not allow a second look for further debridement of necrotic tissue that is not apparent during the initial procedure (2). However, we believe that if the wound looks clean, with relatively minimal tissue damage, good vascularity, and no severe infection, the objective of surgery has been achieved. Furthermore, if the patient's condition is stable and the patient does not appear ill from sepsis and has normal systemic and metabolic capabilities, the surgeon could choose to close the wound primarily (14) over suction drainage, as a single procedure. The drains are usually left in place for 4 to 5 days.

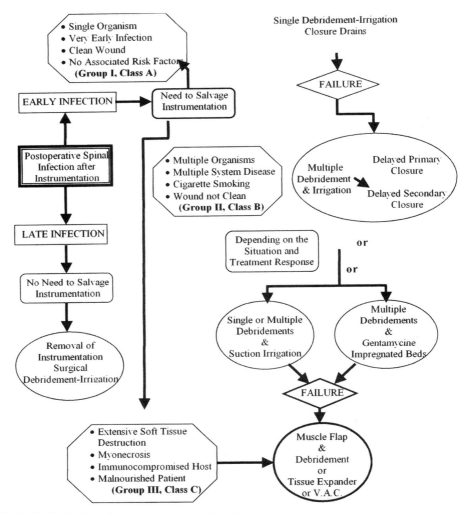

FIG. 11.2. Guidelines for management of early postoperative infection after instrumentation From ref (1), with permission from Marcel Dekker Inc.

Instead of the method outlined, the surgeon may elect the option of packing the wound open with gauze, soaked preferably in half-strength Dakin's solution. The surgeon may repeat the same procedure every 48 hours until the wound is clean, and then as needed every 4 to 5 days (this may be done on the wards under good analgesia-sedation preparation) until the formation of granulation tissue. This process requires an average of four to six sessions.

When the wound is suitable for secondary closure, the surgeon either elects to manage the wound by means of primary delayed closure (Fig. 11.3) or allows it to heal by secondary intent. The dressings are changed frequently on the ward or at home, until the wound eventually heals spontaneously by secondary intention (Fig. 11.4). Because this method, however, is a long, disabling, and expensive process (93), most surgeons prefer a delayed primary surgical closure, after the formation of good granulation tissue.

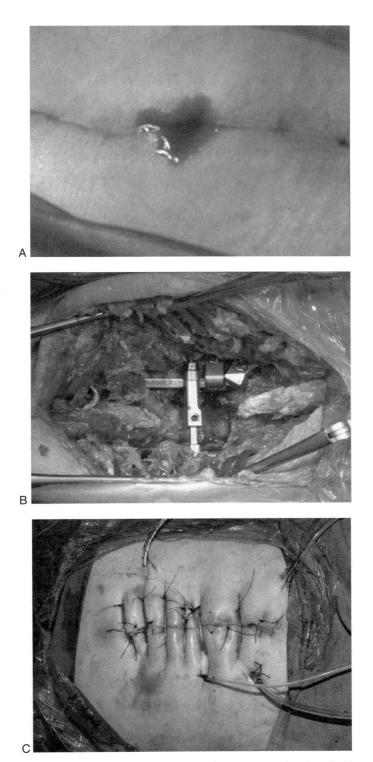

FIG. 11.3. A: Serosanguinous discharge on the fifth postoperative day. **B:** Note, after meticulous surgical debridement and irrigation, absence of pus. **C:** Primary wound closure over four suction drains. From ref (1), with permission from Marcel Dekker Inc.

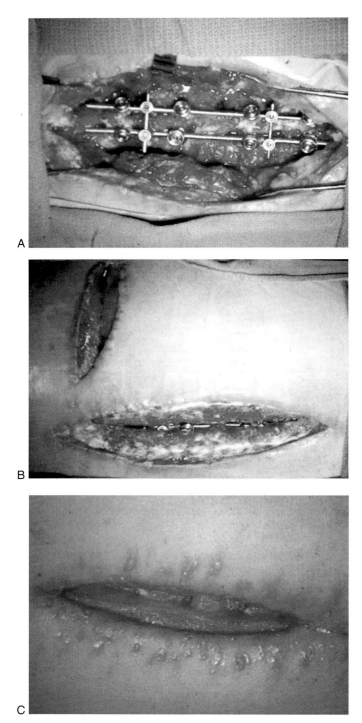

FIG. 11.4. A: Infection of an instrumented thoracic spine surgery in a 60-year-old female patient, treated by serial surgical debridement/irrigation. **B:** The surgeon elected treatment by means of secondary intention closure. Note healthy granulation tissue creeping to cover the entire spine and instrumentation 4 weeks later. **C:** Almost complete healing of the wound is seen in 8 weeks. Although it took a long time, the results were excellent. Fusion was successful and because instrumentation was prominent under the skin, it was removed uneventfully 2 years later. From ref (1), with permission from Marcel Dekker Inc.

A culture should be done at each successive debridement for adjusting the antibiotics because of the potential for flora changes in the wound (14). The timing of wound closure depends on different parameters such as erythrocyte sedimentation rate, white blood count, nutritional status, fever, and overall appearance of the wound. The status of the wound is assessed according to the presence or absence of necrotic tissue, persistence and aggressiveness of infection, and presence of granulation tissue. Local bacterial counts are a good indicator that the wound can be managed with a more definitive procedure such as closure or reconstruction with muscle flaps (93). In terms of available reports, vigorous debridements in the operating room with general anesthesia, appropriate antibiotic coverage, and delayed primary (20) or secondary (99) intent closure (depending on the virulence of infection) can be successful, with no necessity to remove the instrumentation (2,34,100).

Failure of debridement to control infection was reported in 28% of cases in one study (19) and in 18% in another study (2). Both cases were treated successfully by removing the instrumentation in the first case and using muscle flaps to salvage the instrumentation in the second situation.

Repeated debridements and delayed primary closure, overall, constitute a simple surgical technique, but when it is used indiscriminantly for all types of deep wound infection, we have observed complications in 68% of cases, including seroma/hematoma, persistence of infection, and wound dehiscence (93). This procedure, when used for early instrumented spinal infections with relatively minimal tissue damage and especially after noninstrumented surgeries, has an excellent rate of successful outcome (14,70,101). We have treated several cases successfully in this fashion, especially when the procedure was carried out early (within 5 to 10 days).

This record is highlighted with the following example of a 65-year-old retired policeman suffering from chronic low back pain and onset of right sciatica associated with weakness of dorsiflexion of the foot in the past 6 months, with gradual deterioration to complete incapacity. He was treated in the local hospital with analgesics, nonsteroidal antiinflammatory drugs, and complete bed rest with bathroom use for 3 weeks. The patient had well-controlled diabetes mellitus. He was transferred to our institution, where imaging studies revealed a right lateral stenosis at the L4-L5 and L5-S1 levels and grade I L4-L5 degenerative spondylolisthesis. He had microdecompression of the right L4-L5 and L5-S1 regions, foraminotomy, and laminotomy. Unfortunately, there was no substantial relief of his pain except some improvement of the right foot dorsiflexion. Postoperative conservative treatment with the administration of a tapering dose of methylprednisolone (Medrol Dosepak) over 5 days, ranging from 24 mg on day 1 to 8 mg on day 5, failed to relieve the pain, and on the sixth postoperative day he underwent a complete L4 laminectomy, partial bilateral L3-L5 laminectomy, wider L4-L5 and L5-S1 right foraminotomies, transpedicle instrumentation from L3 to the sacrum, and intertransverse compound bone graft. He had an excellent response to this treatment. On the fifth postoperative day while he was getting ready to be discharged from the hospital, he had an asymptomatic serosanguinous discharge. ESR was 106 mm/h, WBC was 14,230, and CRP level was 6.34. The diagnosis of a potential infection was made, and the patient had surgical debridement and irrigation, under general anesthesia, with 6 L of normal saline solution containing 80 mg of gentamycin and 500 mg/L fucidic acid. Because the wound was clean at the end of the procedure, with no excessive necrotic tissue, and the Gram stain finding was negative (the patient was class I and group I), he was treated with primary closure over suction drains (Fig. 11.3) that remained in place for 3 days. As an adjunctive to the antibiotics the patient received during the procedure, he was given 500 mg vancomycin IV for 4 days and 750 mg cefuroxime IV for 3 days. The patient had an uneventful and complete recovery and was treated with culture result–directed antibiotics. The risk factors in this patient were prolonged hospitalization with bed rest (>3 weeks), previous surgery, administration of steroids, and comorbid diabetes mellitus.

We share with others (17) the opinion that the benefits of early surgical intervention of suspected spinal instrumented infections, with aggressive debridement and irrigation, outweigh the risk of delaying surgery even if surgery yields no evidence of infection (Fig. 11.2 outlines the guidelines in an algorithmic approach).

Constant Closed Antibiotic Irrigation-Suction Technique

After a thorough debridement and irrigation, as described earlier, the surgeon inserts the irrigation suction device. This consists primarily of inflow catheters and outflow drains that are usually placed both deep and superficial with respect to lumbosacral fascia, and, if required, an additional irrigation-suction system is placed in the donor bone graft site (16). Antibiotics are added to the irrigation bags. The surgeon may also choose to achieve this effect by using a single-inflow Jackson-Pratt drain and close the skin over single-outflow hemovac drains (14).

The inflow-outflow tubes are sutured to the skin. The fascia is closed with several non-absorbable interrupted number 0 sutures. The skin is closed with number 0 retention sutures and watertight running 3-0 nylon (16).

The rate of irrigation is usually maintained at a continuous flow ranging from 25 to 150 mL/h, depending on the severity of the infection. The irrigation system is usually placed for 5 to 7 days, and the drainage tubes are kept in place for an additional day (16). The irrigant of 1 L of normal saline solution contains 500 mg of vancomycin and 1,000 units of heparin. Successful outcome resulting from this treatment has been reported by several authors (14,16,17,92,95,102,103). Thalgott and associates (14) advocate combining this method with two or three previous surgical debridements. Risk of Pseudomonas sp. superinfection is a serious drawback of this treatment (104,105).

Muscle Flaps

When infected wounds involve exposed bony spine or hardware, the optimal goal for successful closure is a two-layered well-vascularized closure. The deep layer is made up of muscle and then covered with the skin (106). For this reason, muscle flaps are preferred to random and fasciocutaneous flaps in this situation (107–111).

Muscle flap coverage of infected instrumentation in the extremities has become a standard practice, and, with some guidelines and experience, the surgeon can easily apply this principle to the spine (93,106,112). Animal model studies and clinical research have demonstrated the superiority of muscle flaps in inhibiting bacterial growth and promoting wound healing by providing well-vascularized tissue for delivery of antibiotics, immune cells, and oxygen (107,108,109,111,113,115).

Muscle flaps are indicated for extensive wounds when primary closure is not possible, such as in the so-called hostile back (116) (Fig. 11.5). This term describes the most complex back wounds, which are characterized by a large surface area defect (>200cm^2), exposed hardware, and a history of complex infection (other conditions also may be responsible, such as postradiation necrosis). This also may be associated with other problems such as an osteodestructive process, spinal instability, multiple failed attempts at reconstruction (116), and, at worst, a cerebrospinal fluid leak. We found that the average wound length for muscle flap coverage spans about five to six vertebral bodies (except in scoliosis surgery). In our experience, muscle flaps can cover any defect in the spine.

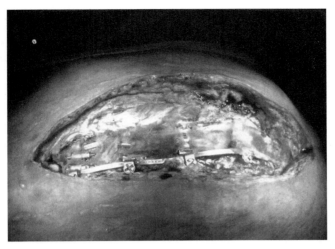

FIG. 11.5. Hostile wound infection. Note wide complete wound dehiscence, with extensive necrotic tissue without evidence of granulation tissue. From ref (1), with permission from Marcel Dekker Inc.

Many different methods for managing infected wounds using various muscle flaps have been reported. Latissimus dorsi, trapezius, gluteus maximus, and paraspinous muscles with their associated fasciocutaneous flaps have been described as bipedicle or unipedicle advancement, rotation, turnover, and free island flaps. These have been used individually or in combination (117).

In our experience, a higher complication rate was found in wounds closed in a delayed primary fashion (68%) than in those reconstructed with muscle flaps (20%) (93). For this reason, we have started using a paraspinous sliding flap as a primary reconstruction for infected spinal instrumentation in the lumbar region, after the initial two or three surgical debridements.

Postoperative infection with extensive deep wound myonecrosis, deep space infection, exposed hardware, bone, and dura mater is amenable to muscle flap reconstructive surgery with a predictable excellent outcome (for controlling the infections). This is performed either as a single one-stage surgery (115), after repeated debridements (2), or as a salvage procedure when other methods have failed (2,14,119).

Postoperative spinal infection after instrumentation complicated by dehiscence, a large defect, and cerebrospinal fluid (CSF) leak is a serious and potentially life-threatening complication, which fortunately is rare. These cases can also be managed satisfactorily with muscle flap reconstruction (85,106,117,120). One of our patients treated with spinal instrumentation developed spinal infection, wound dehiscence, and CSF leak and eventually died.

Flap Selection

Flap selection for spinal wound reconstruction is based on the anatomical location of the lesion. Cervical, thoracic, and upper lumbar spinal wounds can be reconstructed with trapezius and latissimus muscles. Lower lumbar spinal wounds are best reconstructed with gluteus maximus flaps, bilateral bipedicled skin flaps (121), and free latissimus dorsi

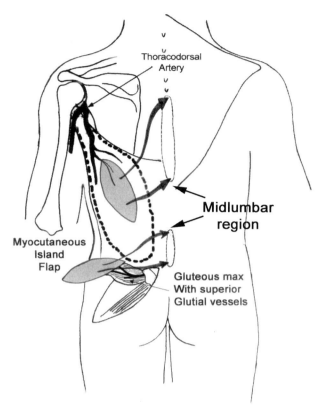

Thoracodorsal
Artery

**Midlumbar
region**

Myocutaneous
Island
Flap

Gluteous max
With superior
Glutial vessels

FIG. 11.6. Illustration demonstrating selection of muscle flaps. Latissimus dorsi flap is indicated for the upper lumbar and mainly thoracic spine regions. Lower lumbar wounds are reconstructed with gluteus maximus flap. The flap is advanced through a subcutaneous tunnel to reach the intended target. This skin muscle flap can also be used to patch dural defect. Midlumbar wounds are inferior to arc rotation for latissimus and superior to gluteus muscle. For this level we advocate the use of paraspinous muscle.

muscle flaps (119). Upper lumbar spine and especially the mid- and lower lumbar spine are best reconstructed with turnover paraspinous muscle flaps (106) or bipedicle sliding paraspinous muscle flaps (93) (Fig. 11.6). Large midline back defects may require multiple flaps such as paraspinous muscles combined with latissimus or gluteus muscles (106,117).

Gluteus Maximus Muscle

The gluteus maximus muscle flap is useful for the lowermost region of the spine (lumbosacral region). Either the entire gluteus maximus (122) or the superior portion can be used as a turnover flap (114,118,123). It is important to preserve function on the inferior portion of the gluteus maximus in ambulatory patients (118), so the superior one-half segment of this muscle is used. Usually the patients do not have subjective symptoms related to removal of the superior portion of the gluteus maximus (119). The surgeon first dissects it off the posterior iliac crest, then separates it from the underlying gluteus medius muscle, and finally raises and turns it about 160 degrees to move it from the greater trochanteric region to the inferior lumbar and sacral region. One should take care not to damage its vascular pedicle while maneuvering the flap (118,119). Deep epithelialized myocutaneous turnover of a gluteus maximus island flap based on the superior gluteal vessels has been successfully used for closure of a CSF leak (117).

Trapezius Muscle Flap

The trapezius muscle flap is usually indicated for lesions in the upper thoracic and cervical region (120). The vascular pedicle enters the muscle about 7 to 8 cm lateral to the seventh cervical spinous process. The surgeon elevates the muscle off the paraspinous musculature and divides it on its lateral aspect and, under direct vision, carries out the dissection with the vascular pedicle remaining on the medial segment of the muscle and then transports it proximally. One complication of this technique is a shoulder drop.

Latissimus Dorsi Flap

The latissimus dorsi muscle flap is indicated for reconstruction or hardware coverage of thoracic or upper lumbar spinal wounds. Because the pedicle of the latissimus dorsi is in the axillary region, the arc of rotation of the latissimus dorsi muscle precludes its use for reconstruction of mid- and lower lumbar lesions (119,124) (Fig. 11.6).

Depending on the situation, the surgeon either dissects the latissimus dorsi muscle from the underlying paraspinal muscles and transposes it as an island based on the thoracodorsal vessels or chooses to turn over the muscle based on its segmental perforators along the spine (125,126). This turnover or reverse latissimus flap is not a reliable option for wound closure after spinal procedures because the spinal perforators may have been divided for a previous spinal instrumentation exposure.

Free Flaps

The free flap method is usually indicated when the local tissue conditions are very poor and spine fusion is not performed. The superior gluteal muscle (126) or the latissimus muscle (119), with its overlying soft tissues, is commonly harvested for this technique and, in general, has been used for reconstructing lumbar wounds. The muscle flaps can be anastomosed to different vessels such as local lumbar perforators, the 11th intercostal, the superior gluteal vessels, and local lumbar perforators. The 11th intercostal vessels may be too small to match the diameter of the thoracodorsal vessels (119). The superior gluteal vessels are short, and, for that reason, reversed saphenous vein grafts are required when using these recipient vessels for anastomoses to the free muscle flap (119). One of the problems of using local perforators to anastomose the flap is the great difficulty encountered when dissecting out these donor vessels adjacent to the spine. After stabilization procedures, these target vessels are rarely available (116,119,127,128). An alternative method is to use interposition of long vein grafts such as the saphenous or cephalic vein (116) (as long as 28 cm) to anastomose the flap either to the thoracodorsal vessels or to the femoral artery or external carotid.

Paraspinal Muscle Flaps

Local paraspinous muscles neighboring the spine can be used (106) to provide muscle coverage in the lumbar region, which is involved in most spinal surgery (129). The medially based turnover paraspinous muscle flaps (106) may not be an option for spinal wound

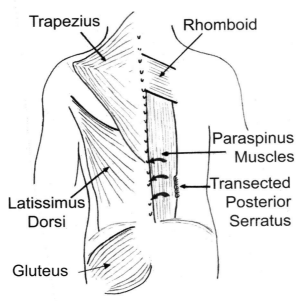

FIG. 11.7. Diagram of paraspinal muscles on patient's right side, located deep to trapezius, rhomboid, latissimus dorsi, posterior inferior serratus, and thoracolumbar fascia. The little arrows indicate the advancement of the paraspinous muscle flap, which is particularly useful for midlumbar region.

reconstruction after posterior spinal instrumentation procedures because the medial paraspinous perforators may have been divided and sacrificed. The paraspinous muscles are also known as the erector spinae muscles, which include the longissimus, iliocostalis, and spinalis portions. The erector spinae muscles were also formerly called the sacrospinalis muscles (130). The paraspinous muscles are located deep in the latissimus dorsi muscles and thoracolumbar fascia, originate inferiorly from the spinous processes and the iliac crest, and insert superiorly into the posteriomedial aspect of the ribs (Fig. 11.7).

For the paraspinal muscle advancement flap, the paraspinous muscles are found by incising the thoracolumbar fascia medially and then elevating them from the underlying serratus posterior inferior muscles. The portion of the paraspinous muscle required for bone or hardware coverage is released from its origin on the spine. Then this portion of the paraspinous muscle is bluntly elevated from the multifidus muscle, transverse processes, intertransversarii muscles, and transversalis fascia, from the medial to the lateral direction. This blunt dissection allows for mobilization and advancement of the paraspinous muscles in the medial direction while preserving its lateral perforator vessels (93) (Fig. 11.8). Sometimes perforator vessels, which enter the muscle along its deep surface, limit muscle advancement to the midline, necessitating ligation of the medial column of perforator vessels. Because the blood supply to the paraspinous muscle is segmental, and is therefore a type IV muscle, the integrity of the superior and inferior muscle continuity must be preserved (114). Therefore, only the medial column of perforators corresponding to the area requiring muscle elevation and advancement is ligated with impunity (93). The muscle bodies are sutured in the midline. Then the skin adjacent to the defect is undermined, medially advanced, and approximated over closed suction drains. We recommend use of several drains for closed suction (about five to six) strategically located for a prolonged period (usually 10 days).

Clinical Manifestation

The clinical manifestation of delayed spinal infection after instrumentation is milder than that of early infections. Characteristically, it has an indolent nature and a paucity of diagnostic criteria (150) that cause delay in diagnosis. Incisional swelling or drainage may develop after several months of nonspecific symptoms (3). In terms of available reports, increased back pain (60% of cases) (28), especially after a prolonged period of normal postoperative recovery, is a good diagnostic clue, particularly when combined with an elevated ESR. In 78% to 87.5% of patients, the average elevation of ESR ranged from 39 to 57 mmHg/h (3,28). According to one report, mild elevation of WBC (usually high range of normal 9,000 to 12,000) was noted in 25% of patients (3).

A high pseudoarthrosis rate, ranging between 20% and 62% (2,27,89) of cases, has been observed. This suggests an association between pseudoarthrosis and delayed spinal infection (3). Although whether pseudarthrosis may be a contributing factor for late infection has not been established with certainty, reports (143,151) indicate a correlation between instrumentation loosening and late infections.

TREATMENT

Most authors advocate surgical debridement and irrigation, as well as removal of instrumentation, in the treatment of delayed spinal infections, with high rate of success (21,28,146). In this situation, the hardware is typically covered with glycocalix, an avascular enveloping polysaccharide resistant to both antibiotics and the host's immune system. Stability for the spine is not a major concern, as it is in the early postoperative infections, and therefore removal of hardware is thought to be an important aspect of the treatment in this situation (28).

ADJUNCTIVE TREATMENT

Antibiotics

Administration of antibiotics alone in the management of infected spinal surgery after instrumentation is not effective in the majority of cases (29,104,152). In this situation, it is our strong opinion that surgical debridement is the definitive treatment, and administration of antibiotics can be considered an adjunctive therapy. However, for noninstrumented spinal infections, the mainstay of treatment is the administration of intravenous antibiotics. One may select a combination of intravenous vancomycin and oral rifampin as the antibiotic of choice (16,153) until specific tissue cultures results and antibiotic sensitivity are available. The duration of intravenous antibiotics may be individualized according to the severity of infection from 1 to 6 weeks and then followed by a course of oral antibiotics for approximately another 6 weeks. When a prolonged use of intravenous antibiotics is needed to facilitate early discharge from the hospital, a Groshong or Hickman intravenous catheter insertion is required. In general, for class B or C patients (see Thalgott and coworkers' classification), a 6-week course of parenteral antibiotics followed by an additional 6 weeks of oral antibiotics administration is usually given (14).

Hyperalimentation

Hyperalimentation is advocated in group II and group III infections in order to improve the host response (14).

PREVENTION OF "REVERSIBLE" RISK FACTORS

Close attention should be paid to the perioperative risk factors of patients undergoing spinal surgery, particularly when instrumentation is being used. It behooves the surgeon, before undertaking major elective spinal surgery, to deal first with risk factors that can be controlled, the so-called reversible risk factors:

- The patient should be encouraged to quit smoking (14,16).
- Steps should be taken to minimize OR contamination (154). Proper sterile OR techniques should be followed, traffic in the OR should be minimized, and access doors should be kept closed. Filtered air should be exchanged at a rate of 25 times per hour (26). Laminar airflow systems may play a role in spine surgery as they do in hip surgery.
- The surgeon should treat intercurrent infection and use prophylactic administration of antibiotics (155). The role of prophylactic antibiotics in spinal surgery is well established. The recommended administration is just before the induction of anesthesia and continued for at least 24 hours after surgery. Poor penetration of cefalozin (a first-generation cephalosporin) and oxacillin was demonstrated in animal experiments (156,157), suggesting the uncertainty of their therapeutic effect. Certainly supplemental intraoperative antibiotics should be administered in more lengthy operations. For cases without a suspected potential concomitant infection, first- or second-generation cephalosporins have proved cost effective.

Animal experiments (158) have demonstrated the efficacy of prophylactic antibiotics for spinal instrumentation and arthrodesis and have also shown that a single preoperative dose of cefazolin was as effective as 48-hour postoperative administration of cefazolin in eradicating wound infections.

This conventionally accepted method has been challenged for disc surgery. Animal experiments (159) demonstrated that intervertebral disc penetration may not be achieved 2 hours after an IV bolus injection, suggesting it would be safer to administer prophylactic antibiotics at least 60 minutes before surgery. A retrospective study of a large number of posterior fusions (7,000 cases) revealed that prophylactic administration of antibiotics significantly reduced the rate of postoperative infection from 4.4% to 1.2% (92). Similar findings have been reported by others (105), who were able to decrease the rate of infection from 7% to 3.6% after Harrington instrumentation. Another large series confirmed this practice by demonstrating a drop in the infection rate from 9.3% to 1% (56) when prophylactic antibiotics were administrated.

In another relatively large prospective clinical study, it was noted that the patients who had spinal instrumentation and received three doses of 2 g/day cefamandole after surgery for 3 days had a rate of early and late postoperative infection of only 0.6% (103).

One clinical study (63), using a different method of prophylactic administration of antibiotics, reported a dramatic drop in postdiscectomy infections, from 3.7% to 0%. In this study, a collagenous sponge containing gentamycin was placed in the discectomy region. Bactericidal gentamycin levels in the drainage fluid could be detected 48 to 72 hours after surgery (160), indicating the effectiveness of this method. Other prophylactic techniques include the following:

- An irrigant solution containing a mixture of neomycin, 5% bacitracin (25,000 units/L), and polymixin (25 mg/L) was proved sufficient to eradicate 19 commonly found strains of gram-negative and gram-positive pathogens common in orthopedic surgery (161), thus rendering this solution ideal for wound irrigation. This is a relatively safe usage, although one case of anaphylaxis has been reported in a patient who had been previously exposed to the same irrigant (162).

- It has been conventionally accepted that avoiding certain pitfalls during a posterior surgical procedure may contribute to a reduction in the surgical risks for infection (16,154). This includes careful dissection of the ligamentous attachments of the paraspinal muscles (decreases tissue necrosis and blood loss), intermittent release of paraspinal muscle refractors (reduces hypoperfusion and alleviates muscle ischemia), meticulous hemostasis, insertion of surgical drains (eliminates hematoma), and meticulous wound closure (eliminates dead space and provides an airtight barrier against bacterial infiltration).
- When a procedure that requires two surgical approaches (anterior and posterior) is anticipated to take a long time and will be performed in one sitting, the surgeon may decrease the risk factor for infection by performing a two-stage procedure on two different days.
- Because the anterior approach is associated with diminished risk factors for development of infection after spinal instrumentation (16), it is preferable to use an anterior rather than a posterior approach, provided both exposures are equally effective for the given type of spinal surgery.
- Close attention should be given to the preoperative nutritional status of patients undergoing lumbar spinal surgery. Patients with suboptimal nutritional parameters should have supplementation and replenishment before elective surgery (30).
- In paraplegic patients, because of potentially gram-negative microorganism and polybacterial contamination of the wound, more targeted preventive strategies such as broad-spectrum antibiotics with activity against gram-negative organisms should be used for prophylaxis (19), coupled with impermeable wound dressings and other hygiene measures (19).

SUMMARY

Postoperative spinal infections carry a great cost, both medically and socioeconomically, and the surgeon must consider and minimize the risks of such infection. Preventive measures should be instituted before and during the surgical intervention.

If, however, infection occurs despite prophylaxis, treatment should be instituted quickly and aggressively to prevent or reduce sequelae. Antibiotic therapy, which may take the form of intravenous, intramuscular, or oral administration or placement of antibiotic-impregnated beads, is the first line of defense after noninstrumented procedures, although debridement may also become necessary. In cases of infection that follow spinal instrumentation, debridement is the initial approach and antibiotic therapy is the adjunctive step. Antibiotic therapy should be designed with the infecting organism(s) in mind. Late postinstrumentation infection may necessitate removal of the instrumentation along with debridement. Closure of wounds after infection may be accomplished by delayed primary closure or closure by secondary intention. In some cases, muscle flaps may be required for reconstruction.

REFERENCES

1. AG Hadjipavlou, I Gaitanis, P Katonis, J Simmons. Postoperative infections of the spine and treatment options. In JH Calhoun, JT Meder eds. Musculoskeletal infections. New York: Marcel Dekker:379.
2. MA Weinstein, JP McCabe, FP Cammisa JR. Postoperative spinal wound infection: a review of 2,391 consecutive index procedures. J Spinal Disord 13:422-6, 2000.

3. RW Viola, HA King, SM Adler, CB Wilson. Delayed infection after elective spinal instrumentation and fusion: a retrospective analysis of eight cases. Spine 20:244-50, 1997.

4. JE Jensen, RG Jensen, TK Smith, DA Johnston, SJ Dudrick. Nutrition in orthopaedic surgery. J Bone Joint Surg 62A:1263-972, 1982.

5. BE Dall, DE Rowe, WG Odette, DH Batts. Postoperative discitis: diagnosis and management. Clin Orthop 224:138-46, 1987.

6. F Postacchini, G Ginotti, D Perugia. Post-operative intervertebral discitis: evaluation of 12 cases and study of ESR in the normal postoperative period. Ital J Orthop Traumatol 19:57-69, 1993.

7. AM Frank, AE Trappe. The role of magnetic resonance imaging (MRI) in the diagnosis of spondylodiscitis. Neurosurg Rev 13:279-83, 1990.

8. TS Lindholm, P Phylkkanen. Discitis following removal of the intervertebral disc. Spine 7:618-22, 1982.

9. S Pilgaard. Discitis (closed space infection) following removal of lumbar intervertebral disc. J Bone Joint Surg 51A:713-16, 1969.

10. J Puranen, J Makela, S Lahde. Postoperative intervertebral discitis. Acta Orthop Scand 55:461-5, 1984.

11. D Stolke, V Seifert, U Kunz. Die postoperative discitis intervertebralis lumbalis: Eine ubersicht uber einen 15-jahresitraum und 7493 operationen. Z Orthop Ihre Grenzgeb 126:666-70, 1988.

12. ME Jimenez-Mejias, JD Colmenero, FJ Sanchez-Lora, J Palomino-Nicas, JM Reguera, JG Heras, et al. Post-operative spondylodiskitis: etiology, clinical findings, prognosis, and comparison with nonoperative spondylodiskitis. Clin Infect Dis 29:339-45, 1999.

13. JS Thalgott, HB Cotler, RC Sasso, H LaRocca, V Gardner. Postoperative infections in spinal implants: classification and analysis—a multicenter study. Spine 16:981-4, 1991.

14. W Calderon, N Chang, S Mathes. Comparison of the effect of bacterial inoculation in musculocutaneous and fasciocutaneous flaps. Plast Reconstr Surg 77: 785, 1986.

15. PJE Cruse, R Ford. A five-year prospective study of 23,649 surgical wounds. Arch Surg 107:206-10, 1973.

16. AD Levi, CA Dickman, VK Sonntag. Management of postoperative infections after spinal instrumentation. J Neurosurg 86:975-80, 1997.

17. JB Massie, JG Heller, JJ Abitbol, D McPherson, SR Garfin. Postoperative posterior spinal wound infections. Clin Orthop 284:99-108, 1992.

18. JW Perry, J Montgomerie, S Swank, DS Gilmore, K Maederi. Wound infections following spinal fusion with posterior segmental spinal instrumentation. Clin Infect Dis 24:558-61, 1997.

19. PD Sponseller, DM LaPorte, MW Hungerford, K Eck, KH Bridwell, LG Lenke. Deep wound infections after neuromuscular scoliosis surgery: a multicenter study of risk factors and treatment outcomes. Spine 25:2461-6, 2000.

20. JL Stambough, D Beringer. Postoperative wound infections complicating adult spine surgery. J Spinal Disord 3:227-85, 1992.

21. C Wimmer, H Gluch, M Franzreb, M Ogon. Predisposing factors for infection in spine surgery: a survey of 850 spinal procedures. J Spinal Disord 11:124-8, 1998.

22. H Malamo-Lada, O Zarkotou, N Nikolaides, M Kanellopoulou, D Demetriades. Wound infections following posterior spinal instrumentation for paralytic scoliosis. Clin Microbiol Infect. 5(3):135-9, 1999.

23. AC Labbe, AM Demers, R Rodrigues, V Arlet, K Tanguay, DL Moore. Surgical site infection following spinal fusion: a case-control study in a children's hospital. Infect Control Hosp Epidemiol 24(8):591-95, 2003.

24. SD Glassman, JR Dimar, RM Puno, JR Johnson. Salvage of instrumental lumbar fusions complicated by surgical wound infection. Spine 21:2163-9, 1996.

25. MA Ritter. Surgical wound environment. Clin Orthop 190:11-13, 1984.

26. MA Ritter, HE Eitzen, JB Hart, ML French. The surgeons garb. Clin Orthop 153:204-9, 1980.

27. AG Gristina, Y Shibata, G Giridhar, A Kreger, QN Myrvik. The glycocalyx, biofilm, microbes, and resistant infection. Semin Arthroplasty 5(4): 160-70, 1994.

28. BS Richards. Delayed infections following posterior spinal instrumentation for the treatment of idiopathic scoliosis. J Bone Joint Surg 77A:524-9, 1995.

29. JG Heller. Postoperative infection of the spine. In: RH Rothman, FA Simeone, eds. The spine. 3d ed. Philadelphia: WB Saunders, 1992:1817.

30. JD Klein, LA Hey, CS Yu, BB Klein, FJ Coufal, EP Young, LF Marshall, SR Garfin. Perioperative nutrition and postoperative complications in patients undergoing spinal surgery. Spine 21:2676-82, 1996.

31. JD Klein, SR Garfin. Nutritional status in the patients with spinal infection. Orthop Clin North Am 27:33-6, 1996.

32. WP Piotrowski, MA Krombhol, B Muhl. Spondylodiscitis after lumbar disc surgery. Neurosurg Rev 17:189-93, 1994.

33. JA Bendo, J Spivak, R Moskovich, M Neuwirth. Instrumented posterior arthrodesis of the lumbar spine in patients with diabetes mellitus. Am J Orthop 29(8):617-20, 2000.

34. Perry M. Erythrocyte sedimentation rate and C-reactive protein in the assessment of suspected bone infection-are they reliable indices? J R Coll Surg Edinb 41: 116-8, 1996.

35. L Sanzen, M Sundberg. Periprosthetic low-grade hip infections. Erythrocyte sedimentation rate and C-reactive protein in 23 cases. Acta Orthop Scand 1997; 68: 461-5, 1997.

36. LY Shih, JJ Wu, DJ Yang. Erythrocyte sedimentation rate and C-reactive protein values in patients with total hip arthroplasty. Clin Orthop 225: 238-46, 1987.

37. B Jonsson, R Soderholm, B Stromqvist. Erythrocyte sedimentation rate after lumbar spine surgery. Spine 16:1049-50, 1991.
38. KP Schulitz, J Assheuer. Discitis after procedures on the intervertebral disc. Spine 19:1172-7, 1994.
39. U Thelander, S Larsson. Quantitation of C-reactive protein levels and erythrocyte sedimentation rate after spinal surgery. Spine 14:400-4, 1992.
40. CE Clark, LH Shufflebarger. Late-developing infection in instrumented idiopathic scoliosis. Spine 24(18):1909-12, 1999.
41. BS Richards. Delayed infections following posterior spinal instrumentation for the treatment of adolescent idiopathic scoliosis. J bone Joint Surg (Am) 77:524-9, 1995.
42. P Grane, A Josephsson, A Seferlis, T Tullberg. Septic and aseptic post-operative discitis in the lumbar spine-evaluation by MR imaging. Acta Radiol 39:108-15, 1998.
43. SL Rothman. The diagnosis of infections of the spine by modern imaging techniques. Orthop Clin North Am 27:15-31, 1996.
44. A Hadjipavlou, F Cesani-Vazquez, J Villaneuva-Meyer, JT Mader, JT Necessary, W Crow, RE Jensen, G Chaljub. The effectiveness of gallium citrate Ga 67 radio-nuclide imaging in vertebral osteomyelitis revisited. Am J Orthop 27:179-83, 1998.
45. CJ Palestro, CK Kim, AJ Swyer, et al. Radionuclide diagnosis of vertebral osteomyelitis: indium-111-leukocyte and technetium-99 m-methylene diphosphonate bone scintigraphy. J Nucl Med 32: 1861-5, 1991.
46. R Lisbona, L Rosenthall. Observations on the sequential use of 99m Tc-phosphate complex and 67 Ga imaging in osteomyelitis, cellulitis and septic arthritis. Radiology 123:123-9, 1977.
47. R Lisbona, V Derbekyan, J Novales-Diaz, A Veksler. Gallium-67 scintigraphy in tuberculous and nontuberculous infectious spondylitis. J Nucl Med 34:853-9, 1993.
48. Y Sugawara, TD Gutowski, SJ Fisher, et al. Uptake of positron emission tomography tracers in experimental bacterial infections: a comparative biodistribution study of radiolabeled FDG, thymidine, L-methionine, 67Ga-citrate, and 125I-HSA. Eur J Nucl Med 26: 333-41, 1999.
49. S Yamada, K Kubota, R Kubota, et al. High accumulation of fluorine-18-fluorodeoxyglucose in turpentine-induced inflammatory tissue. J Nucl Med 1995; 36: 1301-6, 1995.
50. F De Winter, F Gemmel, C Van De Wiele, B Poffijn, D Uyttendaele, R Dierckx. 18-fluorine fluorodeoxyglucose positron emission tomography for the diagnosis of infection in the postoperative spine. Spine 28(12):1314-9, 2003.
51. SC Dickhaut, JC DeLee, CP Page. Nutritional status: importance in predicting wound healing in amputations. J Bone Joint Surg 66A: 71-5, 1984.
52. BA Feed, M Corliss, RS Bergman. Serum albumin levels and total lymphocyte a predictors of morbidity and mortality in patients undergoing abdominal surgery (abstract). J Parenter Enteral Nutr 6:584, 1982.
53. RD Zoma, RD Sturrock, WD Fisher, PA Freeman, DL Hambleden. Surgical stabilization of the rheumatoid spine: a review of indications and results. J Bone Joint Surg 696:8-12, 1987.
54. D Bontoux, L Codello, F Debiais, G Lambert de Cursay, I Azais, M Alcalay. Infectious spondylodiscitis. Analysis of a series of 105 cases. Rev Rhum Mal Osteoartic 59(6):401-7, 1992.
55. E Meys, X Deprez, PH Hautefeuille, et al. Place des spondylodiscitis iatrogénies parmi les spondylodiscites à germes banals: 136 cas observés entre 1980 et 1989. Rev Rhum Mal Osteoartic 58 :839-46, 1991.
56. NH Horwitz, JA Curtin. Prophylactic antibiotics and wound infections following laminectomy for lumbar disc herniation. J Neurosurg 43:727-31, 1975.
57. WA Dauch. Infection of the intervertebral space following conventional and microsurgical operation on the herniated lumbar intervertebral disc: a controlled clinical trial. Acta Neurochir 82:43-9, 1986.
58. G Bonaldi, G Belloni, D Prosetti, L Moschini. Percutaneous discectomy using Onik's method: 3 years' experience. Neuroradiology 33:516-9, 1991.
59. JL Schaffer, P Kambin. Percutaneous posterolateral lumbar discectomy and decompression with a 6.9-millimeter cannula. Analysis of operative failures and complications. J Bone Joint Surg 73A(6):822-31, 1991.
60. RD Fraser, OL Osti, B Vernon Roberts. Diskitis after discography. J Bone Joint Surg 698:26-35, 1987.
61. RD Fraser. Chymopapaine for the treatment of intervertebral disc herniation: the final report of a double-blind study. Spine 1:815-8, 1984.
62. M Klinger. Spondylitis: a complication following lumbar disc operations. Adv Neurosurg 10:394-9, 1982.
63. V Rohde, B Meyer, C Schaller, W Hassler. Spondylodiscitis after lumbar discectomy: incidence and a proposal for prophylaxis. Spine 23:615-20, 1998.
64. Levi AD, Dickman CA, Sonntag VK. Management of postoperative infections after spinal instrumentation. J Neurosurg 86(6):975-80, 1977.
65. J Puranen, J Makela S Lahde. Postoperative intervertebral diskitis. Acta Orthop Scand 55:461-5, 1984.
66. CE Rawlings, RH Winkins, HA Gallis, JL Goldner, R Francis. Post-operative intervertebral disc space infection. Neurosurgery 13:371-5, 1983.
67. AG Hadjipavlou, JT Mader, JT Necessary, AJ Muffoletto. Hematogenous pyogenic spinal infection and their surgical management. Spine 25:1668-79, 2000.
68. RA Deyo, DC Cherkin, JD Loeser, SJ Bigos, MA Ciol. Morbidity and mortality in association with operations on the lumbar spine. The influence of age, diagnosis, and procedure. J Bone Joint Surg (Am) 74 (4):536-43, 1992.
69. RD Fraser, OL Osti, B Vernon-Roberts. Iatrogenic discitis: the role of intravenous antibiotics in prevention and treatment. An experimental study. Spine 14:1025-32, 1989.

70. AG Hadjipavlou. The management of postoperative pyogenic infection of the spine. The 10th University Congress of Osteosynthesis. Patras, Greece, March 22-24, 2001.
71. O Svensson, PA Parment, G Blomgren. Orthopaedic infections by Serratia marcescens: a report of seven cases. Scand J Infect Dis 19: 69-75, 1987.
72. NP Warren, RR Coombs. Delayed Serratia marcescens osteomyelitis following a gunshot injury. Injury 22: 493-4, 1991.
73. E Bouza, M Garcia de la Torre, A Erice, et al. Serratia bacteremia. Diagn Microbiol Infect Dis 7: 237-47, 1987.
74. A Dominguez, JR Arribas, MD Folgueira, et al. Nosocomial bacteremia caused by Serratia marcescens: analysis of 44 cases. Enferm Infect Microbiol Clin 8: 553-9, 1990.
75. DE Fry, RV Fry, DM Shlaes. Serratia bacteremia in the surgical patient. Am Surg 53: 438-41, 1987.
76. RI Haddy, BL Mann, DD Nadkarni, et al. Nosocomial infection in the community hospital: severe infection due to Serratia species. J Fam Pract 42: 273-77, 1996.
77. B Henry, C Plante-Jenkins, K Ostrowska. An outbreak of Serratia marcescens associated with anesthesia agent propofol. Am J Infect Contr 29: 312-5, 2001.
78. C Wetanakunakorn. Serratia marcescens: a review of 44 episodes. Scand J Infect Dis 21: 477-83, 1989.
79. WL Yu, CW Lin, DY Wang. Serratia marcescens bacteremia: clinical features and antimicrobial susceptibilities of the isolates. J Microbiol Immunol Infect 1998; 31: 171-9, 1998.
80. AG Hadjipavlou, IN Gaitanis, CA Papadopoulos, PG Katonis, GM Kontakis. Serratia spondylodiscitis after elective lumbar spine surgery: a report of two cases. Spine 27(23):E507-512, 2002.
81. M Liebergall, G Chaimsky, J Lowe, et al. Pyogenic vertebral osteomyelitis with paralysis: prognosis and treatment. Clin Orthop 269:142-50, 1991.
82. S Arya, W Crow, A Hadjipavlou, H Nauta, A Borowski, L Vierra, E Walser. Percutaneous transpedicular management of discitis. J Vase Interv Radiol 7(suppl):921-7, 1996.
83. S El-Gindi, S Afer, M Salama, J Andrew. Infection of the intervertebral disc space after operation. J Bone Joint Surg 586:114-6, 1976.
84. GA McCain, M Harth, A Bell, TF Disney, T Austin, E Ralph. Septic discitis. J Rheumatol 8:100-9, 1981.
85. SS Ramasastry, B Schlechter, M Cohen. Reconstruction of posterior trunk defects. Clin Plast Surg 22:167-85, 1995.
86. R Roy-Camille, G Saillant, C Mazel. Internal fixation of the lumbar spine with pedicle screw plating. Clin Orthop 203:7-17, 1986.
87. AM Borowski, WN Crow, AG Hadjipavlou, G Chaljub, J Mader, F Cesani, E van Sonnenberg. Interventional radiology case conference: The University of Texas Medical Branch: percutaneous management of Spondylodiscitis. Am J Roentgenol 170:1587-92, 1998.
88. A Hadjipavlou, WN Crow, A Borowski, JT Mader, A Adesokan, RE Jensen. Percutaneous transpedicular discectomy and drainage in pyogenic Spondylodiscitis. Am J Orthop 27:188-97, 1998.
89. AS Baker, RG Ojemann, MN Swartz, EP Richardson Jr. Spinal epidural abscess. N Engl J Med 293:463-8, 1975.
90. LE Weiss, AR Vaccaro, G Scuderi, M McGuire, SR Garfin. Pseudoarthrosis after postoperative wound infection in the lumbar spine. J Spinal Disord 10:482-7, 1997.
91. DM Abbey, DM Turner, JS Warson, TC Wirt, RD Scalley. Treatment of postoperative wound infections following spinal fusion with instrumentation. J Spinal Disord 8:278-83, 1995.
92. JE Lonstein. Management of musculoskeletal infections. Philadelphia: WB Saunders, 1989:243-9.
93. B Wilhelmi, N Snyder, T Colquhoun, A Hadjipavlou, L Philips. Bipedicle paraspinous muscle flaps for spinal wound closure: an anatomic and clinical study. Plast Reconstr Surg 106:1305-11, 2000.
94. WR MacAusland, RG Eaton. Management of sepsis following intramedullary fixation for fractures of the femur. J Bone Joint Surg 45A: 1643-53, 1963.
95. RB Keller, AM Pappas. Infection after spinal fusion using internal fixation instrumentation. Orthop Clin North Am 3:99-111, 1972.
96. JH Moe. Complications of scoliosis treatment. Clin Orthop 53:21-30, 1967.
97. G Cierny, JT Mader, JJ Penninck. A clinical staging system for adult osteomyelitis. Contemp Orthop 10:17-37, 1985.
98. BD Rosestein, FC Wilson, CH Funderburk. The use of bacitracin irrigation to prevent infection in postoperative skeletal wounds. J Bone Joint Surg 71A:427-30, 1989.
99. G Szoke, G Lipton, F Miller, K Dabney. Wound infection after spinal fusion in children with cerebral palsy. J Pediatr Orthop 18:727-33, 1998.
100. R Picada, RB Winter, JF Lonstein, F Denis, MR Pinto, MD Smith, JH Perra. Postoperative deep wound infection in adults after posterior lumbosacral spine fusion with instrumentation: incidence and management. J Spinal Disord 13:42-45, 2000.
101. PD Dernbach, H Gomez, J Hahn. Primary closure of infected spinal wounds. Neurosurgery 26:707-9, 1990.
102. K Ido, K Shimzu, Y Nakayama, J Shikata, M Matsushita, T Nakamura. Suction/irrigation for deep wound infection after spinal instrumentation: a case study. Eur Spine J 5:345-9, 1996.
103. C Wimmer, M Nogler, B Frischhut. Influence of antibiotics on infection in spinal surgery: a prospective study of 110 patients. J Spinal Disord 11:498-500, 1998.
104. J Lonstein, R Winter, J Moe, D Gaines. Wound infection with Harrington instrumentation and spine fusion for scoliosis. Clin Orthop 96:222-33, 1973.

105. EE Transfeldt, JE Lonstein. Wound infections in elective reconstructive spinal surgery. Orthop Trans 9:128-9, 1985.
106. LA Casas, VL Lewis Jr. A reliable approach to the closure of large acquired midline defects of the back. Plast Reconstr Surg 84:632-631, 1989.
107. JP Anthony, SJ Mathes, BS Alpert. The muscle flap in the treatment of chronic lower extremities osteomyelitis. Plast Reconstr Surg 88:311-8, 1991.
108. W Calderon, N Chang, SJ Mathes. Comparison of the effect of bacterial inoculation in musculocutaneous and fasciocutaneous flaps. Plast Reconstr Surg 77:785-94, 1986.
109. N Chang, SJ Mathes. Comparison of the effect of bacterial inoculation in musculocutaneous and random-pattern flaps. Plast Reconstr Surg 70:1-10, 1982.
110. SJ Mathes, F Nahai. A systemic approach to flap selection. In: SJ Mathes, F Nahai, eds. Clinical applications for muscle and musculocutaneous flaps. St Louis: Mosby, 1982:1-358.
111. RC Russell, DR Graham, AM Feller, EG Zook, A Mathur. Experimental evaluation of the antibiotic carrying capacity of a muscle flap into a fibrotic cavity. Plast Reconstr Surg 81:162-70, 1988.
112. ME Manstein, CH Manstein, G Manstein. Paraspinous muscle flaps. Ann Plast Surg 40:458-62, 1998.
113. I Eshima, SJ Mathes, P Paty. Comparison of the intracellular bacterial killing activity of leukocytes in musculocutaneous and random-pattern flaps. Plast Reconstr Surg 86(3):541-7, 1990.
114. SJ Mathes, BS Alpert, N Chang. Use of the muscle flap in chronic osteomyelitis: experimental and clinical correlation. Plast Reconstr Surg 69:815-29, 1982.
115. RC Murphy, MC Robson, JP Heggers, M Kadowski. The effect of microbial contamination on musculocutaneous and random flaps. J Surg Res 41:75-80, 1986.
116. JW Few, JR Marcus, MJ Lee, S Ondra, GA Dumanian. Treatment of hostile midline back wounds: an extreme approach. Plast Reconstr Surg 105:2448-51, 2000.
117. C Hill, M Riaz. A new twist to the myocutaneous turnover flap for closure of a spinal defect. Plast Reconstr Surg 102:1167-1160, 1998.
118. JR Wendt, VO Gardner, JI White. Treatment of complex postoperative lumbosacral wounds in nonparalyzed patients. Plast Reconstr Surg 101(5):1248-53, 1998.
119. HC Chen, HH Chen, WJ Chen, YB Tang. Chronic osteomyelitis of the spine managed with a free flap of latissimus dorsi: a case report. Spine 21:2016-8, 1996.
120. AE Seyfer, AS Joseph. Use of trapezius muscle for closure of complicated upper spinal defects. Neurosurgery 14:341-5, 1984.
121. TS Moore, TM Dreyer, AG Bevin. Closure of large spina bifida cystica defects with bilateral bipedicle musculocutaneous flaps. Plast Reconstr Surg 73:288-92, 1984.
122. JO Stallings, JR Delgado, JM Converse. Turnover island flap of gluteus maximus muscle for the repair of sacral decubitus ulcer. Plast Reconstr Surg 54:52-4, 1974.
123. SJ Mathes, LO Vasconez, MJ Jurkiewitz. Extensions and further applications of muscle flap transposition. Plast Reconstr Surg 60:6-12, 1977.
124. J Bostwick III, M Scheflan, F Nahai, MJ Jurkiewitz. The "reverse" latissimus dorsi muscle and musculocutaneous flap: anatomic and clinical considerations. Plast Reconstr Surg 65:395-9, 1980.
125. TR Stevenson, RJ Rohrich, RA Pollock, RO Dingman, J Bostwick. More experience with reverse latissimus dorsi musculocutaneous flap: precise location of blood supply. Plast Reconstr Surg 74:237-43, 1984.
126. T Fujino, T Harashina, F Aoyagi. Reconstruction for aplasia of the breast and pectoral region by microvascular transfer of a free flap from the buttock. Plast Reconstr Surg 56:178-81, 1975.
127. GR Evans, GP Reece. Lower back reconstruction: an approach to wound closure in the cancer patient. Plast Reconstr Surg 96:635-42, 1995.
128. P Giesswein, CG Constance, DR Mackay, EK Manders. Supercharged latissimus muscle flap for coverage of the problem wound in the lower back. Plast Reconstr Surg 94:1060-3, 1994.
129. DA Capen, RR Calderon, A Green. Perioperative risk factors for wound infections after lower back fusions. Orthop Clin North Am 27:83-6, 1996.
130. CD Clemente. Anatomy: a regional atlas of the human body, 3d ed. Baltimore: Urban & Schwarenberg, 1987.
131. RS Stahl, FD Burstein, JV Lieponis, MJ Murphy, JM Piepmeier. Extensive wounds of the spine: a comprehensive approach to debridement and reconstruction. Plast Reconstr Surg 85:747-53, 1990.
132. A Harle, R VanEnder. Management of wound sepsis after spinal fusion surgery. Acta Orthop Belg 57:242-6, 1991.
133. D Seligson, S Metha, K Voos, SL Henry, JR Johnson. The use of antibiotic-impregnated polymethylmethacrylate beads to prevent the evolution of localized infection. J Orthop Trauma 6:401-6, 1992.
134. KJ Paonessa, WJ Hostnik, BM Zide. Use of tissue expanders for wound closure of spinal infections or dehiscence. Orthop Clin North Am 27(1):155-70, 1996.
135. C Radovan. Tissue expansion in soft tissue reconstruction. Plast Reconstr Surg 74:482-90, 1984.
136. B Bucalo, WH Eaglstein, V Falanga. Inhibition of cell proliferation by chronic wound fluid. Wound Rep Regen 1:181-6, 1996.
137. MJ Morykwas, LC Argenta, EI Shelton-Brown, et al. Vacuum assisted closure: a new method for wound control and treatment-Animal studies and basic foundations. Ann Plast Surg 38: 553-62, 1997.
138. LC Argenta, MJ Morykwas. Vacuum-assisted closure: A new method for wound control and treatment: clinical experience. Ann Plast Surg 38: 563-76, 1997.

139. MJ Yuan-Innes, CL Temple, MS Lacey. Vacuum-assisted wound closure a new approach to spinal wounds with exposed hardware. Spine 26:E30-3, 2001.
140. T Müllner, L Mrkonjic, O Kwasny, et al. The use of negative pressure to promote the healing of tissue defects: a clinical trial using the vacuum sealing technique. Br J Plast Surg 50: 194-9, 1997.
141. MS Heggeness, SI Esses, T Errico, HA Yuan. Late infection of spinal instrumentation by hematogenous seeding. Spine 18:492-6, 1993.
142. C Wimmer, H Gluch. Management of postoperative wound infection in posterior spinal fusion with instrumentation. J Spinal Disord 9:505-8, 1996.
143. K Soultanis, G Mantelos, A. Pagiatakis, PN Soucacos. Late infection in patients with scoliosis treated with spinal instrumentation. Clin Orthop 411:116-23, 2003.
144. SH Davne, DL Myers. Complications of lumbar spinal fusion with transpedicular instrumentation. Spine 17(suppl):S184-9, 1992.
145. JM Davis, B Wolff, TF Cunningham, L Drusin, P Dineen. Delayed wound infection. An 11-year survey. Arch Surg 117:113-7, 1982.
146. J Dubousset, H Shufflebarger, D Wagner. Late "infection" with Cotrel-Dubousset instrumentation. Orthop Trans 18:121, 1994.
147. BS Richards. Delayed infections following posterior spinal instrumentation for the treatment of adolescent idiopathic scoliosis. Presented at the annual meeting of the Scoliosis Research Society, Portland, Oregon, 1994.
148. MH Heggeness, SI Esses, T Errico, HA Yuan. Late infection of spinal instrumentation by hematogenous seeding. Spine 18:492-97, 1993.
149. AG Gristina, J Kolkin. Current concepts review: total joint replacement and sepsis. J Bone Joint Surg (Am) 67:264-70, 1985.
150. L Schofferman, J Zucherman, J Schofferman, K Hsu, H Gunthorpe, G Picetti, N Goldthwaite, A White. Diphtheroids and associated infections as a cause of failed instrumented stabilization procedures in the lumbar spine. Spine 16:356-8, 1991.
151. CB Tribus, KE Garvey. Full-thickness thoracic laminar erosion after posterior spinal fusion associated with late-presenting infection. Spine 28(10):E194-7, 2003.
152. JG Heller, SR Garfin. Postoperative infection of the spine. Semin Spine Surg 2:268-82, 1990.
153. RF Gagnon, GK Richards, R Subang. Experimental staphylococcus epidermidis implant infection in the mouse. Kinetics of rifampin and vancomycin action. ASAIO J 38:M596-9, 1992.
154. JG Heller, MJ Levine. Postoperative infection of the spine. Semin Spine Surg 8:105-14, 1996.
155. RL Rimoldi, W Haye. The use of antibiotics for wound prophylaxis in spinal surgery. Orthop Clin North Am 27:47-52, 1996.
156. FJ Eismont, SW Wiesel, CT Brighton, RH Rothman. Antibiotic penetration into rabbit nucleus pulposus. Spine 12:254-6, 1987.
157. MJ Gibson, MRK Karpinski, RCB Slack, WA Cowlishaw, JK Webb. The penetration of antibiotics into the normal intervertebral disc. J Bone Joint Surg 698:784-6, 1987.
158. JP Guiboux, B Ahlgren, J Patti, M Bernhard, M Zervos, H Herkowitz. The role of prophylactic antibiotic in spinal instrumentation: a rabbit model. Spine 23:653-6, 1998.
159. BL Currier, K Banovac, FJ Eismont. Gentamycin penetration into normal rabbit nucleus pulposus. Spine 19:2614-18, 1994.
160. C von Hasselbach. Klinik und pharmakokinetik von kollagen-gentamycin als adjuvente Lokaltherapie knocherner infektionen. Ulfallchirurg 92:459-79, 1989.
161. DD Scherr, TA Dodd. In vitro bacteriological evaluation of the effectiveness of antimicrobial irrigating solution. J Bone Joint Surg A:119-22, 1976.
162. PA Netland, JE Baumgarmer, BT Andrews. Intraoperative anaphylaxis after irrigation with bacitracin: a case report. Neurosurgery 21:927-8, 1987.
163. JM Tambornino, EN Armbrust, JH Moe. Harrington instrumentation in correction of scoliosis. J Bone Joint Surg 46A:313-23, 1964.
164. DB Levine, RL Wilson, JH Dohedry. Surgical management of idiopathic scoliosis: a critical analysis of 67 cases. Clin Orthop 52:34-47, 1971.
165. JP Kostuik, J Israel, JE Hall. Scoliosis surgery in adults. Clin Orthop 93:225-34, 1973.
166. SM Swank, DS Cohen, JC Brown. Spine fusion in cerebral palsy with L-rod spinal instrumentation: a comparison of single and two-state combined approach with ielke instrumentation. Spine 14:1750-3, 1979.
167. S Swank, JE Lonstein, JH Moe, RB Winter, DS Bradford. Surgical treatment of adult scoliosis. J Bone Joint Surg 63A:268-87, 1981.
168. RE McCarthy, RD Peek, RT Morrissy, AJ Hough Jr. Allograft bone in spinal fusion for paralytic scoliosis. J Bone Joint Surg 68A:370-5, 1986.
169. R Louis. Fusion of the lumbar and sacral spine by internal fixation. Clin Orthop 203:28-33, 1986.
170. LJ Micheli, JE Hall. Complications in the management of adult spinal deformities. In: CH Epps Jr, ed. Complications in orthopaedic surgery. Vol. 2. 2d ed. Philadelphia: JB Lippincott, 1986:1227-9.
171. BL Alien Jr, RL Ferguson. The Galveston experience with L-rod instrumentation for adolescent idiopathic scoliosis. Clin Orthop 229:59-69, 1988.
172. J Zuckerman, K Hsu, A White, G Wynne. Early results of spinal fusion using variable spine plating system. Spine 13:570-9, 1988.

173. KR Gurr, PC McAfee. Cotrel-DuBousset instrumentation in adults: a preliminary report. Spine 13:510-20, 1988.
174. JS Thalgott, H LaRocca, M Agei, AP Dwyer, BE Razza. Reconstruction of the lumbar spine using AO DCP plate fixation. Spine 14:91-5, 1989.
175. TS Whitecloud III, JC Butler, JL Cohen, PD Candelora. Complications with the variable spinal plating system. Spine 14:472-6, 1989.
176. SI Esses, BL Saches. Complication of pedicle screw fixation. 1991 North American Spine Society Meeting, Keystone, Colorado, August 1991.
177. J Kretzler, J Banta. Wound infections following spinal fusion surgery: transactions of the 1991 meeting of the Pediatric Orthopaedic Society of North America. J Pediatr Orthop 12:264, 1992.
178. U Aydinli, O Karaeminogullari, K Tiskaya. Postoperative deep wound infection in instrumented spinal surgery. Acta Orthop Belg 65:182-7, 1999.
179. RL Wright. Septic complications of neurological spinal procedures. Springfield, IL: Thomas, 1970.
180. PC Leung. Complications in the first 40 cases of microdiscectomy. J Spinal Disord 1:306-10, 1988.

12

Epidural Fibrosis
in the Failed Spine

Erdal Coskun

INTRODUCTION

Back pain is a common health problem, and one of its main causes is lumbar disk herniation. Lumbar disc surgery is successful in 75% to 92% of patients. The remaining 8% to 25% have either residual or recurrent low back pain and radiculopathy. Failed back surgery syndrome (FBSS) is a clinical condition in which patients undergo one or more surgical procedures for lumbosacral disease and obtain unsatisfactory long-term relief of symptoms, with persistent or recurrent low back and/or leg pain. This syndrome is characterized by a constellation of pain, dysfunction, psychological disturbances, and incapacitation from low back and/or leg pain. Although FBSS is usually due to improper diagnosis and surgery, other important causes are iatrogenic instability, lateral and central spinal stenosis, arachnoidities, recurrent disc herniation, and epidural fibrosis. Patients with recurrent disc herniation tend to show improvement, whereas those with scar formation (i.e., those in whom no recurrent disc herniation or other cause was found for the recurrent or persistent back or leg pain) tend to show little improvement (3,7,10–13,29,30,31).

Lumbar epidural fibrosis is increasingly recognized as responsible for persistent low back pain. The reported incidence of epidural fibrosis ranges from 10% to 75%. Approximately 10% to 24% of all cases of FBSS are the result of epidural fibrosis. Although discectomy after hemilaminectomy always produces some fibrosis, the association between epidural fibrosis and recurrent pain after lumbar discectomy is controversial. The diagnosis of epidural fibrosis can be done radiologically. Unfortunately, there is no direct correlation between the radiological and clinical findings. There is no explanation for why epidural fibrosis of the same radiological appearance and localization is associated with incapacitating pain in some patients and not in others. The role of epidural fibrosis as a cause of FBSS is the subject of continuing debate among spinal surgeons, mainly because of the multiple factors involved in the pathogenesis of this condition (1,3,8,10,12–14,19,26,31,34,40).

ETIOLOGY

Postoperative epidural fibrosis is a manifestation of the normal process of wound repair after lumbar spine surgery (8,9,14,18,34,39). The formation of scar tissue takes place from 6 weeks to 6 months after laminectomy (33,34). Tulberg et al. found some scar tissue in all patients 1 to 2 months after surgery for lumbar disc herniation (39). The amount of scar tissue decreases during the first year after surgery, but some scar tissue persists in most cases (23,29).

The main question is the source of epidural fibrosis. The exact pathogenesis of epidural fibrosis has not been established. There are several ideas.

1. Key and Ford were the first to describe nerve root entrapment by scar tissue after lumbar laminectomy (21). They theorized that annulus fibrosus was the source of the postlaminectomy scar tissue. This type of epidural fibrosis is usually located anteriorly.

2. In an experimental study, when autologous intervertebral disc material was embedded into the epidural space, the epidural fat tissue was penetrated by newly formed vessels and developed an inflammatory reaction (28). Retained fragment may provoke develop epidural fibrosis. Herniation may be surrounded by scar tissue. In spite of the presence of enhancement in epidural mass, a recurrent or residual disc herniation may still occur.

3. However, even when nucleotomy is not performed on some patients, posteriorly located epidural fibrosis may occur following surgical laminectomy. LaRocca and McNabb in a canine model described the epidural scar tissue as the "post laminectomy membrane" (22). Their study indicated that fibroblasts forming the epidural scar came from the damaged erector spinal muscles overlying the laminectomy site.

4. During a posterior approach of the lumbar spinal canal, arterial bleeding from the paravertebral muscles and epidural venous bleeding are the most important reasons for epidural hematoma. Epidural hematoma occurs in the path of surgical dissection, and even if it does not compress the dural sac, it can be a cause of epidural fibrosis. The hematoma is absorbed and gradually replaced with granulation tissue originating from the fibrous layers of the periosteum and within the deep surface of the paravertebral muscles. This granulation tissue matures into a dense fibrotic tissue that may extend into the neural canal and adhere to the dura mater and nerve roots.

5. Excessive cautery of epidural veins inhibits the nutrition of the nerve roots and causes intraneural fibrosis, epidural fibrosis, and arachnoiditis.

6. The mechanisms of fibrosis may be related to persisting cotton debris from sponges used during the operation. This debris may act as a fibrogenic stimulus. In one study, examination of the biopsy specimens revealed marked collagen proliferation (17). Small areas of focal inflammatory cell infiltration and dilated veins are observed. These chronic inflammatory cell infiltrates are found only in material obtained from patients who underwent previous surgery. They have not been found in proliferating scar tissue from patients who have not had any invasive procedure. When this material was examined by polarized light microscopy, areas of chronic inflammatory cell infiltrations were observed, concentrated around deposits of birefringent crystalline material. By means of a series of histochemical stains and enzyme digestion using celluloses, the author's group has shown that this crystalline material is identical to fragmented cotton debris from surgical swabs and patties as well as to fragmented pure cellulose. These findings suggest that various types of surgical dressing used during the operative procedure will liberate cotton dust into the wound. In our study, the high rate of metal artifacts was thought to be dust from the lower quality surgical tools we had to use (i.e., periost elevator) (7,10,18). This dust may persist and act as a fibrogenic stimulus, leading to the development of excessive scar tissue.

7. During removal of herniation or insertion of a cage system, excessive dural retraction, aggressive endplate curettage, and facet removal lead to epidural fibrosis by excessive inflammatory response.

8. Persistence of the fibrinolytic defect is associated with failure to clear the fibrin. This fibrinolytic defect appeared attributable to disproportionate increases in circulating

plasminogen activator inhibitor-1 levels. This may interfere with the diffusion of oxygen and nutrients into the tissues and provoke inflammation (9,18). Clinical features were slightly worse in patients with radiological epidural fibrosis, whereas the frequency of radiological abnormalities, including epidural fibrosis, was higher in patients with fibrinolytic abnormalities.

9. Considering the fact that epidural fibrosis is not only caused by surgeons' manipulation, bleeding, or dural tears, but also by permanent irritation due to instability, a spinal fusion procedure is likely to be more successful than a neurolysis in cases where true recurrent herniation or a new herniation is excluded (13).

Possible mechanisms for recurrent pain caused by epidural fibrosis include nerve root irritation, nerve root entrapment, anoxia of perineural and intraneural fibrosis, direct dural compression, and restriction of nerve root mobility, which increases susceptibility to small recurrent disc herniations and osteophyte formation. Postoperative epidural scar situated in critical proximity with lumbar nerve root may induce dynamic neural tension, particularly during repeated movement (10,14,18,29,34,41). Spinal nerve roots and dorsal root ganglia are particularly sensitive to mechanical deformation. Even very low pressure may impair the overall nutritional transport to the nerve roots (32). Goddard and Rein documented an average excursion of 3 mm for the intratechal portion of L5 nerve root, whereas for the S1 nerve root this value ranged between 4 and 5 mm (15). If there is a disc herniation smaller than this value with epidural fibrosis, this situation even without significant compression can cause entrapment neuropathy. The combination of epidural fibrosis and segmental micro-instability can be responsible for back pain or sciatic pain.

RADIOLOGICAL DIAGNOSIS

Identification of fibrosis as the cause of recurring lumbar or sciatic pain requires the existence of a good clinical history, selective physical examination, and radiological evaluation of the patient. Distinction between scar and disc can be carried out with myelography, computed tomography (CT), and magnetic resonance imaging (MRI). Myelography is neither sensitive nor specific for differentiation of scar formation and disc herniation (1,3,8,26,33,34,37,39).

It is difficult to establish fibrosis as the cause of FBSS because there are no characteristic CT findings to distinguish normal postoperative fibrosis from fibrosis that could cause symptoms of nerve root entrapment (1,8). In 1982, Schurbiger et al. described contrast enhancement scar tissue by CT (37). The degree of fibrosis is classified as low (+), medium (++), and high (+++) on CT images (1,7). Low-degree fibrosis is present in one slice on CT scan at the disc space level or two slices and involves less than half of the epidural space circumference. Medium-degree fibrosis is present in two slices and involves more than half of the epidural space circumference in at least one slice or present in three slices and involves less than half of the epidural space circumference. High-degree fibrosis is present in three slices and involves more than half of the epidural space circumference at least in one slice or is present in four slices or more. Braun et al. have found enhanced CT to be more accurate than unenhanced CT in differentiation of disc and scar (4). Contrast-enhanced CT has an accuracy of 67% to 100% in distinguishing scar from disc (1,4,37). Cervellini has found that high-degree fibrosis was more common in asymptomatic patients and there was no significant difference in the prevalence of scar tissue in patients with persistent symptoms, compared with postsurgery without complaint (8). They suggest that it should not be considered as a frequent cause of FBSS. In another study, the intraoperative findings have been compared with CT findings, and correct diagnosis has been found in 74% with contrast CT, in 43% with noncontrast CT (4). Ebeling et al. found 43% true recurrent herniations and 23% new herniations at different levels and epidural fibrosis in 5% of the patients at the time of first revision (11).

MRI is the most used imaging technique in differentiating postoperative fibrosis from recurrent disc herniation, although CT and myelography can be useful in some cases (1). MRI without contrast is at least equivalent to contrasted CT. The interpretation of non-contrast MRI using high-field-strength sagittal T1-weighted spin-echo and sagittal and axial proton density and T2-weighted images obtained 94% to 97% accuracy (6,30). This accuracy is related to the partial overlap in imaging characteristics of scar and recurrent herniated nucleus pulposus (6). Epidural fibrosis is seen consistently to enhance immediately after the injection of contrast material. Gadolinium-enhanced MRI has been founded to be 96% accurate in differentiating scar tissue from disc (26,33–35). Scar tissue enhances even several years after surgery. However, no relationship was found between the degree of contrast enhancement of scar and vascular density. Multiple small capillaries and tight and loose junctions between the endothelial cells have been demonstrated (33). Gap junction status and extracellular space size are more important than vascular density in predicting the degree of enhancement (6). The breakdown of the blood-nerve barrier, which can be demonstrated by MRI, may be caused by contrast enhancement (19). The contrast agent transgresses the endothelium through "leaky" intercellular junctions and areas of endothelial discontinuity (33).

The percentage of scar is hyperintense on long TR/TE images. The mechanism for hyperintensity of scar on T2-weighted images could be related to an increase in spin density relative to dense fibrosis or peripheral annulus (because of vascularity) (6,7). T2-weighted MRI is highly accurate in diagnosing recurrent disc herniation (94% to 97%) (30). On the basis of imaging results alone (without consideration of its invasive nature and significant additional cost), the routine use of gadolinium-enhanced MR imaging in the evaluation of postdiscectomy patients is not indicated (30). In addition, the use of intravenous contrast medium to differentiate epidural fibrosis from recurrent disc herniation has its pitfalls. A chronic recurrent disc herniation may develop enhancing peridisc inflammatory change, and the epidural scar may fail to enhance. Initially, the scar is in the form of soft, well-vascularized granulation tissue. Eventually, the scar contracts and vascularity reduces (41).

Epidural fibrosis is isointense or hypointense relative to intervertebral disc on T1-weighted MRI. Epidural fibrosis tends to form a curvilinear pattern surrounding the dural tube and is fairly homogeneous. It leads to retraction of the dural tube toward the side of soft tissue. Axial sections provided an excellent description of amount of scar tissue and reliable determination of the presence or absence of mass effect. The presence or absence of mass effect is not a diagnostic criteria. In spite of the presence of enhancement in epidural mass, a recurrent or residual disc herniation may still be present. Recurrent herniated disc material is isointense compared to the intervertebral disc on T1-weighted images, and appearance on T2 images vary from low-signal intensity to high-signal intensity. It tends to have a polypoid configuration with a smooth outer margin and does not enhance within the first 10 to 20 minutes following administration of contrast material (6,7,33,34).

For the purposes of epidural fibrosis identification, only the axial T1-weighted images with and without contrast may be utilized. The amount of epidural fibrosis is examined on contrast-enhanced MRI in axial slices subdivided into four spatial quadrants (34,35,40).

The amount of epidural fibrosis is graded on a scale of 0 to 4 for each quadrant at each imaging slice encompassing the operative level:

0 no/trace scar
1 >0% and 25% quadrant filled with scar
2 >25% and ≤50% quadrant filled with scar
3 >50% and ≤75% quadrant filled with scar
4 >75% and ≤100% quadrant filled with scar

Scar scored as 0 or 1 was characterized as minimal; what scored 2 or 3 was characterized as moderate; and a score of 4 was considered extensive. Ross et al. also presented a score to quantify the extent of epidural scarring on MR images (34). They defined a lesion as "extensive" if 75% of the quadrant of the spinal canal was filled with scar.

DIFFERENTIAL DIAGNOSIS

Pain seen immediately after discectomy would most probably indicate surgical failure (i.e., wrong level, a retained disc fragment, or inadequate decompression). The pain occurring 1 year or more after surgery results from a recurrent herniation at the same level or new site, probably indicating the need for a second operation. Another group of patients are the ones who initially report little or no pain but who gradually develop activity-related pain several months after surgery. Those patients are difficult to diagnose and treat. The combination of epidural fibrosis, local arachnoiditis, and segmental micro-instability with irritation of nerve roots can be responsible for their complaints. Spinal surgeons believe epidural fibrosis contributes to recurrent radicular pain without reherniation, but this connection has remained speculative (3,7,10,31,34,37,40). There are two controversial groups related to the role of epidural fibrosis in FBSS. The first group suggested that pain induces epidural fibrosis. According to the other group, pain is not related to epidural fibrosis.

Marron et al. suggested that back pain evaluations with MRI scar score of 6 months evaluation that increased amount of scar were predictive of increase of low back pain (26). North et al. reported that favorable outcomes for the patients they evaluated were associated with absence of epidural fibrosis requiring surgical lysis (31). Ross et al. found that patients with extensive epidural fibrosis were 3.2 times more likely to experience recurrent radicular pain than those with less extensive scarring (34). They suggested a correlation between the extent of epidural fibrosis and the level of postoperative complaints. However, 87.3% of their patients with extensive epidural fibrosis on MRI were asymptomatic.

Jinkins et al. suggested that fibrosis in the epidural space may be less important in the pathogenesis of FBSS (19). Annertz et al. also found no differences regarding the amount of epidural fibrosis between patients with radicular pain and patients with nonradicular pain (3). There is no explanation for why epidural fibrosis of some radiological appearance and localization is associated with incapacitating pain in one patient and not in another (3). Coskun et al. have found different degrees of epidural fibrosis on MRI in their patients, but there was no relationship between the severity of epidural fibrosis and pain scores or disability scores (10). Because of the role of psychological factors in postoperative pain and disability, they have advised that psychological evaluation should be included in the assessment of FBSS. For that reason, this group suggested epidural fibrosis might be considered a radiological entity that is not correlated with patients' complaints (3,8,19,40).

Spinal canal diameter measurements and functional lumbar spinal plain X-ray has to be performed to exclude instability and narrow spinal canal. Pain experience of patients is composed of their organic and psychosomatic state. Therefore, personality and behavioral patterns should be evaluated with psychological tests in these patients (10,12,13,29,31).

TREATMENT

There is currently no effective medical or surgical therapy for epidural fibrosis. The goal of treatment is to minimize the epidural fibrosis. The main measurements are prevention, epidural lysis, and medical and surgical treatment. The most important factors to prevent a failed back syndrome related to epidural fibrosis is to use a nontraumatic surgical technique. Although creation of a small surgical wound, meticulous technique to minimize tissue damage, and good hemostasis are the most accepted measures to avoid this devastating complication, symptomatic epidural fibrosis may nonetheless develop in many cases.

The main sources of epidural fibrosis are fibrogenic stimuli such as a residual disc fragment, fibroblast from damaged paravertebral muscle, and fibrin from hematoma (8,9,16,18,23,41). The purpose of the preventive treatment should be to clear the fibrogenic stimulus (16,41). The meticulous microsurgical technique reduces possibility of retained fragment and surgical trauma. Therefore, the amount of anterior epidural fibrosis may be minimized. Although the transplantation of autologous fat graft has many advantages such as the prevention of postoperative epidural fibrosis and bleeding, later fibrosis developed in the fat graft may provoke excessive epidural fibrosis (27). Moreover, dislocation of free fat graft may happen. Irrigation of epidural space to remove foreign material or toxins may also reduce it. Antiinflammatory drugs of both nonsteroidal and steroidal forms have been used to prevent epidural fibrosis. Nonsteroidal antiinflammatory drugs (NSAIDs) inhibit the synthesis of prostaglandin that could decrease the inflammatory response by controlling the hyperplasia of fibrocytes and formation of granulation. As a result, amount of fibrotic tissue could be reduced (16). Hemostatic agents reduce amount of fibrin at the space of the operation (9). Urokinaz, which is a fibrinolytic agent, may provide rapid clearance of the blood from the epidural area. Thus the probability of permanent epidural fibrosis may be reduced (36). The topical thrombolysis with rt-PA after spinal surgery may come to play an important role in the prevention of epidural fibrosis and arachnoiditis (20). Songer et al. reported that sodium hyaluronate reduced fibroblast invasion and retarded fibrosis (38).

A number of investigators have studied the effectiveness of various treatments for preventing epidural fibrosis. A large variety of materials have been used to prevent or reduce scar formation as mechanical barriers to limit tethering of neural elements. They include biological (fat graft), soft nonbiological (absorbable gelatine sponge, bone wax), solid nonbiological (polymethylmetacrylate, membranes, polytetrafluoroethylene), and viscous materials (collagen-based sealant, hyaluronic acid, carboxymethylcellulose, carbohydrate polymer, ADCON-L) (2,14,22,24,27,29,34,41). The results of these studies have demonstrated only moderate success in the inhibition of epidural fibrosis. Some have been applied in humans, and spinal membranes and bioabsorbable adhesion barrier gels are the most widely accepted materials in current practice, although each is associated with certain drawbacks such as requiring repeated surgery and significant expense.

Applications of a spinal membrane or ADCON-L gel are the most common procedures for preventing epidural fibrosis in current practice. ADCON-L is an effective antifibrotic agent. It is biologically active and blocks the ingrowth of fibroblasts from surgically detached muscle (14). The gel is absorbed in 1 month. The application of the gel may be safe in the presence of dural incisions, even when they are not identified during surgery. Because these materials are foreign implants and expensive or require additional time and surgical measures, however, they are usually used only in cases with symptomatic epidural fibrosis. Thus the major drawback of these procedures is that they require a second surgical intervention associated with an even higher complication rate than the first.

The medical treatment consists of bed rest, nonsteroidal antiinflammatory drugs, myorelaxant, and antidepressant medication. In chronic pain, antidepressant treatment with seratonin reuptake inhibitors alleviates the pain threshold of patients. In addition, it provides a more stable patient psychologically. Gabapentin has also established a favorable safety profile and been shown to be effective in various animal models and human studies of chronic neuropathy pain (5). Clinicians should consider gabapentin as a pharmacological treatment alternative in the management of FBSS caused by epidural fibrosis.

Spinal cord stimulation is another choice in intractable pain. Spinal cord stimulation should be undertaken as a late or last resort, after acceptable alternative treatments have been exhausted. In FBSS, for example, surgical options should have been exhausted (although one may consider that reoperation offers lower yield and greater potential risks in some cases) (12,31).

There is an associated high complication rate seen with revision spinal surgery, in particular the increased occurrences of dural tears, nerve root injury, and bleeding. Reoperation with the intention of excising this fibrosis tissue after procedure gives rise to a poor surgical result and further scarring. Repeated surgery for fibrosis has only a 30% to 35% success rate, whereas 15% to 20% of patients report worsening of their symptoms (1,12–14,29,31). The disappointing results are twice as high in multiply revised patients without spinal fusion as in patients in whom a spinal fusion finally was performed (13).

Epiduroscopy is available for visualization of the epidural space and of value in the diagnosis of spinal epidural fibrosis. Epidural adhesiolysis with epiduroscopy is an interventional technique based on the premise that the three-dimensional visualization of the contents of the epidural space provides the physician with the ability to visualize the structures directly, perform appropriate adhesiolysis, and administer drugs specifically to the target (25). The symptom-free period is shorter than 6 months. There are still marked limitations to epiduroscopy due to technical problems. These must be minimized.

SUMMARY

Scar is an inevitable accompaniment of lumbar disc surgery. Fibrosis can cause compression or tethering of the nerve root and has been implicated as one of the reasons for FBSS. Separating epidural fibrosis from recurrent disc prolapses is crucial because patients with the former are expected to benefit from further surgery. MRI with contrast provides an excellent view of scar tissue. However, routine use of gadolinium is unnecessary in postoperative MRI of the lumbar spine by high-resolution MRI. High-resolution T_2-weighted MRI may be the procedure of choice for evaluation of postoperative recurrent low back and leg pain. The relationship between epidural fibrosis and pain is still obscure.

There is currently no effective medical or surgical therapy for epidural fibrosis. The goal of treatment is to minimize epidural fibrosis. The main measurements are prevention, epidural lysis, and medical and surgical treatment. The mechanical tethering of nerve roots or the dura mater by the epidural adhesions may be a contributing factor for a significant subset of a patient's complaints. The interposing materials to prevent the formation and adherence of the tissue to the neural elements are of importance in improving surgical outcome. The evaluation and correction of psychological disturbances are the most important component of treatment.

REFERENCES

1. Albeck MJ, Wagner A, Knudsen LL. Contrast enhanced computed tomography and magnetic resonance imaging in the diagnosis of recurrent disc herniation. Acta Neurochir (Wien) 138: 1256-60, 1996.
2. Alkalay RN, Kim DH, Urry DW, Xu J, Parker TM, Glazer PA. Prevention of postlaminectomy epidural fibrosis using bioelastic materials. Spine 28: 1659-65, 2003.
3. Annertz M, Jönsson B, Strömqvist B, Hotas S. No relationship between epidural fibrosis and sciatica in the lumbar postdiscectomy syndrome. A study with contrast-enhancement magnetic resonance imaging in symptomatic patients Spine 20: 449-3, 1995.
4. Braun IF, Hofman JC, Davis PC, Landman JA, Tindall GT. Contrast enhancement in CT differentiation between recurrent disk herniation and postoperative scar: prospective study. AJR 145: 785-90, 1985.
5. Braverman DL, Slipman CW, Lenrow DA. Using gabapentin to treat failed back surgery syndrome caused by epidural fibrosis. A report of 2 cases. Arch Phys Med Rehabil 82: 691-3, 2001.
6. Bundschuh CV, Stein L, Slusser JH, Schinco FP, Ladaga LE, Dillon JD. Distinguishing between scar and recurrent herniated disk in postoperative patients: value of contrast-enhanced CT and MR imaging. AJNR. Am J Neuroradiol 11: 949-58, 1990.
7. Bundschuh CV, Modic MT, Ross JS, Masaryk TJ, Bohlman H. Epidural fibrosis and recurrent disk herniation in the lumbar spine: MR imaging assessment. AJR 150: 923-32, 1988.
8. Cervellini P, Curri D, Volpin L, Bernardi L, Pinna V, Benedetti A. Computed tomography of epidural fibrosis after discectomy: a comparison between symptomatic and asymptomatic patients. Neurosurgery 23: 710-3, 1988.
9. Cooper RG, Mitchell WS, Illingworth KJ, Forbes WS, Gillespie JE, Jayson MI. The role of epidural fibrosis and defective fibrinolysis in the persistence of postlaminectomy back pain. Spine 16: 1044-8, 1991.
10. Coskun E, Süzer T, Topuz O, Zencir M, Pakdemirli E, Tahta K. Relationships between epidural fibrosis, pain, disability, and psychological factors after lumbar disc surgery. Eur Spine J 9: 218–23, 2000.
11. Ebeling U, Reichenberg W, Reulen HJ. Results of microsurgical lumbar discectomy: review of 485 patients. Acta Neurochir 81: 45-52, 1986.
12. Fiume D, Sherkat S, Callovini GM, Parziale G, Gazzeri G. Treatment of the failed back surgery syndrome due to lumbo-sacral epidural fibrosis. Acta Neurochir Suppl (Wien) 64: 116-8, 1995.
13. Fritsch EW, Heisel J, Rupp S, The failed back surgery syndrome reasons, intraoperative findings, and long-term results: A report of 182 operative treatments. Spine 21: 626-33, 1996.
14. Geisler FH. Prevention of peridural fibrosis: current methodologies. Neurol Res 21 Supp 1: 9-22, 1999.
15. Goddard MD, Reid JD. Movement induced by straight leg raising in the lumbosacral roots, nerves, and pleksus, and in the intrapelvic section of the sciatic nerve. J Neurol Neurosurg Psychiatry 28: 12-18, 1965.
16. He Y, Revel M, Loty B. A quantitative model of post-laminectomy scar formation. Effects of a nonsteroidal anti-inflammatory drug. Spine 20: 557-63, 1995.
17. Hoyland JA, Freemont AJ, Denton J, Thomas AMC, McMillan JJ, Jayson MIV. Retained surgical swab debris in post-laminectomy arachnoiditis and peridural fibrosis. J Bone Joint Surg 70: 659-62, 1988.
18. Jayson MIV The role of vascular damage and fibrosis in the pathogenesis of nerve root damage. Clinical Orthop 279: 40-8, 1992.
19. Jinkins JR, Osborn AG, Garrett Jr D, Hunt S, Story JL. Spinal nerve enhancement with Gd-DTPA: MR correlation with the postoperative lumbosacral spine AJNR 14: 383-94, 1993.
20. Kemaloglu S, Ozkan U, Yilmaz F, Nas K, Gur A, Acemoglu H, Karasu H, Cakmak E. Prevention of spinal epidural fibrosis by recombinant tissue plasminogen activator in rats. Spinal Cord 41: 427-31, 2003.
21. Key JA, Ford LT. Experimental intervertebral disc lesions. J Bone Joint Surg Am 30A: 621–30, 1948.
22. Kim KD, Wang JC, Robertson DP, Brodke DS, Olson EM, Duberg AC, BenDebba M, Block KM, Dizerega GS. Reduction of radiculopathy and pain with oxiplex/SP gel after laminectomy, laminotomy, and discectomy: a pilot clinical study. Spine 28: 1080–7, 2003.
23. LaRocca H, Macnab I. The laminectomy membrane: studies in its evolution, characteristics, effects and prophylaxis in dogs. J Bone Joint Surg 56: 545-50, 1974.
24. Liu S, Boutrand JP, Tadie M. Use of a collagen-based sealant to prevent in vivo epidural adhesions in an adult rat laminectomy model. J Neurosurg. 94 (Suppl 1): 61-7, 2001.
25. Manchikanti L, Singh V. Epidural lysis of adhesions and myeloscopy. Curr Pain Headache Rep 6: 427-35, 2002.
26. Maroon JC, Abla A, Bost J. Association between peridural scar and persistent low back pain after lumbar discectomy. Neurol Res 21 (Suppl 1): S43-6, 1999.
27. Martin-Ferrer S. Failure of autologous fat graft to prevent postoperative epidural fibrosis in surgery of lumbar spine. Neurosurgery 24: 718-21, 1989.
28. Minamide A, Tamaki T, Hashizume H, Yoshida M, Kawakami M, Hayashi N. Effects of steroid and lipopolysaccharide on spontaneous resorption of herniated intervertebral discs. An experimental study in the rabbit. Spine 15: 870-76, 1998.

29. Mohsenipour I, Daniaux M, Aichner F, Twerdy K. Prevention of local scar formation after operative discectomy for lumbar disc herniation. Acta Neurochir 140: 9-13, 1998.
30. Mullin WJ, Heithoff KB, Gilbert TJ Jr, Renfrew DL. Magnetic resonance evaluation of recurrent disc herniation: is gadolinium necessary? Spine 25: 1493-99, 2000.
31. North RB, Campbell JN, James CS, Conover-Walker MK, Wang H, Piantadosi S, Rybock JD, Long DM. Failed back surgery syndrome: 5-year follow-up in 102 patients undergoing repeated operation. Neurosurgery 28: 685-91, 1991.
32. Olmarker K, Rydevik B. Pathophysiology of sciatica. Orthop Clin North Am 22: 223-34, 1991.
33. Ross JS, Delamarter R, Hueftle MG, Masaryk TJ, Aikawa M, Carter J, VanDyke C, Modic MT. Gadolinium-DTPA-enhanced MR imaging of the postoperative lumbar spine: time course and mechanism of enhancement. AJR Am J Roentgenol 152: 825-34, 1989.
34. Ross JS, Roberston JT, Frederickson RCA, Petrie JL, Obuchowski N, Modic MT, Tribolet N. Association between peridural scar and recurrent radicular pain after lumbar discectomy: magnetic resonance evaluation. Neurosurgery 38: 855-63, 1996.
35. Ross JS, Obuchowski N, Modic MT. MR evaluation of epidural fibrosis: proposed grading system with intra- and inter-observer variability. Neurol Res 21 (Suppl 1): 23-26, 1999.
36. Selçuklu A, Pasaoglu A, Akdemir H, Kurtsoy A, Patiroglu TE. Urokinase for control of scar formation after laminectomy. Spine 18: 165-8, 1993.
37. Schubiger O, Valavanis A. CT differentiation between recurrent disc herniation and postoperative scar formation: the value of contrast enhancement. Neuroradiology 22: 251-54, 1982.
38. Songer MN, Ghosh L, Spencer DL. Effects of sodium hyalutonate on peridural fibrosis after lumbar laminectomy and discectomy. Spine 15: 550-4, 1990.
39. Tulberg T, Rydberg J, Isacsson J. Radiographic changes after lumbar discectomy. Spine 18: 843-50, 1993.
40. Vogelsang JP, Finkenstaedt M, Vogelsang M, Markakis E. Recurrent pain after lumbar discectomy: the diagnostic value of peridural scar on MRI. Eur Spine J 8: 475-9, 1999.
41. Wujek JR, Ahman S, Harel A, Maier KH, Roufa D, Silver J. A carbohydrate polymer that effectively prevents epidural fibrosis at laminectomy sites in the rat. Exp Neurol 114: 237-45, 1991.

13

The Failed Perfect Surgery

Jean Charles Le Huec, A. Mehbod, and S. Aunoble

Multiple variables contribute to the success or failure of an operation. Generally speaking, the three most important variables are the indication for surgery, the surgical technique itself, and the postoperative function of the surgical intervention. These factors are usually interdependent. The scenario of good indication, good technique, and good postoperative functioning usually leads to good clinical results. This is exemplified by a patient with advanced degeneration of one level of the spine who receives a one-level discectomy and bone grafting that eventually fuses and leads to a good clinical result. This is a perfect surgery.

On the contrary, in a failed surgery, the surgical intervention leads to poor clinical results. This situation can occur when the indication for surgery and/or the surgical technique is poor. An example may be a patient who undergoes a multilevel spine fusion with poor technique leading to pseudarthrosis and poor clinical results.

However, occasionally one is faced with scenarios that are absurd. Different situations, such as the following, can occur:

- The indication for surgery, technique, and radiological results were all good, but the postoperative function of the intervention is poor. This is the case in many papers where no explanation is found to understand poor results when indication, technique, and radiological results seem to be perfect. Unknown factors have to be considered. Sometimes those factors are demonstrated with accuracy through a global analysis of the spine like Lazennec (1), who showed in his series of lumbar arthrodesis that the poor results were correlated with an imbalance of the spine.

- Another situation is exemplified by a patient who undergoes a one-level decompression and fusion for spondylolisthesis and who has a pseudarthrosis with good clinical results. This occurred in one of the most important studies published to date where Sidhu and Herkowitz (2) reported on patients after posterolateral fusion for degenerative spondylolisthesis with 85% good or excellent clinical results and only a 45% fusion rate. One may view this as ridiculously unreasonable, but we have to accept the fact that this absurd perfect failed surgery does exist. We must try to understand the exact pain generator because the aim of the surgery was to help the patient suffer less pain.

- It is rare to have a bad surgical technique and a good clinical result, but this can occur. In motion technology surgery, there have been reports of total disc arthroplasties of the lumbar spine with no motion and excellent outcome (3). It is also amazing to see papers on disc arthroplasties showing excellent results with less than 3 degrees of motion, which in other situations is considered an argument to assess a good fusion on dynamic X-rays (2) (Fig. 13.1). Histories of implant migration are well known without clinical consequences. However, the early and midtime clinical results can be good but

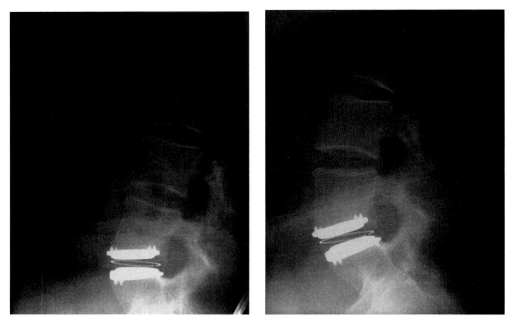

FIG. 13.1. No motion on dynamic X-rays and perfect clinical outcome using a totisc replacement.

sometimes the late follow-up is bad or fair. Placebo effect has to be considered when functional results are evaluated.
• The idea of perfect failed surgery has no rationale. It is a divorce between the indication and the technique and its function. It is not the rule but the exception, although it continues to be observed in clinical practice.

REFERENCES

1. Lazennec JY, Ramare S, Arafati N, et al. Sagittal alignment in lumbosacral fusion: relations between radiological parameters and pain. Eur Spine J 2000;9:47-55.
2. Sidhu KS, Herkowitz HN. Spinal instrumentation in the management of degenerative disorders of the lumbar spine. Clin Orthop 1997;335:39-53.
3. Huang RC, Girardi FP, Cammisa FP Jr, et al. Long-term flexion-extension range of motion of the prodisc total disc replacement. J Spinal Disord Tech 2003;16:435-40.

14

Imaging of the Failed Spine

Johan W. M. Van Goethem, Özkan Özsarlak, Maes Menno,
J. Randy Jinkins, and Paul M. Parizel

INTRODUCTION

Low back and radicular pain, widespread complaints in modern society, are in part adverse effects resulting from present-day lifestyles (1). Genetic factors also play an important role in the development of back pain. Low back and radicular pain taken together are a leading cause of disability and result in a substantial loss of productivity. The prevalence of low back pain varies from 7.6% to 37% among different populations (2). Most episodes of low back pain are mechanical in origin and resolve within a 12-week period (3). Recent studies, however, suggest that low back pain may persist for longer periods of time in a large number of patients but that patients eventually stop seeking medical help. The overwhelming majority of low back pain patients, therefore, in all probability undergo a nonoperative form of self-treatment.

Several imaging techniques are available to the medical imaging specialist, all of which may be helpful in the diagnostic work-up of patients with low back pain. However, some techniques are preferable, depending on several factors. Although costly diagnostic imaging should only be undertaken with a clear indication, advanced diagnostic imaging studies (i.e., everything other than conventional radiography) can play an important role in the optimal selection of treatment in patients with persistent low back pain who are clinically suspected of having disc herniation (4). Some investigators suggest that surgery should not be performed unless a diagnostic imaging study demonstrates nerve root compromise (5). Others have concluded that surgical success is likely only in patients in whom symptoms, physical findings, and imaging results are consistent (6).

In general, surgery for lumbar disc herniation relieves pain in most patients, producing good long-term outcome in almost 90% of subjects (7). Repeat surgery, however, is less successful, with only 60% to 82% of patients with recurrent disc herniation improving after surgery (8–10). In patients who only have epidural scar tissue on serial imaging studies, the success rate of reintervention is as low as 17% to 38% (9,11). The obvious solution for this problem is to avoid when possible the initial operation that may ultimately lead to a less than satisfactory result, and thereby not create a clinical situation that requires repeat surgery.

IMAGING OF THE FAILED SPINE

The Failed Back Surgery Syndrome

Despite the relatively loose application of criteria for judging operative success, lumbosacral spinal surgery has been so often unsuccessful in the past (range: 10% to 40%)

that failed back surgery is now labeled as a clinical syndrome: the failed back surgery syndrome (FBSS). FBSS is characterized by intractable pain and various degrees of functional incapacitation following spinal surgery. The major identifiable causes of FBSS include recurrent/residual disc herniation, arachnoiditis, radiculitis, spinal or spinal neural foraminal stenosis, and failure to identify the structural source(s) of pain correctly (12).

The severity of recurrent symptoms has not been shown to correlate with the amount of epidural scar tissue (13,14). The management of patients with FBSS remains a difficult problem (15), but the presence of recurrent or residual disc herniation generally is thought to be an indication for repeat surgical intervention (16–18). The differentiation of scar tissue and recurrent/residual disc herniation maybe achieved with relatively high accuracy on IV contrast-enhanced CT, but it is even better and more clearly distinguished on IV contrast-enhanced MRI (18–19).

Nevertheless, when a residual disc herniation is present, one should keep in mind that it is not necessarily responsible for the patient's complaints (20). Moreover, herniated disc fragments, especially when extruded into the central spinal canal, as is often the case in the postoperative phase, can regress spontaneously chiefly by means of phagocytosis (20,21).

Recurrent Disc Herniation

The imaging differentiation between recurrent or residual disc herniation and epidural fibrosis can usually be made according to existing criteria (16,18,19), including on the one hand obliteration of the epidural fat by uniformly enhancing epidural fibrosis in the anterior, lateral, and posterior epidural space in the instances of epidural fibrosis (Figs. 14.1 and 14.2), or on the other hand by early central nonenhancement in cases of recurrent/residual disc herniation (Fig. 14.2). It is especially the latter finding that we believe is most important in differentiating between the two conditions. Because MRI is more sensitive in detecting abnormal contrast enhancement, as compared to CT, MRI is the imaging method of choice in accurately evaluating patients suffering from the FBSS.

Epidural Fibrosis

As already mentioned, the lack of early central contrast enhancement in cases of recurrent disc fragments and the homogeneous enhancement pattern of scar tissue have been claimed to be the major differentiating criteria. The vascularized granulation tissue surrounding and often penetrating into the substance of disc herniations represents a normal reactive response (i.e., the body's attempt to destroy or resorb the herniation) and can complicate the differentiation of disc herniation and isolated scar formation.

The association of scar tissue with minor deformations of the dural sac (i.e., mass effect) does not necessarily imply pathological scar tissue formation (22). This accompanying deformation of the dural sac usually diminishes within 6 months of surgery. However, deformation of the dural sac (i.e., more than 10% area loss of central spinal canal in the axial plane) accompanying epidural scar tissue is considered a relatively abnormal finding when found 6 months or later after surgery. Nevertheless, what effect this epidural scarring has on clinical signs and symptoms is not known, and many researchers believe there is no clear relationship between epidural fibrosis and patients' complaints (13,14).

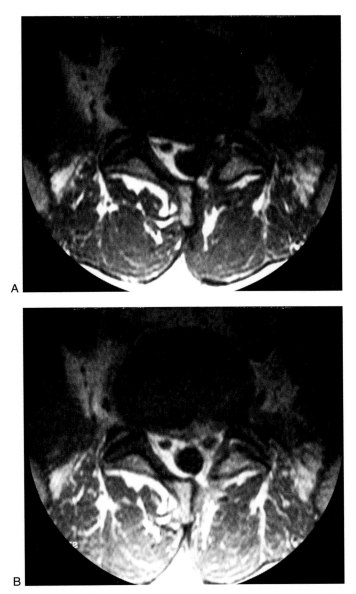

FIG. 14.1. Normal postoperative T1-WI before (**A**) and after (**B**) IV gadolinium enhancement. The axial T1-WI before gadolinium administration shows an effacement of the normal high-fat signal in the epidural space on the left, resembling the preoperative state. After gadolinium enhancement, however, there is generalized enhancement in this region indicating (normal or at least expected) epidural fibrosis.

COMPLICATIONS OF SURGERY

Hematoma

Although uncommon, symptomatic postoperative hemorrhage typically presents hours to days following the spinal surgical procedure. MRI will show mixed blood breakdown products and is more sensitive than CT for the detection of the hematoma as well as its

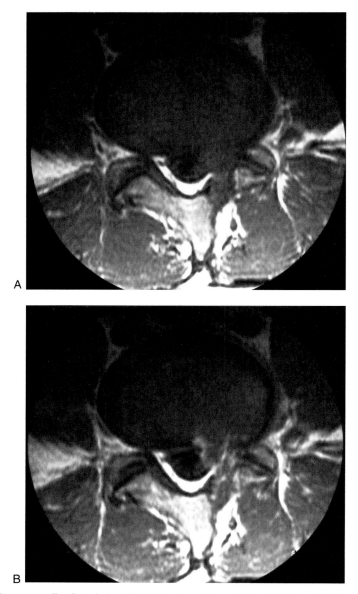

FIG. 14.2. Recurrent disc herniation: T1-WI before (**A**) and after (**B**) IV gadolinium enhancement. The images show a large, centrally nonenhancing mass in the anterior epidural space. This is a typical example of a recurrent/residual disc herniation. The peripheral rim enhancement, which represents normal or expected postoperative fibrous granulation tissue, is almost always seen.

extent. Some hematomas may reach rather large sizes and can extend into the central spinal canal to compress the cauda equina. Such cases potentially constitute medical crises requiring emergency surgical evacuation.

Spondylodiscitis

Spondylodiscitis, or discitis combined with vertebral osteomyelitis, is a relatively uncommon complication of lumbar disc surgery. Postoperative spondylodiscitis occurs in

0.1% to 3% of patients according to various reported series (23,24). Although the incidence of postoperative infection may be progressively decreasing due to better technical and prophylactic measures, it has not been completely eliminated. Disc space infection in such cases is probably due to direct intraoperative contamination (25). Most frequently the infection is caused by Staphylococcus epidermidis or Staphylococcus aureus (26). Spondylodiscitis is a serious postoperative complication, which may lead to long-lasting and sometimes permanent morbidity (27,28). It is a commonly accepted tenet that early appropriate treatment is capable of shortening the disease course and reducing the severe sequelae of spondylodiscitis. The diagnosis of postoperative spondylodiscitis depends on a combination of clinical, laboratory, and imaging findings. Clinically severe low back pain with or without associated sciatica typically appears 7 to 28 days after surgery (29). Clinical findings and classical screening methods such as white blood cell count, erythrocyte sedimentation rate, and elevated temperature are not reliable, however, and have a high failure rate in suggesting the presence of spondylodiscitis (27,30,31). C-reactive protein (CRP) determinations have proved to be a much more reliable screening test for infectious complications after lumbar disc surgery (32).

Although diagnosing spondylodiscitis with the help of MRI in the nonoperated patient can be quite straightforward, it is typically a more challenging problem in the postoperative spine. The operated disc level always shows more or less extensive changes due to the surgical intervention itself and the accompanying postoperative aseptic inflammatory response (22–26). These alterations may include type 1 (e.g., marrow edema) changes (33) of the adjacent peridiscal vertebral marrow. In addition, normal contrast enhancement can be seen in the intervertebral disk space and along the vertebral endplates postoperatively (34). It should be noted that the disappearance of the "intranuclear cleft" sign (35) is usually not reliable because the surgeon may have resected the nucleus pulposus at the time of the discectomy.

Of all the imaging techniques available, only MRI contributes significantly in establishing the diagnosis of postoperative spondylodiscitis (23). MRI may assist in several ways in making the diagnosis of postoperative septic spondylodiscitis (Fig. 14.3), including the following (36):

- The absence of peridiscal marrow changes (i.e., low signal intensity on T1-WI and high signal intensity on T2-WI) makes the diagnosis of septic spondylodiscitis highly unlikely.
- The same holds true for absence of enhancement of the intervertebral disc space.
- An enhancing soft tissue mass surrounding the affected spinal level in the perivertebral and epidural spaces is highly suggestive of septic spondylodiscitis, requiring further evaluation of such patients.

However, according to some authors, MRI is not reliable by itself in diagnosing (septic) postoperative spondylodiscitis (26,37). If in any given case of suspected postoperative infection MRI is unable to either exclude or affirm septic spondylodiscitis, one should attempt to confirm the diagnosis via percutaneous biopsy. Biopsy of the disc space material and successful isolation of the organism will yield the definitive diagnosis (38). Because fine-needle aspiration is often negative in cases of septic spondylodiscitis (26,39), biopsy with a larger bore nucleotome is recommended (40).

Pseudomeningocoele

Pseudomeningocoeles are CSF-filled collections extending from the central spinal canal into the posterior perispinal soft tissues. These cystic lesions typically develop after inadvertent surgical laceration of the dural sac during surgery or following incomplete

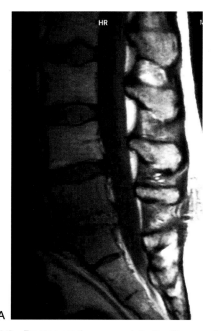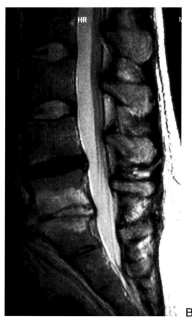

A   B

FIG. 14.3. Postoperative spondylodiscitis: sagittal T1- (**A**) and T2-WI (**B**) and axial T1-WI before (**C**) and after (**D**) IV gadolinium enhancement. The sagittal T1- and T2-weighted images, respectively, show low and high signal intensity changes in the bone marrow of the vertebral bodies adjacent to the operated disc. Although these changes can also be seen in the normal postoperative spine, they are usually less extensive in asymptomatic patients. More typical for infectious spondylodiscitis, as in this proven case of staphylococcus infection, is the enhancing soft tissue mass in the epidural space and around the operated level, as visualized on the axial pre- and postgadolinium images.

closure of the dural sac in cases of intradural surgery. Usually they protrude through a surgical bony defect of the posterior spinal elements to form a cystic lesion with MRI signal intensities comparable to CSF. They are called pseudomeningocoeles because they have no true arachnoidal lining but instead have walls of reactive fibrous tissue.

Pseudomeningocoeles are sometimes incidental imaging findings, causing no symptoms. However, in part because of their mass effect, they may also be responsible for low back pain and even radiating mono- or polyradicular leg pain.

Sterile Radiculitis

On MRI, enhancement of the intrathecal spinal nerve roots of the cauda equina following IV gadolinium administration at a conventional dosage of 0.1 mmol/kg (0.2 cc/kg) is not a normal observation. With frank compression injury (e.g., by posterolateral disc herniation) to spinal nerves and nerve roots, however, this otherwise relatively intact Blood Nerve Barrier (BNB) may break down. The complex and as yet poorly understood sequelae of chronic neural trauma and ischemia are believed to be the cause of the abnormal neurophysiological changes resulting in clinical radiculopathy that may continue long after the disc herniation has been surgically removed (41).

In a published study on asymptomatic postoperative patients, intrathecal nerve root enhancement was seen in 20% of cases 6 weeks after disc surgery, but in only 2% of patients after 6 months (36). In a study of symptomatic postoperative patients, enhancement

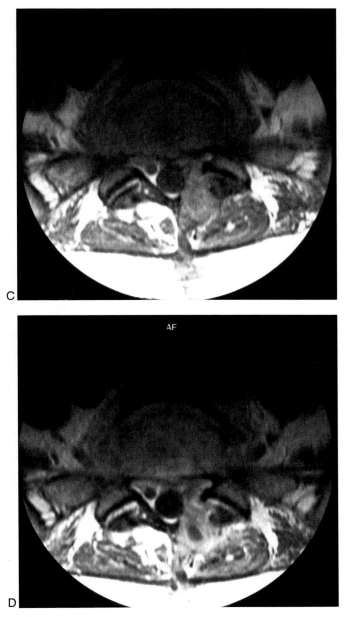

FIG. 14.3. *(continued)*

of spinal nerve roots after IV gadolinium administration was demonstrated at, and extending cranially and caudally away from, the surgical site in the chronic postoperative period (i.e., more than 6 to 8 months after surgery) (41).

Sterile Arachnoiditis

The potential factors inciting chronic sterile spinal arachnoiditis are much debated but include the surgical procedure itself, the presence of intradural blood following surgery, diagnostic lumbar puncture, treated perioperative spinal infection, the previous use of myelographic contrast media (especially older oil-based preparations), and the prior intraspinal injection of anesthetic, antiinflammatory, or chemotherapeutic agents (e.g., steroids, methotrexate). Chronically persistent lumbosacral signs and symptoms in up to 6% to 16% of postsurgical patients may be attributed to sterile arachnoiditis.

The three MRI patterns that have been described in adhesive arachnoiditis include (a) scattered groups of matted or "clumped" nerve roots, (b) an "empty" thecal sac caused by adhesions of the nerve roots to the walls of the thecal sac, and (c) an intrathecal soft tissue "mass" with a broad dural base, representing a large group of matted nerve roots that may obstruct the CSF pathways. These alterations may be either focal or diffuse. Enhancement of the thickened meningeal scarring and involved underlying intrathecal nerve roots on IV gadolinium-enhanced MRI may or may not be observed (41).

The degree of severity of the enhancing and nonenhancing imaging findings in patients with chronic sterile arachnoiditis does not appear to correlate well with the clinical degree of signs and symptoms. The symptoms when present are usually polyradicular, with pain and paresthesias perceived within both lower extremities.

Textiloma

A surgical sponge, or "cottonoid," accidentally left behind in a surgical wound, eventually becomes a textiloma (42). The term "gossybipoma" was used in more dated literature to denote a mass composed of a cotton matrix (43). The foreign body is made of synthetic cottonlike ("cottonoid") fiber ("rayon") with a barium sulphate ($BaSO_4$) marking filament, which is visible on radiographical examination. The pseudotumor consists of the foreign body itself with perilesional reactive changes (i.e., foreign body granuloma).

It is important to emphasize that MRI acquisitions can be confusing and misleading because the most typical sign of a forgotten cottonoid, the filament, is not visible on MRI (44). Indeed this filament consists of barium sulphate, which is neither magnetic nor paramagnetic and therefore causes no visible magnetic trace on an MRI examination. Furthermore, the filament contains very few free protons and thus does not yield a significant MRI signal. After IV gadolinium injection, the lesion shows a moderate degree of peripheral contrast enhancement on T1-WI, believed to be related to an inflammatory foreign body reaction. On T2-WI these lesions are hypointense, presumably reflecting dense fibrous tissue reaction peripherally and central foreign body material absent of mobile hydrogen protons (Fig. 14.4) (45). This also explains the centrally nonenhancing area on the gadolinium-enhanced T1-WI.

Stenosis

Stenosis of the central spinal canal, the lateral recesses of the central spinal canal, and the spinal neural foramen(a) may be a cause of the FBSS. These forms of spinal stenosis may preexist or follow the spinal surgery. When the stenosis follows surgery, it may present years after the surgery as a result of accelerated degeneration of spinal segments above or below a single or multilevel bony segmental spinal fusion. These alterations occur because of increased stresses placed on these segments supra- and subjacent to the fused segment(s) as load sharing is shifted away from the solidly fused levels.

Although published studies have methodological biases and small sample sizes, it appears that the sensitivity and specificity of MRI and CT for depicting spinal stenosis are similar to one another (i.e., true-positive rate of approximately 90%, false-positive

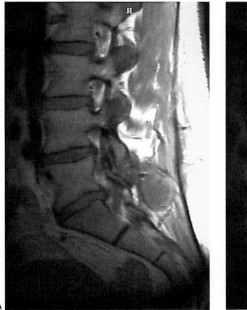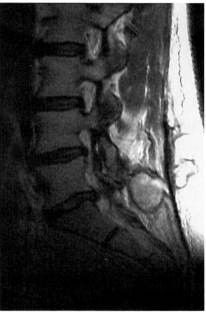

FIG. 14.4. Textiloma: sagittal T1- (**A**) and T2-WI (**B**) and axial T1-WI before (**C**) and after (**D**) IV gadolinium enhancement. A cottonoid that is left behind in the operation wound initiates a marked aseptic inflammatory reaction. These so-called textilomas present as rounded low signal intensity masses on T1- and T2-WI. The center may be of high-signal intensity in some cases on T2-WI due to central cystic/necrotic degeneration. The periphery shows marked enhancement representing the extensive granulomatous reaction.

rate of approximately 10%). Lumbosacral spinal neural foramen narrowing is best imaged with direct sagittal T1-WI. Foraminal narrowing with resultant nerve root impingement due to loss of intervertebral disc space height after complete discectomy is not uncommonly observed. Therefore, some surgeons only resect the visibly herniated or sequestered disc material after blunt enlargement of the rupture site in an attempt to preserve the residual biomechanics of the intervertebral disc. Unfortunately, this also leaves behind a significant amount of nuclear and annular disc material, which may subsequently lead to postoperative reherniation.

IMAGING FOLLOWING INTERVERTEBRAL FUSION AND/OR INSTRUMENTATION

Radiographic Signs of Fusion

The value of obtaining serial conventional radiographs of the spine in the postfusion patient is unclear (46). It has been suggested that radiography underestimates the rate of pseudarthrosis (i.e., nonunited intersegmental bony fusion) when compared with direct observations at the time of surgical reexploration, particularly when a hairline pseudarthrosis is present (47).

Conversely, other authors have contended that conventional radiographs may underestimate the degree of fusion. The referring clinician is sometimes faced with the puzzling contradiction that in a patient who is doing well clinically, the static and dynamic radiological

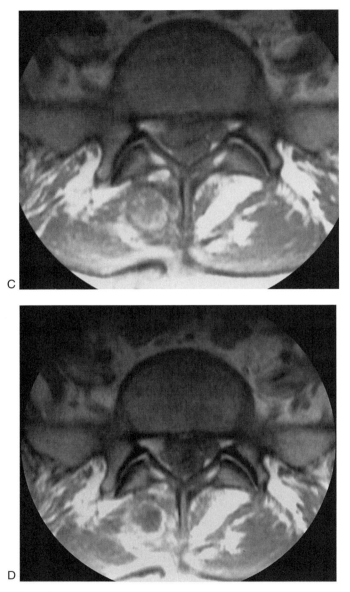

FIG. 14.4. *(continued)*

examinations do not show evidence of bony intersegmental fusion. The reason for this apparent contradiction is believed to be that premineralized osteoid may be functionally fused but may nevertheless appear radiolucent on conventional radiographs (56). The calcification of osteoid typically takes many months to complete. As a general rule, it is accepted that at least 6 to 9 months from the time of surgery are necessary for the development of solid intersegmental fusion to be seen radiographically (50–51).

After mineralization of the osteoid, the bone in the fusion area may appear radiographically more dense than the adjacent otherwise normal vertebral bone. As mature bony trabeculae develop, they bridge the fusion area between the respective native bony structures. This leads to visual obliteration of the cortical vertebral endplates and thus to a loss of the so-called graft-host interface between the implant bone and the native vertebral bone. In some instances, a dense line of sclerotic bone may be an indicator of fusion between the graft material and the host vertebra. A well-documented observation indicating solid intervertebral bony fusion is the resorption of preexistent peridiscal spondylotic spurs, although this may take several months or years to occur. Likewise, bony fusion across the posterior spinal facet joint space is a reassuring sign of functional bony fusion of two segments.

Pseudarthrosis and Other Complications

Late postoperative complications are migration, complete dislodgment, or fracture of implant material. This may contribute to complications such as failure of bony fusion, intersegmental spinal instability caused by fusion failure, and neurological injury (51). On MRI, the presence of an intermediate signal intensity gap between the vertebral body and the (bone) graft on T1-WI is an indicator of pseudarthrosis (47). On T2-WI this is characterized by a region with high signal intensity (Fig. 14.5). Bone graft material can migrate or hypertrophy, resulting in encroachment on the spinal canal or neural foramina. Rarely, the vertebra(e) adjacent to the operated levels may fracture, especially in osteoporotic patients.

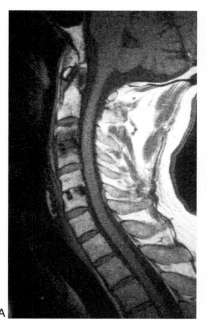
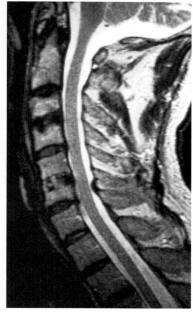

FIG. 14.5. Pseudarthrosis after attempted surgical fusion: sagittal T1- (**A**) and T2-WI (**B**) one year after intervertebral fusion at the C3-C4 and C5-C6 levels. Extensive signal changes are seen in the marrow of the vertebral bodies adjacent to the operated C3-C4 level, with low signal on T1-WI and high signal on T2-WI. These changes represent bone marrow edema. If these are noted later than 6 months after surgery, they are evidence of probable nonfusion or pseudarthrosis in the chronic phase after attempted intersegmental surgical fusion. On the other hand, the C5-C6 level is normal with incorporation of the graft in the C6 vertebral body and partial incorporation in the C5 vertebral body.

A promising application of MRI is in the postoperative evaluation of patients treated with interbody fusion grafts in order to document possible posterior or posterolateral graft extrusion into the central spinal canal or neural foramina, or failure of bony interbody fusion (48). In large published series, the approximate incidence of graft extrusion is estimated to be 2% of cases (48). Posterolateral extrusion of a graft can result in direct nerve root compression, usually characterized by immediate and severe radicular pain.

In the assessment of the postoperative patient after lumbar fusion, comparison with previous imaging examinations is desirable in order to detect subtle changes that may indicate successful bony fusion, or alternatively that may herald an impending complication such as progressive spondylolisthesis (46). Subtle changes on conventional radiography may become more evident on dynamic flexion-extension views or with thin multislice spiral CT images coupled with multidimensional reformatted images. It is important for the clinician to inform the radiologist performing the examination of the type of previous surgical procedure(s) as well as the current clinical syndrome. This may affect the imaging strategy to be followed, and it is important when evaluating the images and in the consideration of supplemental imaging studies. In the postoperative patient with a normal postsurgical clinical course, routine reexploration of the spine is obviously not necessary (54,56). However, in problem patients (e.g., persistent inexplicable pain, symptoms suggesting pseudarthrosis), surgical reexploration may be justified (54).

Radiologists should be familiar with the procedures and the surgical implants used by the surgeons at their various institutions. Obviously, a meaningful postoperative radiological evaluation can be accomplished only when the indications for specific surgical techniques, their radiological appearance postoperatively, and their possible complications are known. Radiologists face continual changes in both surgical technique and instrumentation, and they should be knowledgeable about the devices available and the biomechanical principles that direct their use. A working knowledge of evolving spinal fixation devices and surgical techniques is required in order to identify specific complications. The radiological findings should be discussed in close collaboration with the respective surgical colleagues.

Imaging of Spinal Implants

Spinal fixation devices are used to stabilize the spine, reduce deformities and fractures, and replace abnormal vertebrae (46,49–51). Bony fusion is usually attempted along with placement of metallic surgical instrumentation materials (49–50). The spine is unstable in such patients, and early operative intervention allows rapid mobilization and rehabilitation. Various methods of fusion have evolved and are currently in use. Surgical procedures usually consist of posterior (posterior bony elements) and/or anterior (vertebral body) fixation. However, persistent lumbar instability is a potential clinical problem (52). It is often believed to be the cause of recurrent low back pain in patients who have undergone lumbar fusion (53).

Determining the solidity of the fusion is a difficult problem. For a long time, it was widely accepted that the only way of determining the solidity of lumbar fusion was by surgical exploration (54). This principle is known as Bosworth's dictum (54–56). It was undoubtedly inspired by the limitations of imaging techniques half a century ago, and by the inconsistent and often unreliable results provided by conventional radiography. Routine reexploration for the purposes of determining the status of a surgical fusion is impractical, however, because of the expense and morbidity involved (54).

A variety of radiological methods have been used to evaluate the postoperative spine. These imaging modalities include radiographs (conventional X-rays, polytomograms, biplane stress bending films, stereophotogrammetry, dynamic flexion-extension myelography, and CT-myelography), computed tomography (CT), radionuclide bone scans, and MRI. Medical imaging studies can be divided into two categories, depending on whether they assess either functional or structural integrity of spinal fusions. Most modalities assess structural integrity (radiographs, tomograms, CT, MRI). The purpose of these techniques is essentially to identify the bony continuity of the fusion mass. Conversely, imaging studies that assess functional integrity include any type of dynamic stress films. The purpose here is to demonstrate the presence or absence of motion between previously fused vertebral segments. These studies depend heavily on patient cooperation and may fail to show abnormal motion because of muscle guarding, spasm, or internal fixation (54).

REFERENCES

1. Fengler H, Wagner W. Backache—orthopedic diagnosis and special therapeutic possibilities. Z Arztl Fortibild Jena 1997;90(8):677-85.
2. Borenstein DG. Epidemiology, etiology, diagnostic evaluation, and treatment of low back pain. Curr Opin Rheumatol 1997;9(2):144-50.
3. Borenstein DG. Chronic low back pain. Rheum Dis Clin N Am 1996;22(3):439-56.
4. Ackerman SJ, Steinberg EP, Bryan RN, BenDebba M, Long DM. Persistent low back pain in patients suspected of having herniated nucleus pulposus: radiologic predictors of functional outcome-implications for treatment selection. Radiology 1997;203(3):815-22.
5. Butt W. Radiology for back pain. Clin Radiol 1989;40:6-10.
6. Junge A, Dvorak J. Ahrens S. Predictors of bad and good outcomes of lumbar disc surgery: a prospective clinical study with recommendations for screening to avoid bad outcomes. Spine 1995;20:460-8.
7. Davis RA. A long-term outcome analysis of 984 surgically treated herniated lumbar discs. J Neurosurg 1994;80:415-21.
8. Bernard TN. Repeat lumbar spine surgery. Factors influencing outcome. Spine 1993;18:2196-2200.
9. Fandino J, Botana D, Viladrich A, Gomez-Bueno J. Reoperation after lumbar disc surgery. Results in 130 cases. Acta Neurochir 1993;122:102-4.
10. Herron L. Recurrent lumbar disc herniation. Results of repeat laminectomy and discectomy. J Spinal Disord 1994;7:161-6.
11. Jonsson B, Stromqvist B. Repeat decompression of lumbar nerve roots. A prospective two-year evaluation. J Bone Joint Surg Br 1993;75:894-7.
12. Van Goethem JWM, Parizel PM, van den Hauwe L, De Schepper AMA. Imaging findings in patients with failed back surgery syndrome. J Belge Radiol 1997;80/2:81-4.
13. Cervellini P, Curri D, Volpin L, et al. Computed tomography of epidural fibrosis after discectomy: a comparison between symptomatic and asymptomatic patients. Neurosurgery 1998;23:710-3.
14. Coskun E, Suzer T, Topuz O, Zencir M, Pakdemirli E, Tahta K. Relationships between epidural fibrosis, pain, disability, and psychological factors after lumbar disc surgery. Eur Spine J 2000;9:218-23.
15. Hudgins PA, Clare CE. Radiographic evaluation of the patient with failed back surgery syndrome (FBSS). Cont Neurosurg 1990;12:23.
16. Bundschuh CV, Modic MT, Ross JS, Masaryk TJ, Bohlman H. Epidural fibrosis and recurrent disk herniation in the lumbar spine. AJNR 1998;9:169-78. AJN 150:923-32.
17. Frocrain L, Duvauferrier R, Husson J-L, Noel J, Ramee A, PawlotskyY. Recurrent postoperative sciatica: evaluation with MR imaging and enhanced CT. Radiology 1989;170:531-3.
18. Sotiropoulos S, Chafetz NI, Lang P, et al. Differentiation between postoperative scar and recurrent disk herniation: prospective comparison of MR, CT, and contrast-enhanced CT. AJNR 1989;10:639-43.
19. Bundschuh CV, Stein L, Slusser JH, Schinco FP, Ladaga LE, Dillon JD. Distinguishing between scar and recurrent herniated disk in postoperative patients: value of contrast-enhanced CT and MR imaging. AJNR 1990;11:949-58.
20. Weber H. The natural history of lumbar disc herniation and the influence of intervention. Spine 1994;19:2234-8.
21. Komori H, Okawa A, Haro H, Muneta T, Yamamoto H, Shinomiya K. Contrast-enhanced magnetic resonance imaging in conservative management of lumbar disc herniation. Spine 1998;23:67-73.
22. Van De Kelft E, Van Goethem JWM, De La Porte C, Verlooy J. Early postoperative gadolinium-DTPA-enhanced MR imaging after successful lumbar discectomy. Br J Neurosurg 1996;10(1):41-9.
23. Lindholm TS, Pylkkanen P. Diskitis following removal of intervertebral disk. Spine 1982;7:618-22.
24. Bircher MD, Tasker T, Crawshaw E, Mulholland RC. Discitis following lumbar surgery. Spine 1988;13:98-102.

25. Tronnier V, Schneider R, Kunz U, Albert F, Oldenkott P. Postoperative spondylodiscitis: results of a prospective study about the aetiology of spondylodiscitis after operation for lumbar disc herniation. Acta Neurochir 1992;117:149-52.

26. Grane P, Josephsson A, Seferlis A, Tullberg T. Septic and aseptic post-operative discitis in the lumbar spine-evaluation by MR imaging. Acta Radiologica 1998;39:108-15.

27. Fouquet B, Goupille P, Jattiot F, Cotty P, Lapierre F, Valat JP, Amouroux J, Benatre A. Discitis after lumbar disc surgery, features of "aseptic" and "septic" forms. Spine 1992;17:356-8.

28. Rohde V, Meyer B, Schaller C, Hassler WE. Spondylodiscitis after lumbar discectomy. Spine 1998;5:615-20.

29. Dall BE, Rowe DE, Odette WG, Batts DH. Postoperative discitis. Clin Orthop 1987;224:138-46.

30. Grollmus J, Perkins RK, Russel W. Erythrocyte sedimentation rate as a possible indicator of early disc space infection. Neurochirurgia 1974;17:30-5.

31. Kapp JP, Sybers WA. Erythrocyte sedimentation rate following uncomplicated lumbar disc operations. Surg Neurol 1979;12:329-30.

32. Meyer B, Schaller K, Rohde V, Hassler W. The C-reactive protein for detection of early infections after lumbar microdiscectomy. Acta Neurochir 1995;136:145-50.

33. Modic MT, Steinberg PM, Ross JS, Masaryk TJ, Carter JR. Degenerative disk disease. Assessment of changes in vertebral body bone marrow with MR imaging. Radiology 1988;166:193.

34. Grand CM, Bank WO, Baleriaux D, Matos C, Levivier M, Brotchi J. Gadolinium enhancement of vertebral endplates following lumbar disc surgery. Neuroradiology 1993;35:503-5.

35. Aguila LA, Piraino DW, Modic MT, Dudley AW, Duchesneau PM, Weinstein MA. The intranuclear cleft of the intervertebral disk. Magnetic resonance imaging. Radiology 1985;155:155.

36. Van Goethem JWM, Parizel PM, Van den Hauwe L, Van de Kleft E, Verlooy J, De Schepper AMA. Value of MR imaging in the diagnosis of postoperative spondylodiscitis. Neuroradiology 2000;42:580-5.

37. Schulitz KP, Assheuer J. Discitis after procedures on the intervertebral disc. Spine 1994;19(10):1172-7.

38. Fouquet B, Goupille P, Jattiot F, Cotty P, Lapierre F, Valat JP, Amouroux J, Benatre A. Discitis after lumbar disc surgery. Features of "aseptic" and "septic" forms. Spine 1992:17:356-8.

39. Demaerel P, Van Ongeval C, Wilms G, Lateur L, Baert A. MR imaging of spondylitis with gadopentate dimeglumine enhancement. J Neuroradiol 1994;21:245.

40. Onik G. Automated percutaneous biopsy in the diagnosis and treatment of infectious discitis. Neurosurg Clin N Am 1996;7:145.

41. Jinkins JR. Magnetic resonance imaging of benign nerve root enhancement in the unoperated and postoperative lumbosacral spine. Neuroim Clin N Am 1993;3:525-41.

42. Guiard JM, Bonnet JC, Boutin JP, Plane D, Guilleux MH, Delorme G. Textile foreign body, "Textiloma": CT features. Case Report. Ann Radiol 1988;31:49-52.

43. Williams RG, Bragg DG, Nelson JA. Gossybipoma—the problems of the retained surgical sponge. Radiology 1978;129:323-6.

44. Van Goethem JWM, Parizel PM, Perdieus D, Hermans P, de Moor J. MR and CT imaging of paraspinal textiloma (gossybipoma). J Comput Assist Tomogr 1991;15:1000-3.

45. De Marco K, McDermott M, Dillon W, Bollen A, Edwards M. MR appearance of postoperative foreign body granuloma: case report with pathologic confirmation. AJNR 1991;12:190-2.

46. Parizel PM, Van Goethem JWM, van den Hauwe L, et al. Imaging of spinal implants and radiologic assessment of fusion. In: Szpalski M, Gunzburg R, Spengler M, et al. (eds.), Instrumented fusion of the degenerative lumbar spine: state of the art, questions, and controversies. Philadelphia: Lippincott-Raven, 1996:25-33.

47. Ghazi J, Golimbu CN, Engler GL. MRI of spinal fusion pseudarthrosis. J Comput Assist Tomogr 1992;16:324-26.

48. Coughlan JD. Extrusion of bone graft after lumbar fusion: CT appearance. J Comput Assist Tomogr 1986;10:399-400.

49. Slone RM, MacMillan M, Montgomery WJ. Spinal fixation. Part 1. Principles, basic hardware, and fixation techniques for the cervical spine. Radiographics 1993;13:341-56.

50. Slone RM, MacMillan M, Montgomery WJ, Heare M. Spinal fixation. Part 2. Fixation techniques and hardware for the thoracic and lumbosacral spine. Radiographics 1993;13:521-43.

51. Slone RM, MacMillan M, Montgomery WJ. Spinal fixation. Part 3. Complications of spinal instrumentation. Radiographics 1993;13:797-816.

52. Parizel PM, Ozsarlak O, Van Goethem JWM, van den Hauwe L, et al. The use of magnetic resonance imaging in lumbar instability. In: Szpalski M, Gunzburg R, Pope M (eds.), Lumbar segmental instability. Philadelphia: Lippincott-Raven, 1999:123-38.

53. Lang P, Chafetz N, Genant HK, et al. Lumbar spinal fusion. Assessment of functional stability with magnetic resonance imaging. Spine 1990;15:581-8.

54. Brodsky AE, Kovalsky ES, Khalil MA. Correlation of radiologic assessment of lumbar spine fusions with surgical exploration. Spine 1991;16:S261-5.

55. Cleveland M, Bosworth DM, Thompson FR. Pseudarthrosis in the lumbosacral spine. J Bone Joint Surg 1948;30A(2):302-12.

56. Blumenthal SL, Gill K. Can lumbar spine radiographs accurately determine fusion in postoperative patients? Correlation of routine radiographs with a second surgical look at lumbar fusions. Spine 1993;18:1186-9.

15

Behavioral Aspects of Chronic Back Pain: Contemporary Approaches to Conceptualization and Treatment

Lance M. McCracken

Chronic pain, including pain of a spinal origin, is an important, albeit sometimes vexing, problem. With all of the efforts toward new technologies for chronic pain management by pharmacological, interventional, and surgical means, a simple notion can sometimes get lost. No treatment for chronic pain can claim effectiveness unless it results in some meaningful change in patient behavior. No technology has much to offer the pain sufferer if after treatment patients do not (a) say their pain is no longer the problem it once was, (b) engage more fully in important aspects of their life such as family and work, and (c) alter potentially unhelpful patterns of medication or health care use. Seen in this light, all chronic pain treatment must take behavioral or psychological aspects into account.

PSYCHOLOGICAL APPROACHES TO CHRONIC PAIN

Specific psychological treatment approaches to chronic pain have evolved over the past 40 years. In the 1960s, the operant behavioral approach focused on overt patient behavior, so-called pain behavior, and influences in the patient's environment that might affect the frequency of those behaviors (8). The emphasis tended to be on publicly observable aspects of the pain experience. The 1980s signaled a relative shift in emphasis from the role of the external environment to the patient's internal environment, to the realm of thoughts, cognitive processes, and emotions (20). This approach, referred to as cognitive behavioral therapy (CBT), remains the popular psychological approach to chronic pain today. Although most proponents of this approach advocate behavior change as a means for the pain sufferer to improve, they tend to see thoughts, interpretations, beliefs, and feelings as the primary targets of change efforts. Hence changes in patients' internal, private experiences are seen as the critical route to overall improvements in functioning.

There have been attempts to integrate an understanding of the link between psychology and physiology into the dominant approaches to pain management. These approaches propose a role for predisposing physiological states (diathesis) and psychological influences (stress) on such things as sympathetic arousal and muscle tension in the experience of pain (e.g., 6). These approaches tend to put physiology and pain in a central role as the pathway to disrupted functioning, at least for some patients (5). The relative emphasis in treatment remains on pain reduction.

DO PSYCHOLOGICAL APPROACHES TO CHRONIC PAIN WORK?

There are numerous quantitative and nonquantitative reviews of behavior and cognitive therapies for chronic pain including low back pain patients only (21), or mixed samples of predominantly back pain sufferers, treated in studies where cognitive behavioral therapy is the primary treatment (19) or in multidisciplinary contexts based on cognitive behavioral principles (4,7). Overall behavioral and cognitive therapies clearly and significantly reduce patients' pain, emotional distress, and pain behavior and improve their daily activities (16).

Results from a systematic review by Morley et al. (19) included 25 controlled trials and 1,672 patients. Patients were typically treated in groups for an average of 16 hours. Compared to waiting list control conditions, those in the behavioral and cognitive therapies showed significantly improved pain, mood, cognitive coping and appraisal, pain behavior, and social role performance. The effect sizes were approximately 0.5 in magnitude, or a change in the treated group mean by one half a standard deviation.

Often behavioral and cognitive therapies are combined with physical rehabilitation strategies, interventions to aid return to work, or conservative medical management strategies. These programs, referred to as multidisciplinary or interdisciplinary, include the use of self-management strategies, emphasize restoration of lost functioning, and operate on broadly cognitive behavioral principles. Flor and colleagues (7) conducted a systematic review of 65 studies, including 3,089 chronic pain sufferers treated for an average of 96 hours. Those treated with the interdisciplinary cognitive behavioral approach showed a 68% chance of return to work, 37% reduction in pain, 63% reduction in medication use, and 53% improvement in daily activity. Each of these improvements represented a statistically significant change and was considerably greater than in the control conditions, which generally included unimodal treatments and treatment as usual.

Cutler and colleagues (4) also conducted a quantitative review of multidisciplinary treatment for chronic pain. They focused their review on the outcome of return to work only and found 37 studies that met their inclusion criteria. They showed that multidisciplinary treatment returns 41% of patients to work when considering only patients who were not working prior to treatment. Taking all of their results together they concluded that multidisciplinary treatment doubles a patient's chances for returning to work in comparison to patients who do not participate in these treatments.

The record of behavioral and cognitive therapies is quite remarkable in several respects: (a) the patients treated have often failed numerous other treatment attempts and tend to have long-standing problems, and (b) unlike other treatment approaches these therapies have documented success in the domains of daily activity, health care consumption, and work. Also, these approaches achieve their results at a considerable cost savings in comparison to other treatments, including a net cost savings of thousands of dollars in health care expense in the first year, even when figuring in the cost of treatment (22). There are, however, significant limitations of these approaches in that (a) a significant minority of patients do not gain benefits, (b) there is at least some loss of improvements over time for some patients, and (c) the specific processes by which treatments produce their effects are not clear (16).

NEW FORMULATIONS OF THE PROBLEM OF PAIN

For the past 7 years or so we have been conducting research that questions some assumptions regarding the nature of the problem of chronic pain. One of these assumptions concerns the issue of pain control. Most treatment methods applied to chronic pain are ultimately about reducing pain as an important goal. Even rehabilitation methods are

16

Patient Selection for Surgery

Norbert Passuti, Joel Delécrin, Dominique Brossard, and M. Romih

INTRODUCTION

It has been estimated that 300,000 first-time laminectomies are performed annually in the United States, and as many as 15 % of these patients may have continued or recurrent pain and disability. Failed spine can be due to many problems, and surgical decisions remain difficult. These patients are frequently severely disabled and represent an enormous cost in terms of lost productivity and medical expenditures. Furthermore, Waddell et al. (21) pointed out that the success rate in revision surgery decreases in relation to the number of reinterventions (45% have worse results after four operations), but others authors like Stewart et al. (19) did not find a relationship between the outcome of revision procedures and the number of previous operative procedures or the nature of the previous procedures. So proper patient selection and operative correction of pathological anatomy can result in a dramatic decrease in symptoms and can restore patients to a functional lifestyle.

RESULTS AND COMPLICATIONS FOR LUMBAR SURGERY

Turner et al. (20) analyzed 74 papers to determine the effects of surgery for lumbar spinal stenosis on pain and disability. On average, 64% of patients were reported to have good to excellent outcomes (range: 26% to 100%), but they insisted on the poor scientific quality of the literature and the need for randomized trials with clear outcome assessments. They noted 1% to 27% of complications and 8% of reoperation after laminectomy alone, so they could not come to any conclusions about indications and benefits of fusion to avoid reoperation.

Alastair Gibson et al. (1) did a Cochrane review of surgery for lumbar disc prolapse and degenerative lumbar spondylosis. They analyzed 26 randomized controlled trials for disc prolapse, and reinterventions comprised between 5% and 18%. For degenerative spondylolisthesis, there was strong evidence that instrumented fusion produces a higher fusion rate and does not improve clinical outcomes but can be associated with higher complication rates.

Malter et al. (14), in 1998, observed a cohort of patients in Washington State during a 5-year period. Of 6,376 patients who underwent lumbar surgery, 1,041 (16%) had operations involving fusion. The 5-year reoperation rate for all patients combined was 15%, and reoperations were performed more frequently after fusion (18.2% vs. 14.6%). But randomized trials should be conducted to compare the complications, reoperation rates, and other outcomes associated with fusion and nonfusion lumbar surgery in homogeneous groups of patients.

Hu et al. (10), in 1997, among 4,722 patients revealed 9.5% of reoperation. The rate was not statistically related to diagnosis, type of first operation, complications, length of stay, or comorbid conditions. The only significant predictor of reoperation was age less than 65 years. But after laminectomy alone, 23% of patients had fusion as a second operation and 14% had a discectomy. This study demonstrated that recurrent compression of neurological elements, postoperative instability, and nonunion of lumbar fusion indicated the need for additional surgery. But these different studies mixed and combined different pathologies and different types of surgery.

SPECIFIC ANALYSIS

Österman et al. (15), in 2003, did a retrospective study of patients undergoing two or more reoperations after discectomy. Among 35,309 patients, 14% had at least one reoperation, and 2.3% had two or more reoperations. Most interesting is that patients with one reoperation had a 25% cumulative risk of further surgery in a 10-year follow-up, and reduced risk was seen in patients for whom the first reoperation had been a fusion (relative risk of 0.2%) and patients older than 50 years old. Also risk of reoperations was markedly reduced if the first reoperation had been a spinal fusion (5%).

Katz et al. (11), in 1991, did a study about the outcome of laminectomy for lumbar stenosis among 88 consecutive patients. By the time of the latest follow-up, 23% had a repeat operation because of instability or stenosis. So long-term outcome after decompression for lumbar stenosis suggested that the initial clinical improvement deteriorates over time. Furthermore, Postacchini and Cinotti (16) observed that the regrowth of bone after decompressive laminectomy was more common in patients with degenerative spondylolisthesis who had not had an arthrodesis.

INDICATIONS FOR SURGERY

Generally, the results of surgery for failed back syndrome are poor due to the rate of complications and also the clinical results of the reoperations. Fritsch et al. (8), among 182 revisions done between 1965 to 1990, showed that in 80% of the patients the results were satisfactory in short-term evaluation, decreasing to 22% in long-term follow-up (2 to 27 years), and in multiple revision patients, the rate of epidural fibrosis and instability increased to greater than 50%. Also the rate of disappointing results was twice as high in multiply revised without spinal fusion than in patients in whom a spinal fusion finally was performed. For the authors it was clear that laminectomy performed in primary surgery could be detected as the only factor leading to a higher rate of revisions, whereas a spinal fusion seemed to be more successful in avoiding the release of the fibrosis.

Revision also was associated with specific complications for Dietmar et al. (7). There were 17% of cases with dural tears and 9% with severe bleeding. For Hopp et al. (9) and Sano et al. (18), 15% to 25% of reoperations were concerned with an instability due to preexisting problems such as spondylo or retrolisthesis, traction spurs and facetectomies, or pars excision during the first surgery.

Indications for surgery are related to an multidisciplinary discussion to identify accurately the type of pain, the precise mechanical or nonmechanical causes of radicular pain, scar tissue (arachnoiditis or epidural fibrosis), and psychosocial problems. Of course, these entities will not be improved by any type of additional operations. The most important goal of postoperative imaging is to distinguish scar tissue from treatable entities. For that, unenhanced magnetic resonance imaging (MRI) has been reported to have an accuracy of 76% to 89%. But the diagnostic accuracy of contrast-medium-enhanced MRI approaches 96% to 100%. For us, the images must also be correlated to significant electrophysiological assessments.

For back pain, nonunion of the site of a spinal surgery is difficult to diagnose. Of course, iatrogenic instability caused by overextensive decompression or a postoperative stress fracture of the pars may be easier to diagnose. Plain tomography and computed tomography (axial or three-dimensional reconstructions) may afford increased visualization of a lumbar fusion mass.

SELECTION FOR SALVAGE SURGERY

We must identify treatable mechanical causes like inadequate incomplete surgery (foraminal compression) or technical errors due to screws or cages placed too laterally. We always propose selective periradicular injections, epidural infiltrations, and a lumbar brace. We can observe evaluation of pain analysis with a pantaloon cast.

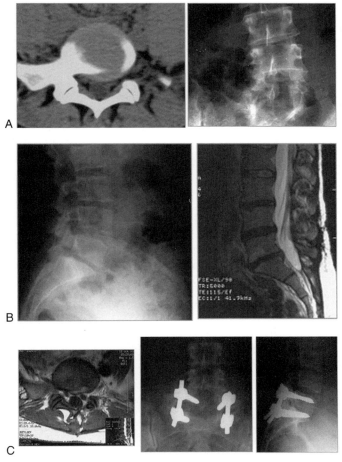

FIG. 16.1. A: A 35-year-old female patient had been operated on 4 years ago for S1 disc prolapse (discectomy). Two years later: reoperation with L5 laminectomy. **B:** She presented severe lumbar and radicular pain ODI: 36. Loss of disc height L5-S1. Modic 2 MRI. **C:** Pantaloon cast and periradicular injection: excellent result. Three years ago: short L5-S1 fusion nondecompression. Excellent result.

- **First situation:** lumbar pain after selective discectomy. The patient presents dynamic root pain without any permanent neurogenic pain; the pantaloon cast can be used, and for Rask et al. (17) this is an effective tool for identifying those chronic low back pain patients who might benefit from a spinal fusion. The use of external spinal fixation should not be used as a predictor of pain relief for lumbar fusion, as shown by Bednar (3), who demonstrated this procedure is not without serious complications.
- In this situation with patients who present a complete loss of disc height with modic 1 or 2 signal at MRI, we propose a single segmental posterolateral fusion, as demonstrated by Stewart et al. (19). He observed among 39 patients who had a reoperation that 72% had a successful outcome. Factors significantly associated with a successful outcome included younger age (p <0.02), working outside of the home (p <0.05), an initial period of improvement after the previous operation (p <0.01), and fusion with instrumentation (p <0.02). Figure 16.1 is an example of a good result after fusion done for failure after discectomies.
- **Second situation:** lumbar pain is associated with radicular pain. For neurogenic root pain, we propose medical treatment and electrostimulation. But for foraminal and lateral stenosis combined with root compression including new disc prolapse, the indication can be lateral decompression associated with transforaminal lumbar interbody fusion. Interbody fusion cages have had a tremendous effect on the treatment of discogenic pain in the postlaminectomy syndrome. The rate of fusion has improved from only

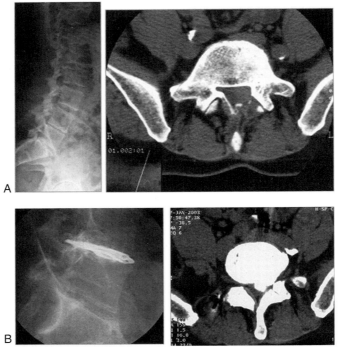

FIG. 16.2. A: Sagittal view CT. Loss of disc height L4-L5. A 53-year-old male patient has been operated on two times at L4-L5 level. He presented combined pain: permanent radicular pain and severe lumbar pain. **B:** We did discogram and CT scan. **C:** MRI with gadolinium confirmed the recurrence of the protrusion and modic 2 signal. **D:** Excellent result. Indication for left TLIF for lateral decompression and circumferential fusion.

17

Yellow Flags: Psychosocial Risk Factors for Chronic Pain and Disability

Gordon Waddell

Selection for surgery rightly focuses on surgical indications and contraindications: specific clinical symptoms and signs with radiological or laboratory confirmation; predictors of surgical outcome; fitness for surgery; risk of complications. Successful surgery depends on accurate diagnosis of a surgically treatable lesion (Table 17.1), efficient surgery, and freedom from complications. This is standard surgical practice.

However, patient-centered outcomes such as pain, disability and (in)capacity for work do not always correlate well with technical surgical outcomes, and it has been known for many years that patient selection is equally important. Wiltse and Rocchio (10) first showed that psychological factors also affect how patients respond to surgery (Table 17.2), and this has since been confirmed for various conservative therapies, all forms of surgery, pain management programs, and rehabilitation (7). It is equally true whether the patient has a clear physical pathology such as a disc prolapse or nonspecific back pain. Nonorganic signs (Table 17.3) provide a simple clinical screen to detect patients who may require more detailed assessment (7,9).

So far, this is standard surgical teaching, but it is worth stopping at this point and considering recent developments in other fields. It is now widely accepted that back pain is

TABLE 17.1. *The importance of accurate diagnosis of a surgically treatable lesion (based on data from Spangfort, 1972)*

Operative Findings	Relief of Sciatica (%)	Relief of Back Pain (%)
Complete herniation	90	75
Incomplete herniation	82	74
Bulging disk	63	54
No herniation	37	43

TABLE 17.2. *Psychological distress predicting symptomatic outcome of chemonucleolysis for disk prolapse (based on data from Wiltse & Rocchio, 1975)*

Preoperative Hs and Hy scores	Excellent or good symptomatic relief (%) on the MMPI*
5+	10
75–84	16
65–74	39
55–64	72
54–	90

*The mean score for normal people is 50.

TABLE 17.3. *Nonorganic signs or behavioral*
responses to examination in low back pain (9)

Tenderness
  • superficial
  • nonanatomic
Simulation
  • axial loading
  • simulated rotation
Distraction
  • straight leg raising
Regional
  • weakness
  • sensory disturbance
Overt pain behavior

a biopsychosocial rather than a purely biomedical condition (Fig. 17.1). Surgery focuses on the biomedical component. But psychosocial issues can also contribute to the development and maintenance of chronic pain and disability and the outcome of treatment, including surgery (7).

Within the past 6 to 7 years, there have been major advances in screening to identify patients at risk of developing chronic pain and disability and long-term incapacity for

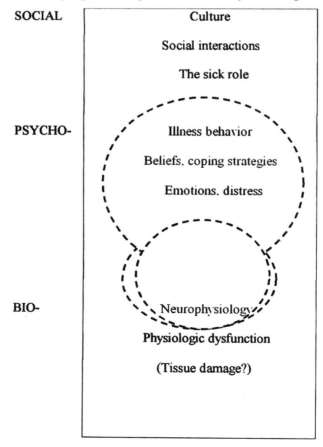

FIG 17.1. A biopsychosocial model of low back pain and disability. Reproduced with permission from G. Waddell, The back pain revolution (2nd ed.), Churchill Livingstone, 2004.

work. Perhaps surprisingly, it appears that standard clinical findings are generally poor predictors, and psychosocial factors perform better. These are the yellow flags: psychosocial factors in the patient or his or her situation that serve as warning signs or predictors that this individual is at increased risk of developing chronic pain and disability. Psychosocial factors not only contribute to the development of chronic pain and disability, they may then continue to act as obstacles or barriers to recovery and return to work. Thus assessment of yellow flags has two goals:

- To identify patients at increased risk of developing chronic pain and disability, so interventions and resources can be directed to them in a timely and cost-effective manner to prevent chronic incapacity.
- To assess obstacles to recovery, in order to plan rehabilitation and return to work interventions.

Kendall et al. (3) introduced the concept of yellow flags in the New Zealand guide to the management of acute low back pain. Their main focus was clinical and psychological, although they also included occupational and compensation elements (Table 17.4).

Main (1,4) further developed the concept of yellow flags and suggested they may be subdivided (Table 17.5). First, Main points out that these are markers of psychosocial dysfunction and not psychiatric illness. To emphasize that distinction, he suggests there should be quite different orange flags for serious psychiatric illness, comparable to the red flags for serious physical disease. Second, he suggests that clinical yellow flags should be distinguished from occupationally focused blue flags. Clinical yellow flags are then the individual psychological range of beliefs and emotional and behavioral responses to pain and disability, recognized as important in pain management and clinical rehabilitation programs. Main characterizes the occupational blue flags as being about *perceptions* of work and relates them to the (largely Scandinavian) literature on psychosocial aspects of work (6). Potentially, at least, yellow and blue flags can be identified, addressed, and modified clinically. Finally, Main suggests there are occupational black flags that are not a matter of perception but are extrinsic to the individual, with the

TABLE 17.4. *Yellow flags: psychosocial risk factors*

When conducting an assessment, it may be useful to consider psychosocial yellow flags (beliefs and behaviors on the part of the patient that predict poor outcomes).

The following factors are important and consistently predict poor outcomes:
- Beliefs that back pain is harmful or potentially severely disabling.
- Fear-avoidance behaviour (avoiding a movement or activity due to misplaced anticipation of pain) and reduced activity levels.
- Tendency to low mood and withdrawal from social interaction.
- Expectation that passive treatments rather than active participation will help.

Suggested questions to the worker with low back pain (to be phrased in your own style):
- Have you had time off work in the past with back pain?
- What do you understand is the cause of your back pain?
- What are you expecting will help you?
- How is your employer responding to your back pain? Your coworkers? Your family?
- What are you doing to cope with your back pain?
- Do you think you will return to work? When?

A worker may be considered to be at risk if:
- There is a cluster of a few very salient factors
- There is a group of several less important factors that combine cumulatively.

The presence of risk factors should alert the clinician to the possibility of long-term problems and the need to prevent their development.

Reproduced with permission from Working Backs Scotland. Adapted from Kendall et al., 1997.

TABLE 17.5. *Signs of psychosocial risk*

Red flags	Warning signs of possible serious physical disease
Orange flags	Warning signs of primary psychiatric illness: psychosis, alcohol and drug abuse
Yellow flags	Iatrogenic factors Beliefs, coping strategies Psychological distress, low mood, illness behavior Willingness and ability to change Family support or reinforcement
Blue flags	Perceived exertion and physical demands of work Attribution to work Job satisfaction Perceptions of work: job stress, high job demand/intensity, monotonous work, low job control, low job clarity, social support.
Black flags	Working conditions and organizational issues Reimbursement, benefits, social policy.

Summarized from CJ Main, CC Spanswick, P Watson P., The nature of disability. In: CJ Main CJ and CC Spanswick (eds.), Pain management: an interdisciplinary approach. Edinburgh: Churchill Livingstone, 2000;89-106.

implication that they cannot be modified or overcome by clinical interventions. These various flags and examples of each are shown in Table 17.5.

We recently carried out a major review for the UK Department of Work and Pensions of screening to identify patients at increased risk of long-term incapacity for work (8). Historically and conceptually, there are two kinds of screening:

1. Administrative/actuarial screening. This forms the basis of the insurance industry. It is largely sociodemographic information, available in an administrative database.
2. Clinical and psychosocial screening. Health care is more interested in how and why some patients develop chronic problems and what can be done about it. This kind of data usually requires more detailed clinical assessment of the individual patient.

TABLE 17.6. *Risk factors for chronic pain and disability*

Sociodemographic risk factors	Clinical and psychosocial risk factors
Gender	Older age (>50-55 years)
Age	Previous history of back pain
Marital/family status (lone parent/young children, partner retired or disabled)	Nerve root pain
Health condition (mental health conditions, musculoskeletal conditions, comorbidities)	Pain intensity/Functional disability
Occupation/Education level	Poor perception general health
Time since last worked	Psychological distress/depression
Occupational status (no longer employed)	Fear avoidance
Local unemployment rate	Catastrophizing Pain behavior Job (dis)satisfaction Duration of sickness absence Occupational status (no longer employed) Expectations about return to work

Reproduced with permission from Royal Society of Medicine Press: G Waddell, AK Burton, CJ Main CJ, Screening to identify people at risk of long-term incapacity for work: a conceptual and scientific review. London: Royal Society of Medicine Press, 2003. www.rsmpress.co.uk/bkwaddell2.htm

Our literature search found much more evidence than originally expected, for both sociodemographic and psychosocial risk factors (Table 17.6). This review also considered the concepts, accuracy, and limitations of screening. All of the material can be downloaded free from the website.

APPLICATION TO SURGICAL PRACTICE

Surgeons do not need to carry out detailed psychosocial assessment in routine surgical patients, but it is important to be aware of such issues. Judicious surgery in carefully selected patients with the correct indications can produce good clinical results, but even then they are not always translated into occupational outcomes (2). Surgery must be set in a broader biopsychosocial perspective, and surgeons should recognize that psychosocial issues can exert a powerful influence on outcomes. Yellow flags are a simple method of screening to alert the surgeon to some patients who need more detailed assessment. At the minimum, surgeons should always consider and be prepared to discuss occupational issues, and not just assume a so-called successful surgical outcome will automatically return the patient to work.

References

1. Burton AK, Main CJ. Obstacles to return to work from work-related musculoskeletal disorders. In: Karwowski W (ed.), International encyclopedia of ergonomics and human factors. Taylor & Francis, 2000;1542-4.
2. Gibson JNA, Grant I, Waddell G. Cochrane reviews on surgery for lumbar disc prolapse and degenerative lumbar spondylosis. In: The Cochrane Library, Issue 1, 1999, Oxford: Update Software. Also published in Spine 1999; 24:1820-32 (update due 2004).
3. Kendall NAS, Linton SJ, Main CJ. Guide to assessing psychosocial yellow flags in acute low back pain. Accident Rehabilitation and Compensation Insurance Corporation and National Advisory Committee on Health and Disability. Wellington, NZ, 1997. www.acc.org.nz.
4. Main CJ, Spanswick CC, Watson P. The nature of disability. In: Main CJ, Spanswick, CC (eds.), Pain management: an interdisciplinary approach. Edinburgh: Churchill Livingstone, 2000;89-106.
5. Spangfort EV. The lumbar disc herniation. A computer aided analysis of 2504 operations. Acta Orthop Scand Suppl 1972; 142:1-95.
6. Vingard E, Nachemson A. Work-related influences on neck and low back pain. In: Nachemson A, Jonsson E (eds.), Neck and back pain: the scientific evidence of causes, diagnosis and treatment. Philadelphia: Lippincott, Williams & Wilkins, 2000;97-126.
7. Waddell G. The back pain revolution (2nd ed.). Churchill Livingstone, 2004.
8. Waddell G, Burton AK, Main CJ. Screening to identify people at risk of long-term incapacity for work: a conceptual and scientific review. London: Royal Society of Medicine Press, 2003. www.rsmpress.co.uk/bkwaddell2.htm.
9. Waddell G, McCulloch JA, Kummel E, Venner RM. Non-organic physical signs in low back pain. Spine 1980; 5:117-25.
10. Wiltse LL, Rocchio PD. Pre-operative psychological tests as predictions of success of chemonucleolysis in the treatment of the low back syndrome. J Bone Joint Surg 1975; 57A:478-83.
11. Working Backs Scotland. www.workingbacksscotland.com.

18

Physical Therapy, Reconditioning, and Learning How to Move Again

Florian Brunner, Sherri Weiser, and Margareta Nordin

International task forces have established the importance of physical activity for those who suffer from chronic low back pain. Physical activity has been defined as work activities, exercise, sports, and recreation. Randomized controlled trials have addressed the importance of movement and exercises in failed back surgery with less convincing results. Even less is known about chronic neck pain and the importance of activity.

Qualitative studies may be helpful in explaining the link between physical exercise and important outcomes. Beaton et al. has proposed a model of the meaning of recovery in patients with work-related upper limb disorders using qualitative methods (grounded theory). The patient's perception of "being better" was highly contextual. "Being better" was reflected in positive changes in the state of the disorder (resolution), the ability to adjust life to accommodate normal activities with the disorder (readjustment), or the ability to accept life with the disorder (redefinition).

Walker et al. studied the experience of chronic back pain patients seeking help from a pain clinic using a qualitative phenomenological approach. Five major themes were identified: the pain takes over, a sense of loss, being in the system, the patient does not understand, and coming to terms. The patients felt trapped by the medical, legal, and social system that rendered them powerless, helpless, and angry. Once this occurs, recovery becomes very difficult.

The largest misconception in treating spine patients is that alleviation of pain solely will return the patients to usual prepain activity. The pain needs to be addressed as well as psychological and social factors. Learning to move again or regain function for the patient with spine problems is a result of good medical care and the health care provider's ability to remove perceived hurdles for the patient. A major hurdle to movement and exercise seems to be the perceived threat of movement. This can be expressed as fear of pain, fear of reinjury, or fear of permanent damage.

Treatment to reduce fear must include cognitive behavioral techniques that address the perceived threat of movement in combination with progressive exercise and function. These treatments reinforce each other so a reduction in fear will increase movement and a gradual increase in activity will reduce fear. This combination treatment should start immediately when a normal course of recovery is absent.

WHAT IS KINESIOPHOBIA, AND WHAT ARE ITS CONSEQUENCES?

In 1990, Kori et al. described the term "kinesiophobia" (kinesis = movement) as the excessive, irrational, and debilitating fear of physical movement and activity resulting from a feeling of vulnerability to painful injury or reinjury (13). Fear of movement/(re)injury is

TABLE 18.1. *The flag system*

Red Flags	Biomedical factors	Sample signs and symptoms: • Infections • Major trauma • Systemic disease • Cancer • Major neurological compromise
Yellow Flags	Psychosocial or behavioral factors	• Patient believes back pain is harmful or potentially severely disabling • Fear-avoidance behavior • Expectation of passive treatment
Blue Flags	Socioeconomic factors	• Unemployment
Black Flags	Occupational factors	• Work satisfaction • Work characteristics

Reprinted with permission from Main CJ, Williams AC. Musculoskeletal pain. BMJ 2002;325:534-7.

associated with avoidance behaviors that increase functional disability in chronic low back pain (24). In this population, pain-related fear also increases the patient's perception of disability (23).

A New Zealand task force recently proposed a flag system to help identify factors associated with poor outcome of low back pain (2). Four groups of risk factors, or "flags," were identified (Table 18.1). In addition to "red flags," which constitute conditions requiring further immediate evaluation and treatment, "blue flags" refer to socioeconomic risk factors such as unemployment, "black flags" represent occupational factors such as work satisfaction, and "yellow flags" focus on the psychological and psychosocial aspects of the disorder. The concept of fear is prominent among these "yellow flags" and refers to the belief that back pain is harmful or potentially severely disabling and one must avoid potentially painful behaviors (2,11,14).

WHAT IS THE FEAR-AVOIDANCE MODEL?

The fear-avoidance model describes how patients avoid normal activities if they believe these activities will provoke pain (25). Vlaeyen et al. postulate two divergent behavioral responses that occur in the face of pain: confrontation and avoidance (24). Avoidance is a possible pathway by which injured patients get caught in a downward spiral of increasing pain and disability. If pain is interpreted as threatening (pain catastrophizing), pain-related fear develops. Pain catastrophizing is assumed to be influenced by negative affectivity and threatening illness information. This leads to avoidance behavior and hypervigilance to bodily sensations followed by disuse, depression, and disability. These factors will maintain the pain experiences, thereby fueling the vicious circle of increasing fear and avoidance. In contrast, patients who do not perceive pain as threatening rapidly confront their daily activities, leading to a fast recovery (Fig. 18.1).

WHAT ARE THE CONSEQUENCES OF INACTIVITY ACCORDING TO THE FEAR-AVOIDANCE MODEL?

Physical inactivity has physical, psychological, and social consequences. The main physical consequence is the deconditioning of various body systems. This explains why the complaints of chronic pain patients often include the cardiovascular system and why comorbidities are common (6). The basis for the development of a chronic pain syndrome

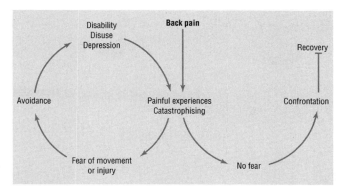

FIG. 18.1. Fear-avoidance model. From Vlaeyen JW et al.: Fear-avoidance and its consequences in chronic musculoskeletal pain: a state of the art. 2000 International Association for the Study of Pain. Reprinted with permission from Elsevier Science B.V. Main CJ, Williams AC. Musculoskeletal pain. BMJ 2002;325:534-7.

are a decreased aerobic capacity, a reduction in muscle force, insufficient posture, dysbalance of the muscles, demineralization of the bones, adhesion of joint capsules, decrease in stress tolerance of soft tissue, fatigability, and depression (6).

Psychologically, the patient may embark on a series of cognitive and emotional changes that result in chronic pain. In acute pain, nociception is associated with underlying pathology. Unless informed otherwise, patients with benign musculoskeletal conditions may maintain this belief even after the initial pathology is gone. The belief that pain signifies damage prevents them from performing any activity that evokes the pain. In a short period of time, deconditioning occurs, making movement increasingly difficult and painful.

Patients with extreme anxiety or those with few incentives to improve are at risk of succumbing to chronic pain syndrome. Over time, these patients give up their usual social, work, and family roles and identify themselves as permanent patients. Once this change of identity occurs, it is nearly impossible to reverse (29).

WHY IS WADDELL'S BIOPSYCHOSOCIAL MODEL IMPORTANT IN THIS CONTEXT?

For patients with chronic low back pain, the biomedical approach is often insufficient because it only focuses on structural and morphological pathologies. In the biopsychosocial model, introduced by Waddell, pain and pain disability are not only influenced by a possible organic pathology but also by other biological, psychological, and social factors (26). Pain and disability results from a complex interplay of these influences. Both components have the same potential importance. A change in one results in a change in the other. This model has important treatment implications. In addition to treating the physical complaints, psychological and social factors must also be addressed to achieve a successful recovery (Fig. 18.2).

WHAT IS A GOOD OUTCOME FROM THIS PERSPECTIVE?

The goal of treatment is to improve physical performance and decrease possible fear-avoidance behavior. This is done by interfering with the cycle of fear, catastrophizing, activity avoidance, and disability. Successful treatment changes the patient from an

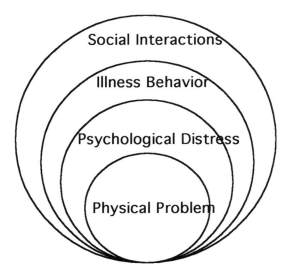

FIG. 18.2. The biopsychosocial model. From Waddell G et al.: Symptoms and signs: physical disease or illness behavior? BMJ Publishing Group. Reprinted with permission from BMJ Publishing Group. Br. Med J (Clin Res Ed) 1984;289:739-41.

avoider to a confronter, finally leading to recovery. A good outcome from this perspective could mean a decrease in pain and an increase in function, but it also includes the patient's subjective evaluation of progress. Function is defined more broadly here and not only means better physical condition but also better psychological and social health.

HOW DOES THE PATIENT DEFINE RECOVERY FROM MUSCULOSKELETAL DISORDERS?

The meaning of recovery to the patient with low back pain is not well studied. However, Beaton et al. have proposed a model of the meaning of recovery in patients with work-related upper limb disorders based on qualitative methods (grounded theory) (5). The patient's perception of "being better" was highly contextual. "Being better" was reflected in positive changes in the state of the disorder (resolution), the ability to adjust life to accommodate normal activities with the disorder (readjustment), or the ability to accept life with the disorder (redefinition). The experience of the disorder can be influenced by factors such as the perceived legitimacy of the disorder in the eyes of others, the patient's definitions of health and illness, and coping styles.

This definition may apply to patients with chronic back pain as well. For a patient with chronic pain, the construct of redefinition is probably the most accurate because no resolution of the disorder has occurred and the patient struggles with a change in his or her identity from a healthy to a sick person (Fig. 18.3).

WHAT IS THE PATIENT'S EXPERIENCE WITH CHRONIC LOW BACK PAIN?

Using a qualitative phenomenological approach, Walker et al. studied the experience in the workers' compensation system of chronic low back pain patients seeking help from

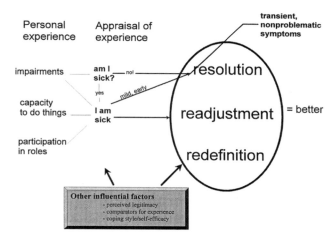

FIG. 18.3. Model for recovery. From Beaton et al.: Are You Better? 2001, American College of Rheumatology. Reprinted with permission from Wiley-Liss, Inc., a subsidiary of John Wiley & Sons, Inc. Arthritis Rheum 2001;45:270-9.

a pain clinic (28). The patients attended two pain clinics in England and were diagnosed with chronic low back pain. Five major themes were identified: "the pain takes over," "a sense of loss," "in the system," "they don't understand," and "coming to terms." The patients felt trapped by the medical, legal, and social systems that rendered them powerless, helpless, and angry. This experience contributes to development of a sick role identity as seen in the "Pain Ladder" (29). The Pain Ladder demonstrates why it is of great importance what patients believe and why attitudes and misunderstandings or miscommunication should be recognized early and addressed promptly.

Patients with chronic low back pain often have negative attitudes toward therapy because they believe it will cause pain or not be successful. This may partly explain the poor outcome with exercise therapy among patients with chronic low back pain. It has been stated that exercise compliance in physical therapy clinics is 50% at most for low back pain patients (3,7). Signs of noncompliance are not showing up for the treatment sessions, only attending periodically, and stopping treatment altogether.

HOW CAN PATIENTS WITH KINESIOPHOBIA BE DETECTED?

Kinesiophobia has been shown to be a predictor of chronic low back pain (19). An in-depth interview at the beginning of the treatment can indicate possible fears related to low back pain. These include fear of movement, fear of damage, fear of pain, fear of permanent disability, and even fear of losing one's job. An interview may be supplemented with the Pain Anxiety Symptoms Scale (PASS) (15), the Tampa Scale for Kinesiophobia (TSK) (13), and the Fear-Avoidance Beliefs Questionnaire (FABQ) (27). They were developed to detect avoidance of behaviors due to fear of pain and its consequences.

It is equally important to detect fear behaviors in physical therapy through the therapist's observation. A therapist with a biopsychosocial perspective may be able to distinguish pain behavior caused by fear from behavior caused by other factors such as mistrust of the therapist. Many patients will state outright that they fear movement and pain. Also, patients who fear movement are usually consistent in their behavior across situations and do better when their fears are alleviated by an explanation of treatment and reassurance from the therapist.

HOW CAN KINESIOPHOBIA BE TREATED?

For some patients who have never had active therapy, kinesiophobia can be successfully treated with exercise alone. Exercise has been proven to be beneficial in all stages of nonspecific low back pain and after surgery (8,9,12,17,22–24). One pathway by which exercise improves outcome is that it allows patients to take some control over their health. Once they observe the benefits of exercise, they become less fearful of movement and resume normal activities. In addition, an increase in a sense of control usually leads to the patient taking more responsibility for recovery.

Although there is sufficient scientific evidence to recommend physical, therapeutic, or recreational exercises (1,21), it remains unclear whether any specific type of exercise is more effective than any other (16–18,20,21). However, to avoid a general deconditioning of the patient, it is recommended the exercise program consist of strengthening, endurance, and stretching. According to the guidelines of the American College of Sports Medicine, an active program should start at 50% of baseline and can be progressively increased (4). The minimum time is three times a week for 6 weeks or every day for 4 weeks. Throughout this period, 1.5 hours to 2 hours per visit should be used for active physical therapy. Benefits only occur if the exercises are done regularly at the right intensity while using proper technique. In addition, to maintain achieved goals, patients must exercise on a regular basis at home after the prescribed training sessions are completed. The exercises should be built into the daily routine. To ensure good compliance and motivation, the exercises must be simple and of short duration. Also, the exercise program should be realistic and tailored to the needs of the individual patient (7).

After the program, the patient should be able to take responsibility for self-care and be motivated to continue with a carefully designed home program. If difficulties occur, follow-up visits may be planned and a psychological intervention may be warranted. Such an intervention usually consists of cognitive-behavioral treatment. This includes relaxation exercises and progressive exposure in a safe environment to the movements or tasks the patients has identified as threatening (22). Although physical and psychological treatments may be used independently, studies show that a combined approach is best (6,10). These approaches complement and reinforce each other in that the reduction of fear leads to an increase in movement, and increased movement reduces fear. When a multidisciplinary approach is used, it is important that health care providers give a unified message to the patient about the back pain, the therapy, and the expected outcome. Consistency among therapists increases patient confidence and reduces ambiguity, both of which decrease fear.

SO WHAT DO WE DO?

A combination treatment consisting of exercise and cognitive-behavioral therapy should start as soon as possible when a normal course of recovery is absent or possible risk factors are identified (19). These risk factors include psychological, behavioral, social, and economic factors (14). These factors should be familiar to physical therapists while monitoring treatment so prompt referrals to a psychologist or appropriate health care provider are made.

Treatment to reduce fear must include cognitive-behavioral techniques that address the perceived threat of movement or pain in combination with progressive exercise and function. As fear is reduced, function improves just like when the patient realizes that activity helps reduce dysfunction, disabling fear and associated avoidance behaviors are diminished. It is only then that a patient can be reconditioned successfully.

TABLE 19.1. *Overview of characteristics of radio frequency (RF) and steroid injection treatments for chronic low back pain*

Treatment	Abbreviation	Target	No. of electrodes or needles	Type of electrode or needle	Sensory and/or motor stimulation	Local anesthesia and/or steroid injection	RF temperature/ duration of lesion	Additional information
RF facet joint denervation	RF-Facet	Medial branch of dorsal ramus	3	22G 10 cm with 5 mm tip	50/2 Hz	0.25–0.5 ml mepi* 2%	80°C/60 sec	
RF disc treatment	RF-Disc	Center of disc	1	20G 15 cm with 10 mm tip	–/2 Hz	No local anesthesia required	80°C/240 sec	Intradiscal antibiotic prophylaxis
RF ramus communicans nerve denervation	RF-RC	Ramus communicans nerve	2	20G 15 cm with 5 mm tip	50/2 Hz	0.5 ml mepi* 2%	80°C/60 sec	
RF sacroiliac joint denervation	RF-SI	Dorsal ramus at sacral level	3 or 4	22G 10 cm with 5 mm tip	50/2 Hz	0.25–0.5 ml mepi* 2%	80°C/60 sec	
RF dorsal root ganglion treatment	RF-DRG	Dorsal root ganglion	1	22G 10 cm with 5 mm tip	50/2 Hz	2–5 ml mepi* 2%	67°C/90 sec	
Therapeutic sacroiliac joint injection	SI-inj	Periarticular space of SI-joint	1	22G 10 cm needle	–/–	2–4 ml bupi† 0.25% + 40 mg MPA‡	—	
Therapeutic epidural injection	Epid-inj	Epidural space	1	22G 10 cm needle	–/–	2–4 ml bupi† 0.25% + 40 mg MPA‡	—	Midline or transforaminal approach
Epidural adhesiolysis (transforaminal)	Epid-Adh	Scar tissue in epidural space	1	22G 10 cm needle	–/–	2 ml bupi† 0.25% + 10 mg MPA‡ + 750 IU hyaluron§	—	Repeated 3–4 times
Epidural adhesiolysis (caudal approach)	Racz	Scar tissue in epidural space	1 + catheter	Tuohy needle + spring guide epidural (Racz-) catheter	–/–	2 ml bupi† 0.25% + 10 mg MPA‡ + 750 IU hyaluron§	—	In addition to foraminal approach

* Mepivacain
† Bupivacain
‡ MPA (methylprednisolone acetate)
§ Hyaluronidase

back pain syndrome (see classification of CLBP). For a specified overview of treatments and techniques used, see Table 19.1.

Baseline and 12-Month Follow-Up Assessment Instruments

Assessment of Pain Intensity

Intensity of pain was measured by a calculation of median values of four successive VAS scores of maximum leg pain (VAS leg, 0–10) and maximum back pain (VAS back, 0–10), based on pain diaries that were completed twice weekly by the patients during 2 weeks before the start of the study (t = 0), until 12 months (t = 12) follow-up. In the back pain group, substantial pain relief had to concern back pain; in the leg pain group, pain relief concerned leg pain.

Assessment of Changes in Pain Behavior

Apart from the visual analogue scales, the pain diary consisted of a physical activities scale (0–30 points). Median values of physical activities and intake of analgesics were calculated in the same way as the VAS.

The Dutch version of the Multidimensional Pain Inventory (MPI) (Dutch-Language-Version; MPI-DLV) was assessed to register psychosocial and behavioral (coping) aspects related to pain (6,7). The MPI assigns individual patients to one of four clusters, that is, Adaptive Coper (AC), Average (AV), Interpersonally Distressed (ID), and Dysfunctional (DYS). It allows distinguishing psychologically "stable" (AC + AV) from "unstable" patients (ID + DYS) (8).

Assessment of Pain Cognitions

A Pain Cognition List (PCL) containing 81 items that are scored 1 to 5 and clustered in five major scales was used to study pain cognitions. The reliability and validity of the PCL was judged sufficient (9). For the purpose of this study we used the following scales: negative self-efficacy (17 items), catastrophizing (17 items), positive expectations, resignation, and faith in health care.

Assessment of Anxiety

The Dutch version of the state-trait anxiety inventory (10) was applied to discriminate between state anxiety and trait anxiety. The scores on both scales extend from 20 to 80 points.

Assessment of Personality Traits

The Dutch Personality Questionnaire contains seven scales: inadequacy, social inadequacy, rigidity, feeling wronged, self-satisfaction, dominance, and self-esteem (11).

Evaluation of Changes in Quality of Life

Quality of life was measured at the start of the study and at 12-month follow-up by the SF-36 questionnaire, containing nine scales (12,13): physical functioning; social functioning; role limitations (physical problem); role limitations (emotional problem); mental health; vitality; pain; general health perception; and health change.

Data Analysis

The present follow-up study was set up in a semiexperimental structured mode to create the opportunity to allow for a maximal discrimination between success versus failure to respond to therapy. Based on frequency tables, constructed for both leg pain and back pain groups in order to get an impression of the distribution of pain intensities (as measured by VAS; Fig. 19.1A,B) at 12 months among patients, it was decided to dichotomize patients according to a VAS improvement. This resulted in three categories, that is, a VAS improvement ≥66% (upper border, i.e., success), a VAS improvement ≤0% (lower border, i.e., failure to improve), and a VAS improvement in between 0 and 66% (intermediate response) (Fig. 19C,D). Because, in our experience, 100% pain relief is hardly ever achieved when treating chronic low back pain patients under the purely somatically oriented conditions of minimally invasive treatment, it was decided that an improvement of >66% would fit with our primary goal.

Under these circumstances, numbers of patients in the success and failure groups turned out to be sufficiently large to allow for statistical analysis. The intermediate group

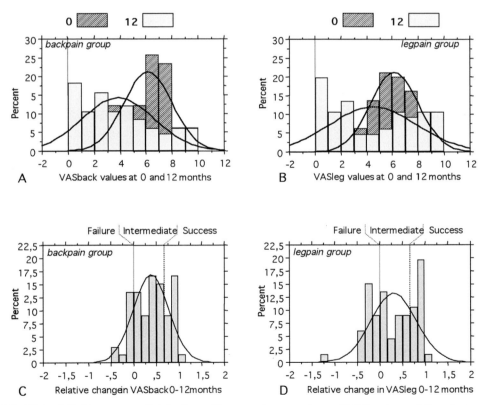

FIG. 19.1. A,B: Frequency distribution with normal comparison of VAS values at the start and at 12 months, with VAS back values for the back pain group (**A**), and VAS leg values for the leg pain group (**B**), respectively. **C,D:** Frequency distribution with normal comparison of relative changes in VAS back (**C**), VAS leg (**D**), respectively, between 0 and 12 months displaying percentages of failure (relative values < = 0), intermediate (relative values >0, <0,66), and success (relative values > = 0.66).

was not considered for statistical analysis other than for control purposes. It was argued that excluding these patients would optimize the chances to detect for an associated effect among the three variables. Pain relief change was considered a semi-independent categorical variable; changes in psychological profile and quality of life were dependent on categorical variables. Because data of the dependent variables were continuous, differences in values between groups at 12 months were assessed by analysis of variances (ANOVA). Success, intermediate, and failure groups were entered as group variables. VAS leg, VAS back, DAS, MED, and the subscales of the MPI, PCL, STAI, and SF-36 were entered as dependent variables.

Correlation between change in VAS (as a continuous variable) and changes in daily activities, analgesics intake, SF-36, and other psychological test outcomes after 12 months were determined with Pearson correlation analysis. Significance levels were set after Bonferroni correction for post hoc comparisons. Because of the large number of tests (about 30) carried out, a Bonferroni correction was used to obtain an overall a of 0.05. This was in line with the number of subscales the three categories were compared for.

P-values of 0.05 or less were defined as statistically significant. P-values between 0.05 and 0.10 were considered as trends.

RESULTS

In both leg pain and back pain groups, data from 132 patients could be analyzed. Data of 14 patients in the leg pain group were incomplete, but because these patients were classified in the "intermediate" groups, these dropouts were not considered relevant to the outcome. It appeared from the constructed frequency tables that, in the leg pain group, 20 patients showed a "successful" response, 25 showed an "intermediate" response, and 21 showed "failure to improve." In the back pain group, these numbers were 18, 36, and 12, respectively, and 15 patients in the intermediate group were excluded for the same reasons as depicted for the leg pain group.

After 12 months of minimally invasive treatment, the back pain group as a whole (n = 66) experienced significant back pain reduction as measured by VAS back, while, similarly, a significant reduction of VAS leg in the leg pain group as a whole (n = 66) appeared. These changes were confirmed by significant decrease in pain intensity as measured by the relevant subscales of the MPI and SF-36. Overall, pain reduction was not accompanied by improvement of psychological distress as measured by MPI, PCL, and STAI. Improvement of quality of life as measured by the "Change in health" subscale of the SF-36 occurred in the leg pain group. A larger improvement of quality of life appeared in the back pain group, where the subscales "physical functioning," "physical limitations," and "change in health" improved.

After dichotomization of patients in both the leg pain and back pain group, differences between "successful" patients (VAS reduction ≥66%) and "failure-to-improve" patients (VAS reduction ≤0%) with regard to VAS, daily activities, analgesics intake, MPI, PCL, STAI, and SF-36 were noticed at 12-month follow-up (Table 19.2). In both groups, "successful" patients performed significantly better than "failure-to-improve" patients. Also "intermediate" patients performed better on a few psychological items and on almost all scales of the SF-36, again both in the leg pain group and back pain group. In both leg pain and back pain groups, VAS-leg and VAS-back reduction were associated, and this was confirmed by a decrease of pain as measured by the relevant subscales of the MPI and SF-36.

Regarding "success" patients as opposed to "failures" in the back pain group, changes in psychological distress were limited to a significant decreased interference of pain with

TABLE 19.2. *ANOVA table for comparison of differences at 12 months between Success (S), Failure (F), and Intermediate (I) group.[#] All data are of 12 months.*

	Leg pain group $F_{(2,63)}$ value°	Mean Diff. S-F	Mean Diff. S-I	Mean Diff. F-I	Back pain group $F_{(2,63)}$ value°°	Mean Diff. S-F	Mean Diff. S-I	Mean Diff. F-I
VAS back					42,046*	−6,042*	−3,528*	2,514*
VAS leg	113,009*	−7,379*	−3,672*	3,707*				
DAS	9,670*	7,054*	5,445*	−1,609	9,518*	9,167*	5,736*	−3,431
MED	3,590	−1,540*	−1,110	0,430	4,128	−1,542*	−1,056	0,486
MPI								
Pain intensity	18,28*	−2,170*	−1,179*	0,991*	11,818*	−2,156*	−1,443*	0,713
Interference	4,705*	−1,333*	−0,702	0,631	12,700*	−2,281*	−1,450*	0,831
Life control	3,275	0,739	0,841	0,102	7,447*	1,840*	1,250*	−0,589
Disturbed mood	2,024	−0,822	−0,584	0,238	6,378*	−1,688*	−1,061*	0,626
Support	0,011	−0,085	−0,024	0,061	0,589	0,640	0,337	−0,302
Punishing response	3,005	−0,917	−0,275	0,642	0,588	−0,567	−0,213	0,353
Caring response	0,037	−0,105	−0,110	−0,005	0,200	0,200	0,279	0,079
Distracting response	0,238	0,175	0,368	0,193	0,387	0,550	0,315	−0,235
General activities	5,323*	0,412	0,878*	0,467	2,294	0,717	0,443	−0,274
PCL								
Negative self-efficacy	4,778*	−9,317*	−8,741*	0,576	13,859*	— 17,863*	−9,529*	8,333*
Catastrophizing	3,193	−9,917*	−4,432	5,485	9,576*	— 21,745*	10,440*	11,306 *
Expectations								
Fault in health care	6,833*	3,871*	1,891	−1,981	3,489	3,422*	1,033	−2,389
STAI								
Trait anxiety	5,635*	−6,411*	−7,751*	−1,340	6,366*	— 11,407*	−7,629*	3,778
SF-36								
Physical functioning	7,513*	28,940*	20,576*	−8,364	10,606*	32,396*	19,777*	−12,619
Social functioning	5,890*	20,387*	22,690*	2,303	6,820*	26,562*	26,741*	0,179
Limitations, physical	10,118*	41,607*	27,011*	−14,596	12,809*	57,812*	42,634*	−15,179
Limitations, emotional	2,922	30,641	25,947	−4,694	3,632	45,973*	17,798	−23,175
Mental health	7,735*	20,067*	20,009*	−0,058	9,310*	26,583*	17,479*	−9,105
Energy and fatigue	3,612	16,190*	13,043	−3,147	15,097*	36,042*	22,946*	−13,095
Pain	9,709*	— 24,927*	— 14,390*	10,536	15,795*	— 34,704*	23,270*	11,434
General health	4,45*	21,048*	5,913	−15,135	10,793*	31,667*	19,929*	−11,738
Health		*	*			*		

[#] For the patients with primarily leg pain, groups were defined as "Success" if VAS-leg reduction 0–12 was ≥ 66%; as "Failure" if VAS-leg reduction (0–12 remained the same or became worse; and as "Intermediate" if VAS-leg reduction 0–12 was between 0% and 66%.

[#] For the patients with primarily back pain, groups were defined as "Success" if VAS-back reduction 0–12 was ≥ 66%; as "Failure" if VAS-back 0–12 remained the same or became worse; and as "Intermediate" if VAS-back reduction 0–12 was between 0% and 66%.

* With post hoc Bonferroni correction, significance level was $p < 0.0167$.

° 14 cases were omitted due to missing values, for SF-36 16 cases ($F_{(2,61)}$ values).

°° 14 cases were omitted due to missing values, for SF-36 17 cases ($F_{(2,60)}$ values).

daily activities (subitem of the MPI) and a decreased negative self-efficacy (subitem of the PCL). In the same back pain group, most notably, differences in SF-36 occurred. A pain reduction as measured by VAS back was associated with a significantly associated increase of physical functioning and health improvement.

Regarding "success" patients in the leg pain group, a sole significant association for VAS-leg reduction was noted with improved life control (subitem of the MPI), and changes in quality of life items were by far more expressed: in 6 out of 9 items on the SF-36 questionnaire, improvements were significantly associated with a VAS-leg improvement, that is, physical and social functioning, physical role limitation, mental health, pain, and health change (Table 19.2).

DISCUSSION

Only one study so far has investigated whether substantial pain relief obtained by a purely medical approach eventually might lead to a resolution of psychological distress and regression of aberrant behavior in chronic spinal pain. In persistent low back pain, psychosocial elements play an important role (14). In this study, we were not able to prove an association between pain relief and subsequent resolution of psychological stress. This is in line with a previous study on cervical RF-DRG applied for chronic cervicobrachialgia (15), but in contradiction to a study on RF-PFD for whiplash patients (1).

Because it has been stated (1,16) that only complete pain relief might be able to resolve psychological distress, it was decided in this study to select, from both leg pain and back pain groups, only those patients exhibiting major improvement of their most invalidating complaint. We agreed to select for less than 100% pain relief for practical reasons. In our experience, contrary to whiplash patients, chronic low back pain patients usually present with pain that is the result of a combination of nociceptive substrates, for instance, the combination of discogenic pain and facettal pain and psychological distress, leading to a complex pain syndrome of a multidimensional character. Because these patients represent the preponderance of chronic low back pain patients, we chose not to select "exceptional" cases because they represent only a small part of the chronic low back pain population treated by pain clinicians (16,17).

No other psychological or surgical therapies were offered during the purely somatic treatment period of 12 months. Further evidence that demonstrated pain relief was caused by minimally invasive treatment comes from the consistently significant association found between VAS decrease and pain decrease, as measured by MPI and SF-36. Additionally, SF-36 improved, most notably the physical items, in 3 in the BP-group, and 6 out of 9 items in the LP-group, respectively, if "success" patients were compared with "failure-to-improve" patients.

The observed differences between leg pain and back pain groups suggest a greater impact of somatic treatment in the leg pain group compared to the back pain group. Thus in accordance with previous studies, a relatively larger somatic impact in low back pain with radicular pain compared to chronic low back pain without radicular component was concluded (14). It is remarkable that in both leg pain and back pain group the observed VAS reduction at 12 months, obtained during minimal invasive treatment, was confirmed by the subscales of MPI and PCL. VAS reduction at 12 months was significantly associated with an improvement of quality of life, the leg pain group improving more than the back pain group. Pain relief as measured by VAS reduction did not lead to a spontaneous resolution of psychological stress. It seems that relief from low back pain, as measured by VAS, results in improvement of quality of life as measured by SF-36, whereas psychological distress remains unchanged, indicating other factors may be responsible for the distress noticed in patients exhibiting chronic low back pain.

REFERENCES

1. Wallis BJ, Lord SM, Bogduk N. Resolution of psychological distress of whiplash patients following treatment by radiofrequency neurotomy: a randomised, double-blind, placebo-controlled trial. Pain 1997; 73: 15-22.
2. Kendal N, Main CI, Linton SI, Vlaeyen JW, Nicholas MK. Reply to Wallis et al., Pain, 73 (1997) 15-22. Pain 1998; 78: 223-5.
3. Thompson EN. Psychogenic pain; in whose mind? Letter to the editor. Re: Kendall et al., Pain, 78 (1998) 223-5. Pain 1999; 82: 109-10.
4. Geurts JW, Wijk van RMAW, Wynne HJ, Hammink E, Buskens E, Lousberg R, Knape JTA, Groen GJ. Radiofrequency lesioning of dorsal root ganglia for chronic lumbosacral radicular pain. A randomised, double-blind, sham lesion-controlled trial. Lancet 2003; 4: 21-6.
5. BenDebba M, Torgerson WS, Long DM. A validated, practical classification procedure for many persistent low back pain patients. Pain 2000; 87: 89-97.
6. Lousberg R, Van Breukelen GJ, Groenman NH, Schmidt AJ, Arntz A, Winter FA. Psychometric properties of the Multidimensional Pain Inventory, Dutch language version (MPI-DLV). Behav Res Ther 1999; 37: 167-82.
7. Turk DC, Rudy TE. Towards an empirically derived taxonomy of chronic pain patients: integration of psychological assessment data. J Consult Clin Psychol 1988; 56: 233-8.
8. Lousberg R, Groenman NH, Schmidt AJ. Profile characteristics of the MPI-DLV clusters of pain patients. J Clin Psychol 1996; 52: 161-7.
9. Vlaeyen JW, Geurts SM, Eck van H, Snijders AM, Schuurman JA, Groenman NH. Pain Cognition List: experimental version. Lisse: Swets & Zeitlinger, 1989.
10. A Dutch version of the Spielberger state-trait anxiety inventory (STAI-DV). Lisse: Swets & Zeitlinger, 1980.
11. Luteijn F, Starren J, Van Dijk H. Nederlandse Persoonlijkheidsvragenlijst. Lisse: Swets & Zeitlinger, 1989.
12. McHorney CA, Ware JE, Raczek AE. The MOS 36-item short-form health survey (SF-36): II. Psychometric and clinical tests of validity in measuring physical and mental health constructs. Med Care 1993; 31: 247-63.
13. Patrick DL, Deyo RA, Atlas SJ, Singer DE, Chapin A, Keller RB. Assessing health-related quality of life in patients with sciatica. Spine 1995; 20: 1899-1909.
14. Ben Debba M, Torgerson WS, Long DM. Personality traits, pain duration and severity, functional impairment, and psychological distress in patients with persistent low back pain. Pain 1997; 72: 115-25.
15. Samwel H, Slappendel R, Crul BJ, Voerman VF. Psychological predictors of the effectiveness of radiofrequency lesioning of the cervical spinal dorsal ganglion (RF-DRG). Eur J Pain 2000; 4: 149-55.
16. Dreyfuss P, Halbrook B, Pauza K, Joshi A, McLarty J, Bogduk N. Efficacy and validity of radiofrequency neurotomy for chronic lumbar zygapophyseal joint pain. Spine 2000; 25: 1270-7.
17. Kleef van M, Barendse GA, Kessels A, Voets HM, Weber WE, de Lange S. Randomized trial of radiofrequency lumbar facet denervation for chronic low back pain. Spine 1999; 24: 1937-42.

20

Spinal Cord Stimulation for Failed Back Surgery Syndrome: Technique, Results, and Cost Effectiveness

Richard B. North

BACKGROUND

In the United States, lumbosacral spine surgery fails to relieve pain in 10% to 40% of cases (1–5). In some patients, the pain persists despite the surgical procedure; in others, it returns. This incidence of failure is sufficiently high that physicians, perhaps inappropriately, named the painful condition failed back surgery syndrome (FBSS). FBSS patients are desperate to relieve their pain, and their physicians try various therapies on a treatment continuum that starts with oral medications and progresses from minimally invasive procedures, such as nerve blocks and steroid injections, to more invasive techniques, such as implantation of spinal cord stimulators and drug delivery systems, and finally to repeated operation. No one approach has worked in 100% of patients, and the best way to reduce the incidence of FBSS will be to improve patient selection for and techniques of lumbosacral surgery.

Reducing the incidence of FBSS, however, will not help the tens of thousands of already affected patients, many of whom become depressed and find their lives complicated by financial difficulties (especially if FBSS interferes with their ability to be gainfully employed) and constricted by pain and disability (6,7).

Our experience of more than three decades with FBSS patients has revealed that many can achieve pain relief through use of an ancient therapy, electrical stimulation, revamped for convenient and controlled delivery with modern technology. Spinal cord stimulation (SCS) provides long-lasting relief without incurring the risks associated with reoperation, subjecting patients to the side effects of medications, or providing merely short-term effects via injections. We have found that compared with patients who undergo repeated operation (8), dorsal root ganglionectomy (9), and radiofrequency facet denervation (10), SCS patients enjoy reduced morbidity and pain and improved neurological function, quality of life, and ability to engage in activities of daily living (11,12). Despite the fact that, in the United States, SCS is most often used to treat FBSS and other investigators have reported similar findings, most clinicians continue to consider SCS a last-ditch treatment offered only when all else fails.

MECHANISM OF ACTION

In 1965, Melzack and Wall published *The Gate Control Theory of Pain,* which provided a theoretical basis for the reports that had persisted from antiquity that electrical stimulation can mitigate pain. The theory proposed that transmission of pain sensations from the dorsal horn in the spinal cord to the brain occurs when an excess of activity among small fiber afferents opens the "gate." (13). This meant that SCS, which selectively depolarizes large fiber afferents in the dorsal columns, could close the pain gate without causing uncomfortable side effects.

The gate control theory, however, does not explain how large fibers signal hyperalgesia, and, in fact, an SCS-instigated frequency-related conduction block might instead interfere with pain signals at the point where dorsal column fibers split off from dorsal horn collaterals. Indeed, validated computer-generated models created to predict the distribution of SCS current flow and voltage gradients in the spinal canal and cord suggest the possible involvement of the dorsal roots and of pathways adjacent to the dorsal columns (14). This would explain the observed preference of SCS patients for a minimum stimulation rate of 25 pulses per second (12).

In addition, experimental studies using clinical-range parameters suggest a pain-relieving role for SCS-instigated changes in the sympathetic nervous system and in GABAergic interneurons (15). This has inspired clinicians to investigate the impact of concomitant treatment with SCS and GABAergic drugs, and preliminary studies indicate that the combination works for patients in whom neither therapy alone had an impact. Two more details that might shed light on the mechanism of action of SCS are that the stimulation alters neurotransmitter metabolite concentrations in cerebral spinal fluid and that the opioid antagonist naloxone does not interfere with SCS efficacy.

OVERVIEW OF THE TECHNIQUE
Patient Eligibility

To be eligible for SCS, our FBSS patients have a history of lumbar spine surgery and persistent or recurrent radicular pain that is refractory to conservative care. SCS can also address coexisting axial low back pain (even though nociceptive or mechanical axial low back pain generally does not respond as well as does neuropathic pain).

We exclude patients with conditions that demand immediate reoperation, such as radiographically confirmed compression of a nerve root causing a disabling neurological deficit or gross instability. As is standard in pain interventions, relative contraindications also include unresolved issues of secondary gain (e.g., an outstanding lawsuit or unresolved workers' compensation claim) or a major untreated psychiatric comorbidity and/or who exhibit inappropriate medication use. Additional contraindications to SCS therapy include uncorrected coagulopathy, untreated sepsis, a patient's inability to cooperate or to control the device, the presence of a demand cardiac pacemaker (without EKG monitoring or changing the pacemaker mode to a fixed rate), and a projected need for the patient to undergo one or more magnetic resonance imaging (MRI) tests.

Screening

As is routine, our SCS patients undergo at least a 3-day trial, most often using a percutaneous temporary electrode (e.g., 3487A Pisces Quad, Medtronic, Inc., Minneapolis, MN). During the procedure, we map the epidural space longitudinally to determine the optimal placement of a permanent implant and to decide exactly which electrode and generator will be most advantageous for the patient.

If the patient had prior spine or peripheral nerve surgery that precludes percutaneous access, we conduct the trial with an insulated electrode that must be placed surgically. These insulated electrodes have the advantage of prolonging battery life and reducing the incidence of side effects, such as pain associated with the recruitment of small fibers in ligamentum flavum.

With either type of electrode, clinicians can use a percutaneous lead that is easily removed at the patient's bedside or a percutaneous extension cable that must be placed and removed in the operating room. Countering this extra expense, the extension cable makes it possible to adapt the temporary electrode for permanent use.

The duration of a trial that depends on percutaneous leads, of course, increases the risk of infection. This risk must be weighed against the desire to continue the trial for a sufficient length of time to obtain accurate results and avoid inappropriate implantation. The increased incisional pain associated with the leads might also confound trial results.

Patients later receive a permanent implant (e.g., 3487A-56 or 3587A Resume electrode, Xtrel or Itrel pulse generator) if they report at least 50% pain relief on standard pain rating measures, with no increase in analgesic intake and improved physical activity appropriate for their neurological status and age.

In the United States, third-party payers require patients to undergo such SCS screening trials before embarking on long-term SCS treatment. Some clinicians meet this requirement by conducting a test stimulation and proceeding immediately to implantation.

A prolonged trial with a temporary percutaneous electrode, however, allows clinicians to assess (a) the efficacy of SCS in a fluoroscopy room (which is less expensive to use than an operating room); (b) the specific effectiveness of a large number of anode and cathode positions and pulse parameters under everyday conditions of activity and posture; (c) additional contact positions, as necessary, which are accessible by incrementally withdrawing the needle at the bedside; and (d) any information that might assist the physician with implantation of the permanent device.

A prolonged trial might permit more thorough assessment of several important outcomes; thus we extend the screening trial beyond 3 days as necessary, on an individual basis. Prolonging the trial, however, might increase the risk that the patient will develop an infection or produce sufficient epidural scar tissue to make permanent implantation in the correct location difficult or impossible.

System Design and Use

Two major types of SCS electrodes are in use: multicontact arrays of electrodes on a single carrier that is inserted percutaneously through a Tuohy needle and insulated "paddles" or "plates" that require laminectomy for placement. Percutaneous placement provides longitudinal access to the spinal canal and, when performed with fluoroscopy, it facilitates optimal positioning. Results with the insulated electrodes compare favorably with those obtained by percutaneous electrodes for low back and lower extremity pain (16) and require only half the battery power. It is more difficult, however, to replace or reposition laminectomy electrodes.

As might be expected, the longitudinal position of an electrode controls the segmental location of the stimulation-induced paresthesia, and bipolar stimulation has the most impact on longitudinal midline fibers. Optimally, the contacts should be separated by 1.4 times the thickness of the meninges and cerebrospinal fluid (6 to 8 millimeters) (14). The appropriate position and spacing of electrodes, however, is determined by individual anatomical features. Instead of broadening the paresthesia, advancing the electrodes cephalad might elicit unwanted local segmental effects because as fibers ascend in the dorsal column, they become thinner and the thickness of the cerebrospinal fluid varies (17).

The bipoles should be closely spaced, with the cathode cephalad. Adding anode(s) cephalad can create a longitudinal tripole (18). Adding anodes lateral to create a transverse tripole should mitigate the recruitment of lateral structures (19).

In FBSS patients with associated axial low back pain, we achieve our most effective results with low thoracic electrode placement and complex electrode arrays (20). In our experience, use of dual electrode percutaneous arrays straddling the midline is inferior to use of a single midline electrode for the treatment of axial low back pain (21). Clinicians report the effective treatment of intractable low back pain, however, with an insulated array of two parallel columns with eight contacts each (22).

After placing the electrode(s), the clinician can program multicontact pulse generators and determine which anodes and cathodes to activate with the patient in the appropriate position. Technical and clinical reliability is enhanced by gating single-channel generators to multiple outputs, creating a "multi-channel" system (12,18).

The number of contacts in an electrode dictates the number of potential cathode and anode combinations (e.g., an array of four contacts has 50 possible cathode/anode combinations; an array of eight has 6,050). When determining the best combination, we must assess the performance of each combination at amplitudes that result in a range of sensation from perception to discomfort. Patients can use a computer with a graphic input device to map their pain and paresthesia and control stimulus amplitude while they rate their pain on a visual analog scale (23,24). This improves the efficacy of the system and, by extending battery life, also increases cost effectiveness.

The two available energy sources for the electrodes are (a) radiofrequency-coupled passive implants that have a long life but require an external antenna, which can cause skin irritation and fluctuations in stimulation amplitude, and (b) implanted pulse generators (IPGs) that are battery operated (battery life depends on the amount of power required for the specific setting and time in use). Patients use either an external magnet to turn IPGs on and off and to make limited adjustments in amplitude or a remote transmitter that permits them to make more complicated adjustments.

Complications

The potential complications of SCS implantation include spinal cord or nerve injury, cerebrospinal fluid leakage, bleeding, and infection. Later, device-related, complications include generator failure, electrode fatigue fracture, electrode migration, and disturbance from exposure to an electromagnetic field.

Infection generally requires removal of the system, which can often be reintroduced after appropriate antibody therapy has eliminated the infection. Equipment failure, of course, requires removal and replacement. Clinicians can sometimes compensate for electrode malposition or migration by adjusting the stimulation parameters; otherwise, the electrode must be removed and repositioned. Because of the growth of scar tissue and other anatomical changes, however, this does not guarantee restoration of successful therapy.

Outcome

Our results show that patients whose FBSS is characterized by root compression and radicular pain and who are appropriate candidates for both SCS and reoperation are significantly more likely to benefit from SCS, especially if they receive SCS before undergoing further operations to correct the FBSS. This is good news because SCS is a minimally invasive, reversible procedure with a very low (and declining) morbidity rate, and

SCS outcomes continue to benefit from technical improvements (12). SCS also offers the advantage of a therapeutic trial before implantation of the stimulating system. Not only is such a trial impossible with reoperation, patient selection for reoperation suffers from the same shortcomings as patient selection for the initial operation—the available prognostic tools, even when used appropriately, are not fail safe. Underscoring this point, a review of preoperative imaging studies and records of FBSS patients showed that many of the initial back operations that caused FBSS were not indicated (25).

We continue to believe SCS should be reserved for appropriate patients who have exhausted all other reasonable therapies, but we no longer include reoperation in that list. Instead of deferring SCS until reoperation fails, we should defer reoperation until SCS fails. Indeed, our results indicate that it is possible that FBSS patients who fail an SCS trial might also fail reoperation.

A 1995 review of the SCS literature concluded that approximately 59% of SCS patients achieve at least 50% pain relief (26). Assuming all of the studies reviewed followed the convention of including results only for patients who passed a screening trial, received a stimulator, and were available for long-term follow-up, this percentage nearly matches our SCS success rate of 60%. Rates reported in the literature on reoperation, with various definitions of success, range from 12% to 100% (5,27–30).

In 1991, we published retrospective reports detailing our 5-year FBSS treatment success rates of 47% for SCS and 34% for reoperation (8,11). Since that time, we have continued to observe better success with SCS than with any other neurosurgical treatment for FBSS, including dorsal root ganglionectomy (9) and radiofrequency facet denervation (10).

Self-selected crossover from one study arm to the other mimics the health-care-seeking behavior of many patients who search for and choose among alternative treatments. Although it seems intuitively more likely that a FBSS patient would be more amenable to an SCS trial than another back operation, all 39 of our patients who refused randomization chose repeated operations even though the average number of prior operations was slightly higher for this group than for the study participants. This might indicate that patients have a certain comfort level with procedures they have experienced in the past and are generally well known among their family and friends. It is much easier for a patient to say he or she is having a back operation (most friends do not ask for further details) than to mention a procedure, such as SCS, which works in mysterious ways and is difficult to describe. Moving SCS up the treatment continuum to a position prior to reoperation and efforts to introduce the procedure to a wider general public would counter this.

It is more difficult to achieve overlap of axial low back pain than of radicular pain with SCS, and some investigators report that axial low back pain is also more difficult to treat with reoperation (30–33). Reported success rates (generally defined as a minimum of 50% pain relief) vary from 12% to 88% at follow-ups of 0.5 to 8 years.

Cost Effectiveness

In 1993, the World Health Organization determined that "SCS appears to be cost-effective versus alternative therapies" (34). For patients with FBSS, most clinicians have considered SCS a last resort to be used only if reoperation is not an option. When reoperation is an option, the cost and risks are similar to those of SCS. As operative techniques improve, however, they often become more expensive. SCS, however, becomes more cost effective as manufacturers improve the equipment and implanters develop techniques to reduce the incidence of electrode migration, increase battery life, and so on.

SCS offers additional advantages that have an impact on cost effectiveness. First, SCS patients undergo a screening trial before the system is implanted. It is impossible to test the effect of an operation without performing the procedure. (We have an indication, however, that patients who fail the SCS screening trial will also fail reoperation, but this requires further investigation.) Second, in a study of selected FBSS patients randomized to SCS or reoperation, significantly more reoperation patients than SCS patients crossed over to the competing arm of the trial after initial treatment or screening (in the case of SCS). This indicates that more of these FBSS patients achieved adequate pain control with SCS than with reoperation as a final treatment.

When we consider cost effectiveness, we must not stop with a determination of the initial cost but also consider which procedure is associated with the most pain-free days, the fewest complications/side effects, the most freedom from medication use, and the biggest reduction in health care use. A 2004 review of the literature on the cost effectiveness of SCS (35) notes that the initial cost of SCS is approximately $10,000 and identifies the sole "full economic evaluation" of the financial impact of SCS (36), which grew out of the investigators' randomized trial of SCS plus physical therapy versus physical therapy alone for complex regional pain syndrome. This analysis revealed that SCS was approximately twice as expensive at 1-year follow-up but would result in an approximate lifetime saving of $60,000 per patient. Comparing SCS with reoperation, of course, would not show such a large 1-year disparity and would, therefore, likely result in an even greater lifetime saving.

SUMMARY

Multiple outcome measures indicate that SCS is a significantly more successful treatment than reoperation for appropriate FBSS patients with primarily radicular pain. Several studies conclude that SCS is a cost-effective therapy and will become even more cost effective as manufacturers continue to improve their designs, in particular the power sources, and as investigators improve implantation techniques and adopt enhanced patient-interactive adjustment methods.

REFERENCES

1. Hirsch C, Nachemson A. The reliability of lumbar disc surgery. Clin Orthop 29:189-95, 1963.
2. Law JD, Lehman RAW, Kirsch WM. Reoperation after lumbar intervertebral disc surgery. J Neurosurg 48:259-63, 1978.
3. Lehmann TR, La Rocca HS. Repeat lumbar surgery: a review of patients with failure from previous lumbar surgery treated by spinal canal exploration and lumbar spinal fusion. Spine 6:615-19, 1981.
4. North RB, Kidd DH, Campbell JN, Long DM. Dorsal root ganglionectomy for failed back surgery syndrome: a five year follow-up study. J Neurosurg 74:236-42, 1991.
5. Wilkinson HA. The failed back syndrome: etiology and therapy (2nd ed.). Philadelphia: Harper & Row, 1991.
6. Arnoff GM, McAlary PW. Multidisciplinary treatment of intractable pain syndromes. Adv Pain Res Ther 13:267-77, 1990.
7. Long DM. The evaluation and treatment of low back pain. In: Hendler NH, Wise TN, Long DM (eds.), Diagnosis and treatment of chronic pain. Boston: John Wright PSG-Inc, 1982.
8. North RB, Campbell JN, James CS, Conover-Walker MK, Wang H, Piantadosi S, Rybock JD, Long DM. Failed back surgery syndrome: five-year follow-up in 102 patients undergoing repeated operation. Neurosurgery 28:685-91, 1991.
9. North RB, Drenger B, Beattie E, McPherson RW, Parker S, Reitz B, Williams GM: Monitoring of spinal cord stimulation evoked potentials during thoracoabdominal aneurysm surgery. Neurosurgery 28:325-30, 1991.
10. North RB, Han M, Zahurak M, Kidd DH. Radiofrequency lumbar facet denervation: Analysis of prognostic factors. Pain 57:77-83, 1994.
11. North RB, Ewend MG, Lawton MT, Kidd DH, Piantadosi S. Failed back surgery syndrome: five-year follow-up after spinal cord stimulator implantation. Neurosurgery 28:692-9, 1991.

12. North RB, Kidd DH, Zahurak M, et al. Spinal cord stimulation for chronic, intractable pain: two decades' experience. Neurosurgery 32:384, 1993.
13. Melzack R, Wall PD. Pain mechanisms: a new theory. Science 150:971, 1965.
14. Holsheimer J, Struijk JJ. How do geometric factors influence epidural spinal cord stimulation? A quantitative analysis by computer modeling. Stereotact Funct Neurosurg 56:234, 1991.
15. Linderoth B, Meyerson BA: Spinal cord stimulation. I. Mechanisms of action. In: Burchiel K (ed.), Pain surgery. New York, Thieme, 1999.
16. North RB, Kidd DH, Olin JC, et al. Spinal cord stimulation electrode design: prospective, randomized, controlled trial comparing percutaneous and laminectomy electrodes. I. Technical outcomes. Neurosurgery 51:381, 2002.
17. Holsheimer J. Effectiveness of spinal cord stimulation in the management of chronic pain: analysis of technical drawbacks and solutions. Neurosurgery 40:990, 1997.
18. North RB, Ewend MG, Lawton MT, et al. Spinal cord stimulation for chronic, intractable pain: Superiority of "multichannel" devices. Pain 44:119, 1991.
19. Holsheimer J, Nuttin B, King GW. Clinical evaluation of paresthesia steering with a new system for spinal cord stimulation. Neurosurgery 42:541, 1998.
20. Barolat G, Massaro F, He J. Mapping of sensory responses to epidural stimulation of the intraspinal neural structures in man. J Neurosurg 78:233, 1993.
21. North RB. Spinal cord stimulation for axial low back pain: single versus dual percutaneous electrodes. Lucerne, Switzerland: International Neuromodulation Society Abstracts, 1998;212.
22. Barolat G, Oakley JC, Law JD. Epidural spinal cord stimulation with multiple electrode paddle leads is effective in treating intractable low back pain. Neuromodulation 4:59, 2001.
23. North RB, Calkins SK, Campbell DS, et al. Automated, patient-interactive, spinal cord stimulator adjustment: a randomized controlled trial. Neurosurgery 52:572, 2003.
24. North RB, Sieracki JM, Fowler KR, et al. Patient-interactive, microprocessor-controlled neurological stimulation system. Neuromodulation 1:185, 1998.
25. Long DM, Filtzer DL, BenDebba M, Hendler NH. Clinical features of the failed-back syndrome. J Neurosurg 69:61-71, 1988.
26. Turner JA, Loeser JD, Bell KG. Spinal cord stimulation for chronic low back pain: a systematic literature synthesis. Neurosurgery 37:1088-96, 1995.
27. Boden SC, Wiesel SW. The multiply operated lumbar spine. In: Rothman RH, Simeone FA (eds.), The spine (3rd ed.). Philadelphia: WB Saunders, 1992;1899-1906.
28. Finnegan WJ, Fenlin JM, Marvel JP, Nardini RJ, Rothman RH. Results of surgical intervention in the symptomatic multiply-operated back patient. J Bone Joint Surg 61:A 1077-82, 1979.
29. Turner JA, Ersek M, Herron L, Haselkorn J, Kent D, Ciol MA, Deyo R. Patient outcomes after lumbar spinal fusions. JAMA 268:907-11, 1992.
30. Waddell G, Kummel EG, Lotto WN, Graham JD, Hall H, McCulloch JA: Failed lumbar disc surgery and repeat surgery following industrial injuries. J Bone Joint Surg 61-A(2): 201-7, 1979.
31. Greenwood J, McGuire TH, Kimbell F. A study of the causes of failure in the herniated intervertebral disc operation. J Neurosurg 9:15-20, 1952.
32. Law JD. Targeting a spinal stimulator to treat the "failed back surgery syndrome." Appl Neurophys 50:437-8, 1987.
33. Ohnmeiss DD, Rashbaum RF, Bogdanffy GM. Prospective outcome evaluation of spinal cord stimulation in patients with intractable leg pain. Spine 21:1344-51, 1996.
34. ECRI. Spinal cord (dorsal column) stimulation for chronic intractable pain. Health Technology Assessment Information Service. Plymouth Meeting, PA: ECRI, 1993.
35. Taylor RS, Taylor RJ, Van Buyten J-P, Buchser E, North R, Bayliss S. The cost effectiveness of spinal cord stimulation in the treatment of pain: a systematic review of the literature. J Pain Symptom Manage 27(4);370-8, 2004.
36. Kemler MA, Furnee CA. Economic evaluation of spinal cord stimulation for chronic reflex sympathetic dystrophy. Neurology 59:1203-9, 2002.

21

A Review of Epiduroscopy and Its Results in Chronic Low Back Pain

Joseph W. M. Geurts

HISTORY

Spinal endoscopy was first performed in 1931 in cadavers by an orthopedic surgeon, Burman, and his pioneering work is considered the beginning of epiduroscopy (1). In 1936, Stern published a paper in which he presented an instrument called the "spinascope" (2). However, it never became clear whether he had used it in a living subject or a patient. The neurosurgeon Pool succeeded in visualizing the lumbosacral nerve roots and their blood vessels in more than 400 patients and published his findings between 1938 and 1942. He used the technique for diagnostic purposes (3,4). Because of the availability of other diagnostic methods, the technique was soon abandoned.

A reappraisal of the technique followed in the 1970s, when Ooi et al. started to use rigid instruments to perform diagnostic spinal endoscopy of the subarachnoideal space in low back pain patients, a technique described as "myeloscopy." Subsequently, observations were made on the congestion and stagnation of blood flow in the cauda equina during straight-leg raising and on the changes of blood flow in the cauda equina and nerve roots during positional changes in lumbar canal stenosis (5–8).

With a rigid scope, Blomberg studied the human anatomy of the epidural space in cadavers (21–26). He performed one clinical study (10 patients) in which a rigid endoscope was used to visualize the epidural space (27) (Personal communication, 1998). From the mid-1980s on, experimental studies were performed on animals (9–13) and human cadavers (9,14–20), some using more flexible fiberscopes.

Igarashi et al. focused on evaluating physiological events in humans. The researchers were able to identify structures in the thoracic and lumbar epidural space (defined as "extradural space") (28,30). Furthermore, they observed changes in epidural structure with increasing age (29), during deep breathing (31), and in pregnant women (31).

Whereas Ooi et al. focused on endoscopic confirmation of *preoperative* diagnosis in patients already scheduled for an operation (5), more recent investigations concentrated on making a diagnosis per se. These were aimed at identifying signs of adhesive arachnoiditis in the epidural and subarachnoideal space, hypothesizing this could be an underlying cause of chronic persistent pain (32–37).

Shimoji et al. (1991) were the first to use small-diameter flexible fiberoptic endoscopes in patients (32). In their study on 10 patients with chronic low back pain, they advocated that for safety reasons patients should be examined awake. Because they observed the patients' pain could be reproduced with gentle manipulation of the endoscope, it was suggested this would be a potentially valuable diagnostic tool (32).

Up to then, most researchers had used rigid scopes or a combination of rigid introducers and flexible endoscopes, which were introduced through the intervertebral spaces

TABLE 21.1. *Overview of indications and results of epiduroscopy*

Authors	Patients (n)	Indication	Scope/guide tube OD (mm)	Epidural medication	Approach	Results
Pool (1938–1942)	>400	Diagnostic examination	Rigid			
Ooi et al. (1973)	25	Diagnostic examination for low back pain	Rigid 2.8/3.1		L3/S1, caudal	
Ooi et al. (1978)	200	Diagnostic examination for low back pain	Rigid 1.9-2.8/-			Some patients improved and experienced less pain
Ooi et al. (1981)	208	Diagnostic examination	Rigid 1.8-2.5/-			
Ooi et al. (1989)	25	Research of spinal canal stenosis	Rigid		L4/L5 or L5/S1 interspace	
Blomberg and Olsson (1989)	10	Research	Rigid			
Shimoji et al. (1991)	10	Diagnostic examination: adhesive arachnoiditis in back and leg pain	Flexible 0.5-0.9-1.4		Tuohy needle; paramedian L5/S1 interspace	In 3 patients immediate pain relief of 100%, 60%, and 40%
Peek et al. (1993)	15	Diagnostic examination: adhesive arachnoiditis	Rigid 2.7/-		Suspected lumbar level	
Schutze and Kurtze (1994)	12	Diagnosis of various pain syndromes	Flexible 0.8	Hustaed needle; lumbar interspaces		
Saberski and Kitahata (1995)	1	Treatment of L5 radiculopathy	Flexible 0.8	80 mg triamcinolon	Sacral hiatus	Successful until after 6 months
Saberski and Brull (1995)	1	Treatment of L4 radiculopathy	Flexible 2.0	methyl prednisolone	Sacral hiatus	Successful until after 6 months
Kawauchi et al. (1996)	36	Diagnostic examination of arachnoiditis in lumbar spinal stenosis	Rigid 1.7		Interspaces between levels L2/S1	
Uchiyama (1998)	18	Diagnosis in various pain syndromes	Flexible 0.5-0.9-1.4			
Igarashi et al. (1998)	113	Research	Flexible 0.7		Tuohy needle; paramedian thoracic or lumbar interspace	

Study	N	Purpose	Catheter	Agent	Needle/technique	Results
Igarashi et al. (1998)	73	Research	Flexible 0.7		Tuohy needle; paramedian L2/L3 interspace	
Eguchi et al. (1999)	7	Diagnosis in patients presenting with spinal cord lesions	Flexible 0.5		Tuohy needle; lumbar interspaces	
Igarashi et al. (1999)	20	Research	Flexible 0.7		Tuohy needle; paramedian interspace	
Igarashi et al. (2000)	73	Research	Flexible 0.7		Tuohy needle; paramedian lumbar interspace	
Raffaeli et al. (1999)	10	Treatment of: 6 failed back surgery 2 sciatica 1 back pain 1 radiculopathy	Flexible 2.5	120 mg "steroid"	8 sacral hiatus 2 Paramedian lumbar interspace	Unclear: some patients seemed to improve temporarily
Richardson et al. (2001)	38	Treatment of: chronic back pain with radiculopathy	Flexible 0.9/2.2	Bupivacaine 0.25% 5 ml, dexamethasone 80 mg; clonidine, 100 mcg	Sacral hiatus	Significant pain reduction at 12-month follow-up in 26 patients

directly into the subarachnoideal canal at the targeted level. The introduction of the scope into the subarachnoideal space provided superb views because all the structures are embedded in cerebrospinal fluid.

More recently, Saberski et al., in two case reports on chronic radiculopathy, suggested a caudal approach to the epidural space via the sacral hiatus, thereby reducing the chances of inadvertent subarachnoid entry and neurological disturbance (38,39). They used a flexible steerable instrument that contained two separate injection ports for saline irrigation, thus allowing clear vision of the epidural space, without the need for a CSF leak. Richardson et al. suggested the use of another port for continuous epidural pressure monitoring during the procedure (40).

Only very recently have two prospective studies appeared on the combined diagnostic and therapeutic use of caudal epiduroscopy in persistent lumbosacral radiculopathy and chronic low back pain (40,41). For a review of spinal endoscopies performed on patients and human volunteers, see Table 21.1.

INDICATIONS

In general, clinical indications for caudal epiduroscopy of the lumbosacral epidural space include diagnosis and treatment of various neurological syndromes that affect the contents of the spinal canal. Presently, interest focuses primarily on the lumbosacral spine, but with new technical developments the thoracic and cervical spine may become accessible by epiduroscopy.

Presently, caudal epiduroscopy of the lumbosacral epidural space by a flexible endoscope may be indicated in the following situations:

- Confirmation of presumed diagnoses that cannot be verified by conventional diagnostic procedures (such as CT, MRI scans), for example (small) tumors, inflammation, or anatomical abnormalities (11,14,32,33,35,36)
- Combined diagnostic and targeted therapeutic procedure, for example in persistent lumbosacral radiculopathy (38–40)
- Support and facilitation of catheter and electrode implantation (15–17,24,34)
- Removal of harmful epidural contents, for example, extradural scar tissue (34), draining of cysts, retrieval of foreign bodies (e.g., torn epidural and spinal catheters) (42)
- Biopsies

BACKGROUND

The Application of Epiduroscopy in Persistent Lumbosacral Radiculopathy

Signs and symptoms of lumbosacral radiculopathy depend on progression, localization, and size of the herniated disc and are likely to affect all tissue components of the nerve root, including the nerve fibers, blood vessels, and connective tissue. It has been demonstrated that minor compression of nerve roots results in edema formation and eventually leads to intraneuronal inflammation and hypersensitivity (43). The combination of inflammation and mechanical pressure is presently believed to be responsible for the pain and nerve root symptoms frequently encountered in radiculopathy from symptomatic herniated lumbar disc disease (44). It has also been suggested that the release of endogenous chemicals from a ruptured disc may increase nerve hyperexcitability, leading to susceptibility to mechanical compression (43,44).

Adhesions can imitate disc compression by infiltration and compression of spinal nerves and pocket formation, prohibiting drainage of inflamed areas and resulting in pain and a slow deterioration of sensory and motor functions. Adhesions or postoperative scar tissue surrounding nerve roots may interfere with their nutrition and blood supply (45) and are potent contributors to radicular pain (45,46). Blood supply to the nerve root, compared to the dorsal root ganglion, is poor, with approximately 75% of nutrition depending on a flow of cerebrospinal fluid (CSF) (47,48). In adhesive arachnoiditis, nutrition of the nerve root becomes critical (45,49). This is probably due to a combination of mechanical constriction of the vessels, leading to intraneuronal edema (47–49) and rapid thrombus formation in intraneuronal capillaries induced by the nucleus pulposus contents (43,44,48–50).

With the considerations just mentioned in mind, adhesiolysis, whether mechanical or chemical, should be aimed at a reduction of mechanical pressure, decreasing irritation of the inflamed nerve root and resulting in restoration of intraneuronal blood flow. This should reinstate the efferent conduction system, which is more affected after compression than in the afferent nerve system (51).

It should be noted that chronic low back pain without radiculopathy is presently not considered a primary indication for therapeutic epiduroscopy. If indicated in low back pain, invasive pain management should primarily focus on a reduction of nociceptive input from mechanical structures like discs, facets, joints, and ligaments.

PATIENT SELECTION

Patients are considered candidates if they present with a chief complaint of sciatic pain of unilateral localization, not responding to conservative treatment, of at least of 3 months' duration. The pain radiation should be restricted to lumbosacral dermatomal patterns. Of course, the patient should be cooperative and indications for surgery should not be present. Preferably, patients should present with a history of previous herniated disc complaints, with or without signs of sensory disturbances. For practical reasons, previous low back fusion surgery is considered a contraindication at present. For safety reasons, epiduroscopy is not considered in patients with micturition problems and deafferentation signs. CT or MRI scan should provide signs of adhesions around the compromised nerve, likely to cause the radicular pain complaints.

After obtaining informed consent, patient work-up consists of diagnostic nerve blocks of the main suspected nerves in separate sessions. A caudography is performed, with the instillation of contrast, in order to outline the region obscured by adhesions and to estimate whether a caudal approach by the epiduroscope is technically feasible. If the entrance to the sacral hiatus is to small or lumbosacral lordosis is too prominent (in the case of spondylolisthesis), epiduroscopy currently is not considered appropriate for technical reasons. In cases of persistent sciatic complaints, even if additional CT and MRI scan have revealed no abnormalities, it can be decided to perform an epiduroscopy procedure for diagnostic purposes.

TECHNIQUE

A flexible fiberscope is routinely used for epiduroscopy via the caudal approach. It is based on fiberoptic cold-light technology. Its main advantages are that the scope is flexible and the working tip can be moved in various directions, thus enlarging the field of view. Other advantages are its small size, which enables a harmless introduction in the "virtual" epidural space. Flexible endoscopes are available with an outer diameter from 4 to 0.5 mm. Because these scopes usually contain one working lumen, which is considerably small, sterilization is often problematic. Recently, a system was developed consisting

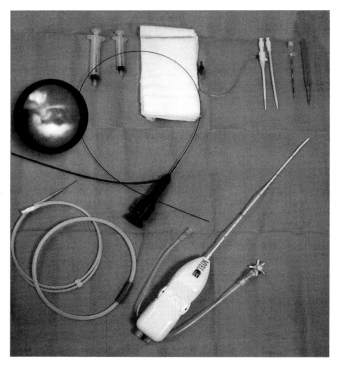

FIG. 21.1. Overview of epiduroscopy instruments.

of a disposable steerable 3.0 mm catheter housing, a 1.2 mm channel for the epiduroscope, and a 1.2 mm channel for the introduction of small working instruments (39). This
steering catheter has a radiopaque tip and shaft. It also contains two side ports to which
a saline flush system and a continuous epidural pressure monitoring system can be connected. The 1.2 mm thick, 800 mm long, flexible fiberoptic endoscope has a high resolution of 10,000 pixels and can be sterilized because it does not contain lumina in itself
(Fig. 21.1). Adjuvants are self-focusing optics with a minimum of 70 degrees field of
view and a 45X optical magnification. The endoscope is connected to a video camera, a
light source, and a monitor.

   Preoperatively, the patient is instructed to not eat or drink. The procedure is carried out
with the patient in the prone position on an X-ray translucent table. Intravenous access,
electrocardiographic, blood pressure, and oxygen saturation monitoring are established.

   If identification of the sacral cornua is problematic, internal rotation of the feet will, by
widening the anal cleft, facilitate identification of the sacral hiatus. The skin and underlying tissue up to the sacral hiatus are anesthetized with a local anesthetic. An 18-gauge
Tuohy needle is advanced 2 to 3 cm into the sacral canal and its position confirmed by
fluoroscopic spread of injected water-soluble contrast medium (iohexol 200 mg/ml;
Omnipaque). Subsequently, a guide wire, introduced through the Tuohy needle, is directed
cranially as close as possible to the target area (as determined by previous diagnostic nerve
blocks and caudogram). Then a small incision is made at the introduction site and with the
guide wire in situ, the needle is replaced by a dilator and introducer sheath. The former is
removed and the side arm of the introducer sheath is left open to allow drainage of surplus
saline. A flexible 0.9 mm (OD) fiberoptic endoscope (magnification X45) is introduced

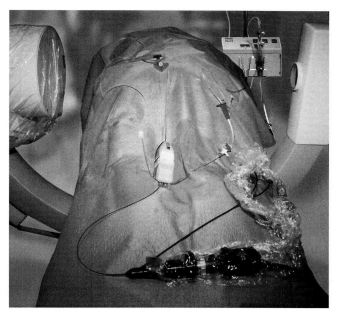

FIG. 21.2. The steerable catheter in situ. The right-sided channel is connected to a fluid instillation system. The left-sided channel is connected to an automatic pressure monitoring system.

through one of two main access ports of a disposable 2.2 mm (OD) steering catheter (Visionary BioMedical Inc.). This steering catheter also contains two side channels for fluid instillation. A standard light source and monitoring system is used. One side channel of the steering catheter is used for an intermittent flush of saline (Fig. 21.2). The other side channel is connected to an automatic monitoring system by means of a standard arterial pressure registration system (AS/3 monitor, Datex, Helsinki, Finland), for continuous registration of epidural/saline delivery pressure. After distension of the sacral epidural space with saline, the steering catheter with the fiberoptic endoscope is slowly advanced to the target area. The epidural space is kept distended with saline, but a pressure limit of 50 to 60 mmHg is set in order to minimize the risks of compromising local perfusion. Total saline volume infusion should not exceed 200 ml. During in vivo experiments in ewes it was found that, after varying cumulative injection volumes, resting pressure rose to 64.1 +/– 17.4 mmHg, to coincide with a peak CSF pressure exceeding 100 mmHg, indicating the compliance of the space had been compromised. If CSF pressure did not exceed 120 mmHg, recovery was without neurological sequelae. Initial decompression seems to occur via leakage into the large sacral root foramina and sheaths (12).

THE IDENTIFICATION OF EPIDURAL STRUCTURES

The following structures in the lumbosacral epidural space can be identified by endoscopy:

1. Epidural fat, which appears as loose, globular, glistening tissue of a yellowish color, with small blood vessels running through it.
2. Spinal dura mater, which is a convex tubular structure, gray-white colored, with blood vessels running on its surface that give it the appearance of a road map.

3. Lumbosacral nerve roots surrounded by their dural sleeve, extending caudodistally toward the intervertebral or sacral foramen. They appear as gray-white tubes with a single blood vessel running typically longitudinally down the center.
4. Ligamentum flavum, situated in the dorsal spinal canal as an arched roof, extending from lamina to lamina.
5. Small arteries, appearing as thin pulsating red threads with a opaque insulation.
6. Epidural venes and venous plexuses are not usually seen because they will collapse with rising epidural pressures during distension of the epidural space.
7. Adhesions, presenting as fibrous bands of tissue, mostly of a white appearance.
8. Inflammation, recognized by its erythematous appearance.

Inadvertent dural puncture shows a quite different view (Fig. 21.3) similar to the descriptions of Ooi et al. (5), who deliberately performed myeloscopy by introducing the endoscope intrathecally by a small incision in the dural sac. They could identify structures in the intrathecal space such as the cauda equina and even intervertebral discs.

CONTRAINDICATIONS FOR CAUDAL EPIDUROSCOPY

In patients with coagulopathy, infection, increased intracranial pressure, space-occupying processes of the central nervous system, and cerebrovascular disease, volumetric caudal injections and epiduroscopy should be avoided (52). Pregnant patients should not be submitted to the procedure, not only because of the harmful effects that radiation has on the developing fetus. Insufficient data exist on physiological changes (i.e., the compliance of the epidural space due to venous congestion prohibiting the instillation of saline) in this patient category. Also, patients with manifest bladder and bowel dysfunction resulting from sacral nerve injury are believed to be at increased risk of aggravation of symptoms during, or after, volumetric injections.

The generation of significant epidural pressures during epiduroscopy could affect local perfusion, or, by cephalad transmission through the CSF, compromise perfusion at more remote cerebral areas. Therefore, extreme care should be taken when performing such a procedure in patients with a low-compliant vertebral canal as, for example, could be expected in older patients and in the presence of central canal stenosis.

COMPLICATIONS

The potential complications of caudal epiduroscopy of the lumbosacral epidural space are similar to those described for conventional epidural injection techniques (53–57):

1. Infections: meningitis, arachnoiditis, epidural abcesses
2. Bleeding: epidural hematoma
3. Visual loss, retinal hemorrhage
4. Nerve root damage, causing paresis, dysesthesia, paresthesia
5. Dural perforation, causing postpuncture headache
6. Inadvertent intrathecal injection of medication
7. Increase of preexistent pain, low back pain
8. Pain at the catheter insertion site, spontaneously resolving within weeks

CONCLUSIONS

There is reason to believe that epiduroscopy by caudal route is a safe and useful technique. The diagnostic and therapeutic possibilities of this technique are still limited.

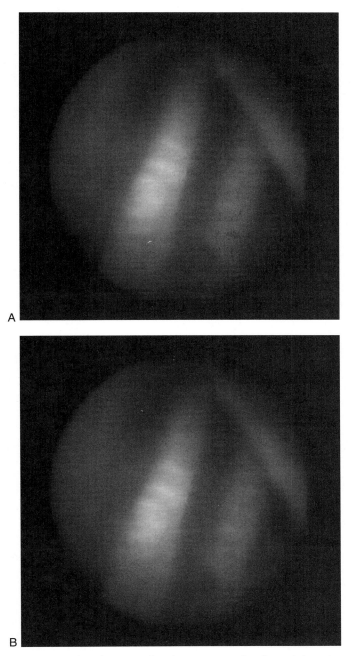

FIG. 21.3. A, B: Intrathecal endoscopy showing nerve roots of caudal equina.

For further improvements, for instance, laser technology that could be used to remove scar tissue, we must wait for more technological progress. The major goal in pain medicine, that is, a search for the main etiology of chronic pain syndromes, may be within reach with epiduroscopy for certain pain syndromes. Especially in patients with chronic low back pain, this is not as simple as it may sound. In fact, the application in low back pain of imaging techniques, that is, computerized tomography (CT) and magnetic resonance imaging (MRI) scanning, have revealed disappointing results so far because of the diagnostic false-positive and false-negative interpretations they lead to. Although, on the one hand, multiple gross disc prolapses can remain entirely asymptomatic, it is not at all unusual to find a patient complaining of well-localized severe radicular pain with no specific change on CT or MRI scan. In this rapidly developing field of modern endoscopy, high-quality three-dimensional color views will greatly improve our insights into the anatomical causes of radiculopathy. The therapeutic possibilities seem very promising, and we are probably not even halfway there in discovering them.

RESULTS

Recently we used targeted methylprednisolone acetate, hyaluronidase, and clonidine injection after diagnostic epiduroscopy for chronic sciatica and prospectively followed up patients for 1 year. Before injection of medication, we evaluated whether abnormalities at the lumbar level as diagnosed by MRI could be confirmed by epiduroscopy.

A flexible 0.9 mm fiberoptic endoscope was introduced through a disposable steering shaft into the caudal epidural space and advanced until the targeted spinal nerve was approximated. Adhesions were mechanically mobilized under direct vision and a mixture of 120 mg methylprednisolone acetate, 600 IU hyaluronidase, and 150 mg clonidine applied locally. Pain scores were measured by Visual Analogue Scale and Global Subjective Efficacy Rating.

Nineteen out of 20 included patients showed adhesions. In 8 patients, of which 6 had never undergone surgery, these were not detected with earlier MRI. Six patients showed concomitant signs of active root inflammation. Of 20 patients treated with a targeted epidural injection, 11 patients (55%) experienced significant pain relief at 3 months. This was maintained at 6, 9, and 12 months for 8 (40%), 7 (35%), and 7 (35%) patients, respectively. Mean VAS (visual analogue scan) at 3 months was significantly reduced (n = 20; ‰VAS = 3.55; p < 0.0001), and this persisted at 12 months (‰VAS = 1.99, p = 0.0073). We concluded that epiduroscopy is of value in the diagnosis of spinal root pathology. In sciatica, adhesions unreported by MRI can be identified. Targeted epidural medication, administered alongside the compromised spinal nerve, results in substantial and prolonged pain relief (58).

REFERENCES

1. Burman MS. Myeloscopy or the direct visualization of the spinal cord. J Bone Joint Surg 1931; 13: 695-6.
2. Stern EL. Spinascope, new instrument for visualizing the spinal canal and its contents. Med Rec (NY) 1936; 143: 31-2.
3. Pool JL. Direct visualization of dorsal nerve roots of cauda equina by means of a myeloscope. Arch Neurol Psychiat (Chicago) 1938; 39: 1308-12.
4. Pool JL. Myeloscopy, intrathecal endoscopy. Surgery 1942; 11: 169-82.
5. Ooi Y, Satoh Y, Morisaki N: Myeloscopy, possibility of observing lumbar intrathecal space by use of an endoscope. Endoscopy 1973; 5: 90-6.
6. Ooi Y, Satoh Y, Hirose K, Mikanagi K, Morisaki N. Myeloscopy. Acta Orthop Belg 1978; 44: 881-94.
7. Ooi Y, Satoh Y, Inoue K, Mikanagi K, Morisaki N. Myeloscopy, with special reference to blood flow changes in the cauda equina during Lasègue's test. Int Orthop 1981; 4; 307-11.

8. Ooi Y, Mita F, Satoh Y. Myeloscopic study on lumbar spinal canal stenosis with special reference to intermittent claudication. Spine 1990; 15(6): 544-9.
9. Heavner JE, Chokhavatia S, Kizelshteyn G. Percutaneous evaluation of the epidural and subarachnoid space with the flexible fiberscope. Reg Anesth 1991;15 (Suppl): 85.
10. Heavner JE, Chokhavatia S, McDaniel K, et al. Diagnostic and therapeutic maneuvers in the epidural space via a flexible endoscope. Abstracts—7th World Congress on Pain 1993; 573-4.
11. Yamakawa K, Kondo T, Yoshioka M, Takakura K. Application of superfine fiberscope for endovasculoscopy, ventriculoscopy, and myeloscopy. Acta Neurochir Suppl Wien 1992; 54: 47-52.
12. Serpell M, Coombs DW, Colburn RW, et al. Intrathecal pressure recordings due to saline instillation in the epidural space. Abstracts—7th World Congress on Pain 1993; 574.
13. Rosenberg PH, Heavner JE, Chokhavatia S. Epiduroscopy with a thin flexible and deflectable fiberscope. Br J Anaesth 1994; 72 (Suppl 1): 74-5.
14. Hertz H, Schabus R, Wunderlich M. [Endoscopy of the spinal canal]. Endoskopie des Spinalkanals—experimentelle Untersuchungen an Leichen. Unfallchirurgie 1985; 11: 275-7.
15. Mollmann M, Holst D, Enk D, Filler T, Lubbesmeyer H, Deitmer T, Lawin P. [Spinal endoscopy in the detection of problems caused by continuous spinal anesthesia]. Spinaloskopie zur Darstellung von Problemen bei der Anwendung der kontinuierlichen Spinalanasthesie. Anaesthesist 1992; 41(9): 544-7.
16. Mollmann M, Holst D, Lubbesmeyer H, Lawin P. Continuous spinal anesthesia: mechanical and technical problems of catheter placement. Reg Anesth 1993; 18(6 Suppl): 469-72.
17. Holmstrom B, Rawal N, Axelsson K, Nydahl PA. Risk of catheter migration during combined spinal epidural block: percutaneous epiduroscopy study. Anesth Analg 1995; 80(4):747-53.
18. Beuls EA, van Mameren H, Vroomen PC. Caudascopic experiences and a new patho-anatomic concept for treatment of sciatica. Minim Invasive Neurosurg 1996; 39: 4-6.
19. Witte H, Hellweg S, Witte B, Grifka J. [Epiduroscopy with access via the sacral canal. Some constructional equipment requirements from the anatomic and biomechanical viewpoint]. Epiduroskopie mit Zugang uber den Sakralkanal. Einige konstruktive Anforderungen an Instrumente aus anatomischer und biomechanischer Sicht. Biomed Tech Berl 1997; 42: 24-9.
20. Jerosch J, Gronemeyer D, Gevargez A, Filler TJ, Peuker ET. [Possibilities of spinal endoscopy within the scope of minimal invasive intervention—an experimental study]. Moglichkeiten der Spinaloskopie im Rahmen der minimal invasiven Intervention—eine experimentelle Untersuchung. Biomed Tech Berl 1999; 44: 243-6.
21. Blomberg R. A method for epiduroscopy and spinaloscopy. Presentation of preliminary results. Acta Anaesthesiol Scand 1985; 29: 113-6.
22. Blomberg R. The dorsomedian connective tissue band in the lumbar epidural space of humans: an anatomical study using epiduroscopy in autopsy cases. Anesth Analg 1986; 65: 747-52.
23. Blomberg RG. The lumbar subdural extraarachnoid space of humans: an anatomical study using spinaloscopy in autopsy cases. Anesth Analg 1987; 66: 177-80.
24. Blomberg RG. Technical advantages of the paramedian approach for lumbar epidural puncture and catheter introduction. A study using epiduroscopy in autopsy subjects. Anaesthesia 1988; 43: 837-43.
25. Blomberg RG. Epiduroscopy and spinaloscopy: endoscopic studies of lumbar spinal spaces. Acta Neurochir Suppl Wien 1994; 61: 106-7.
26. Blomberg RG. Fibrous structures in the subarachnoid space: a study with spinaloscopy in autopsy subjects. Anesth Analg 1995; 80: 875-9.
27. Blomberg RG, Olsson SS. The lumbar epidural space in patients examined with epiduroscopy. Anesth Analg 1989; 68(2): 157-60.
28. Igarashi T, Hirabayashi Y, Shimizu R, Mitsuhata H, Saitoh K, Fukuda H, Konishi A, Asahara H. Inflammatory changes after extradural anaesthesia may affect the spread of local anaesthetic within the extradural space. Br J Anaesth 1996; 77: 347-51.
29. Igarashi T, Hirabayashi Y, Shimizu R, Saitoh K, Fukuda H, Mitsuhata H. The lumbar extradural structure changes with increasing age. Br J Anaesth 1997; 78: 149-52.
30. Igarashi T, Hirabayashi Y, Shimizu R, Saitoh K, Fukuda H. Thoracic and lumbar extradural structure examined by extraduroscope. Br J Anaesth 1998; 81: 121-5.
31. Igarashi T, Hirabayashi Y, Shimizu R, Saitoh K, Fukuda H. The epidural structure changes during deep breathing. Can J Anaesth 1999; 46: 850-5.
32. Shimoji K, Fujioka H, Onodera M, Hokari T, Fukuda S, Fujiwara N, Hatori T. Observation of spinal canal and cisternae with the newly developed small-diameter, flexible fiberscopes. Anesthesiology 1991; 75: 341-4.
33. Peek RD, Thomas JC, Jr., Wiltse LL. Diagnosis of lumbar arachnoiditis by myeloscopy. Spine 1993; 18(15): 2286-9.
34. Schutze G, Kurtze H. Direct observation of the epidural space with a flexible catheter-secured epiduroscopic unit. Reg Anesth 1994; 19(2): 85-9.
35. Kawauchi Y, Yone K, Sakou T. Myeloscopic observation of adhesive arachnoiditis in patients with lumbar spinal canal stenosis. Spinal Cord 1996; 34(7): 403-10.
36. Uchiyama S, Hasegawa K, Homma T, Takahashi HE, Shimoji K. Ultrafine flexible spinal endoscope (myeloscope) and discovery of an unreported subarachnoid lesion. Spine 1998; 23(21): 2358-62.
37. Eguchi T, Tamaki N, Kurata H. Endoscopy of the spinal cord: cadaveric study and clinical experience. Minim Invasive Neurosurg 1999; 42(3): 146-51.

38. Saberski LR, Kitahata LM. Direct visualization of the lumbosacral epidural space through the sacral hiatus. Anesth Analg 1995; 80: 839-40.
39. Saberski LR, Brull SJ. Epidural endoscopy-aided drug delivery: a case report. Yale J Biol Med 1995; 68(1-2): 17-8.
40. Richardson J, McGurgan P, Cheema S, Prasad R, Gupta S. Spinal endoscopy in chronic low-back pain with radiculopathy. A prospective case series. Forthcoming in Anaesthesia.
41. Raffaeli W, Pari G, Visani L, Balestri M. Periduroscopy: preliminary reports—technical notes. The Pain Clinic 1999; 11: 209-12.
42. Manchikanti L, Bakhit CE. Removal of a torn Racz catheter from lumbar epidural space. Reg Anest 1997; 22: 579-81.
43. Olmarker K, Brisby H, Yabuki S, Norborg C, Rydevik B. The effects of normal, frozen and hyaluronidase digested nucleus pulposus on nerve root structure and function. Spine 1997; 22: 471-5.
44. Olmarker K, Myers RR. Pathogenesis of sciatic pain: role of herniated nucleus pulposus, and deformation of spinal nerve root and dorsal root ganglion. Pain 1998; 78: 99-105.
45. Hasue M. Pain and the nerve root. An interdisciplinary approach. Spine 1993; 18: 2053-8.
46. Cornefjord M, Olmarker K, Rydevik B, Nordborg C. Mechanical and biochemical injury of spinal nerve roots. A morphological and neurophysiological study. Eur Spine J 1996; 5: 187-92.
47. Rydevik B, Brown MD, Lundborg G. Pathoanatomy and pathophysiology of nerve root compression. Spine 1984; 9: 7-15.
48. Rydevik B, Holm S, Brown MD, Lundborg G. Diffusion from the CSF as a nutritional pathway for spinal nerve roots. Acta Physiol Scand 1990; 138: 247-8.
49. Kayama S, Konno S, Olmarker K, Yabuki S, Kikuchi S. Incision of the annulus fibrosus induces nerve root morphologic, vascular and functional changes. An experimental study. Spine 1996; 21: 2539-43.
50. Kotani K, Arai I, Mao PG, Konno S, Olmarker K, Kikuchi S. Experimental disc herniation. Evaluation of the natural course. Spine 1997; 22: 2894-9.
51. Rydevik Bl, Pedowitz RA, Hargens AR. Effects of acute, graded compression on spinal nerve root function and structure. Spine 1991; 16: 487-93.
52. Saberski LR. Spinal endoscopy: current concepts. In: Waldman SD, Winnie AP (eds.), Interventional pain management. Philadelphia: WB Saunders, 1996; 137-49.
53. Abram SE, O'Connor ThC. Complications associated with epidural steroid injections. Reg Anesth 1996; 21: 149-62.
54. Purdy EP, Ajimal GS. Vision loss after lumbar epidural steroid injection. Anesth Analg 1998; 86: 119-22.
55. Williams RC, Doliner SJ, Lipton RM, Franz JA, Delaney RD. Retinal hemorrhage as a consequence of epidural steroid injection. Arch Ophthalmol 1996; 114: 362-3.
56. Amirikia A, Scott IU, Murray TG, Halperin LS. Acute bilateral visual loss associated with retinal hemorrhages following epiduroscopy. Arch Ophthalmol 2000; 118: 287-9.
57. Geurts JW, et al. Methylprednisolone acetate/hyaluronidase/clonidine injection after diagnostic epiduroscopy: prospective, 1-year follow-up study. Reg Anest Pain Med 2002: 27: 343-52.

22

Revision Lumbar Fusion

Stephen Eisenstein

A patient returning with back pain after an apparently successful lumbar spinal fusion for pain is one of the most disheartening experiences for the spinal surgeon. There are some well-known causes of relapse of pain, such as adjacent level spondylosis, fixation failure, and late infection, but the presumption must be that there is a pseudarthrosis somewhere in the fusion mass, until proved otherwise. The diagnosis of a pseudarthrosis in itself is fraught with difficulty, and the difficult decision to offer revision surgery is usually made in anticipation of further failure and a high complication rate (1,2). The fact remains that the serious and responsible spinal surgeon must be prepared to accept this challenge as part of the service. A patient with recurrent disabling symptoms and a known technical failure should not be left to suffer without some hope.

Investigations should be repeated if only to eliminate the possibility that the recurrence of pain originates in a degenerating adjacent segment (3). These investigations present another challenge if metal internal fixation of the primary surgery produces a significant artifact on MRI. If there is a major suspicion that the new pain originates in the adjacent mobile segment and MRI is not conclusive, discography may be necessary to prove or exclude the adjacent segment as the source of pain.

The surgeon is then faced with the decision to approach the spine through the previous surgical field or to approach through healthy normal tissue from the opposite direction. The scar tissue of previous posterior surgery provides a relatively avascular bed for new bone graft, and repeat surgery through previous scars frequently results in permanent distressing dysesthesias. It is an attractive proposition to rescue failed posterior fusions through a retroperitoneal anterior approach. The potential vascular, sympathectomy, and retrograde ejaculation complications may be daunting. This is surgery for the experienced anterior surgeon. Likewise, previous anterior surgery will present the surgeon returning there with retroperitoneal fibrosis. The great vessels will be dangerously disguised and immobile. The risk of venous hemorrhage is significant. There is evidence that a fresh-tissue approach is indeed the strategy most likely to succeed for patients who have had no implants (4).

In recent years there would be very few patients without implants of some kind. It is the author's perception that posterior pseudarthrosis in the presence of loose implants is associated with pain far greater than when there are no implants. This perception is based on an experience that began in the era prior to internal fixation. The presence of internal fixation will serve to modify the fresh-tissue strategy: pedicle screw fixation is probably the most common posterior fixation and should be removed in revision surgery because it is almost certainly a cause of persisting pain within a pseudarthrosis. This means a posterior revision will have to follow a primary posterior procedure, and the ideal of a fresh-tissue approach (anterior, in this example) will have to be abandoned. The distal fragment of a broken screw may be left in situ, analogous to an amalgam filling in a tooth. It is tempting, then, having achieved the necessary exposure, to continue with decortication of all exposed bone and to regraft with fresh autogenous bone. If it is felt useful and safe to apply new pedicle screw fixation, previous pedicle entries may be used but tapped to receive larger diameter screws.

The next decision is whether or not to proceed to additional anterior fusion in the hope that anterior strutting with autograft or allograft will increase the likelihood of success (1,5–7). The decision must be tempered by a judgment of the risks of so much surgery as against the benefits to be expected. Some encouragement to settle for posterior revision alone comes from a study that revealed a 77% good or excellent result (3).

The presence of interbody cages in a segment of pseudarthrosis does not imply that these cages must be removed, as recommended for pedicle screw fixation: it is simply too dangerous to neural tissue posteriorly and vascular/retroperitoneal structures anteriorly to be worth the attempt. Failed anterior fusion is rescued with relative ease by posterior fusion with autograft and pedicle screw fixation (8).

The most sophisticated imaging techniques will not clearly define every pseudarthrosis preoperatively. Inevitably there will be occasions where revision surgery is performed for a suspected pseudarthrosis and none can be found after diligent clearance of scar tissue to allow visual confirmation of continuity of graft. Even then, the fusion must be stress-tested under vision because an apparently impressive bar of bone graft may yet have failed to fuse with the relevant vertebra. There need be no embarrassment because second surgery was required to prove a fusion: conveying this information to the patient postoperatively has sometimes produced a spontaneous remission of symptoms in the author's experience.

If internal fixation is present within a surgically proven solid posterior fusion, the advice would be to remove the fixation, usually pedicle screw fixation. On a few occasions in the author's experience, this action has also resulted in a spontaneous remission of pain symptoms (see also Wild et al. [9]), although the general experience has been disappointing. These spontaneous remissions after metal removal remain something of a mystery, and the pain generation has been blamed on some reaction or allergy to the metal under a vague diagnosis of "metallosis." Granulation tissue found in the vicinity of the metal fixation at revision surgery, particularly in respect to stainless steel and chrome cobalt, lent some credence to the concept of metallosis (10,11). Now that titanium is used almost universally, this granulation tissue is rarely evident at revision surgery. Microscopic particles could still be a factor in macrophage activation and inflammation (12), but there is evidence that patients with a solid fusion have negligible levels of particulate matter (13).

REFERENCES

1. Etminan M, Girardi FP, Khan SN, Cammisa FP. Revision strategies for lumbar pseudarthrosis. Orthop Clin N Am 2002; 33:381-92.
2. Whitecloud T, Butler JC, Cohen JL, Candelora PD. Complications with the variable spinal plating system. Spine 1989; 14:472-6.
3. Chen W, Lai PL, Niu CC, Chen LH, Fu TS, Wong CB. Surgical treatment of adjacent segment instability after lumbar spine fusion. Spine 2001; 26:19-24.
4. Jaffray D, Eisenstein S. Repair of pseudarthroses for back pain. Soc Back Pain Res Proc 1990; 53-4.
5. Albert TJ, Pinto M, Denis F. Management of symptomatic lumbar pseudarthrosis with anteroposterior fusion. A functional and radiographic outcome study. Spine 2000; 25:123-9.
6. Buttermann GR, Glazer PA, Hu SS, Bradford DS. Revision of failed lumbar fusions. A comparison of anterior autograft and allograft. Spine 1997; 22:2748-55.
7. Slosar P, Reynolds JB, Schofferman J, Goldthwaite N, White AH, Keaney D. Patient satisfaction after circumferential lumbar fusion. Spine 2000; 25:722-6.

8. McAfee PC, Cunningham BW, Lee GA, Orbegoso CM, Haggerty CJ, Fedder IL, Griffith SL. Revision strategies or salvaging or improving failed cylindrical cages. Spine 1999; 24:2147-53.

9. Wild A, Pinto MR, Butler L, Bressan C, Wroblewski JM. Removal of lumbar instrumentation for the treatment of recurrent low back pain in the absence of pseudarthrosis. Arch Orthop Trauma Surg 2003; (in press).

10. Betts F, Wright T, Salvati EA, Boskey A, Bansal M. Cobalt-alloy metal debris in periarticular tissues from total hip revision arthroplasties: metal contents and associated histologic findings. Clin Orthop 1992; 26:75-82.

11. Takahashi S, Delecrin J, Passuti N. Intraspinal metallosis causing delayed neurologic symptoms after spinal instrumentation surgery. Spine 2001; 26:1495-8.

12. Holgers KM, Thomsen P, Tjellstrom A, Ericson LE. Electron microscopic observations of the soft tissue around clinical long-term percutaneous titanium implants. Biomaterials 1995; 16:83-99.

13. Wang JC, Yu WD, Sandhu HS, Betts F, Bhuta S, Delamarter RB. Metal debris from titanium spinal implants. Spine 1999; 24: 899-903.

23

Treatment Algorithm for the Failed Back Surgery Syndrome

Luc Vanden Berghe

INTRODUCTION

Patients with failed back surgery syndrome (FBSS) present with primarily leg or low back pain, despite previous low back surgery. There are many possible causes for the persisting symptoms and also different types of pain. Treatment of this syndrome presents a challenge to physicians because conservative therapies and repeated surgery are often unsuccessful. Neuropathic pain is often the main cause of this persistent syndrome. In this case, spinal cord stimulation (SCS) may be considered. To address the challenge of managing chronic back and leg pain, an expert consensus group was convened to discuss this problem. The result was a new algorithm for the treatment of chronic pain in patients with FBSS. The use of SCS treatment in patients with FBSS is highlighted in this chapter. Use of these guidelines should allow more rational and straightforward management of this common and clinically—as well as economically—important problem.

Approximately 5% of people experience a new episode of low back pain each year and, over the course of a lifetime, 60% to 85% of people experience at least one episode of low back pain (1–4). With or without treatment, about two thirds of patients return to normal, but a third go on to suffer from a condition that is either chronic or recurs frequently, often with some degree of functional impairment (5,6). Therefore, at any time, a substantial proportion of the population is suffering from troublesome back pain. As a result of this persistent pain, a substantial number of patients will receive, in the first instance, conservative therapies. If these provide inadequate benefits, many will be referred for surgical treatment. About 30% of patients undergoing such lumbosacral surgery "fail," as defined by postoperative persistent or recurrent low back pain, with or without leg pain (7,8). This condition is called the failed back surgery syndrome (FBSS). The treatment of patients with FBSS presents a particular challenge to physicians because there is a wide differential diagnosis, with different types of pain and many treatment options. Some treatment options are beneficial for some problems, but less for others. Reoperation is often unsuccessful (9,10), so these patients may require a multidisciplinary approach to their therapy.

In the face of these challenges to the management of chronic back and leg pain, in particular in patients who have undergone unsuccessful surgery, a workshop was arranged to discuss these problems. The consensus group comprised a multidisciplinary team of experts with wide experience in the fields of pain management and spinal surgery. The objective of the workshop was to discuss and develop treatment algorithms for patients experiencing chronic pain even after technically and anatomically successful spinal surgery related to their specific diagnosis. This patient group might benefit from minimally invasive therapies such as spinal cord stimulation (SCS) and/or intrathecal drug delivery. This chapter provides an overview of the treatment options available for patients with back and leg pain, particularly those with FBSS. Treatment algorithms developed from the data collected and from the panel discussions are presented.

CAUSES OF FBSS

FBSS is defined as persistent or recurrent back and leg pain after technically adequate lumbar spinal surgery (17). The pain can be neuropathic, nociceptive, psychological/ psychogenic, or a combination of these three elements (10a). Neuropathic pain arises from neural tissue injury, whereas nociceptive (mechanical) pain is caused by nonneural tissue injury, such as joint/muscle damage. The causes of FBSS are inappropriate patient selection, irreversible nerve injury with unrealistic expectations, inadequate surgery, recurrent pathology, and failed surgery (28,30).

The most common cause of FBSS is *inappropriate patient selection* (18–21). If the anatomical source of the pain is not clear or if other problems are involved, like psychological problems or compensation, the results of surgery are often poor. The course of low back pain is in many cases benign, and early surgical intervention is often unnecessary and may complicate the condition (9,10).

The second most common cause of FBSS is the persistence of pain resulting from *irreversible nerve injury* and the patient's unrealistic expectations of relief from this pain. Such persistent nerve injury may result from the original cause of the back pain; for example, damage to the dorsal nerve roots by compression from a herniated disc.

A less common cause of FBSS is *inadequate surgery,* for example, persistence of a sequestered disc fragment or of a foraminal or subarticular spinal stenosis (23). A missed far lateral disc herniation is also a possible cause of persisting symptoms. A badly positioned pedicular screw or intervertebral cage, irritating neurological structures, may also cause persisting symptoms.

A cause of recurrent symptoms may be a *recurrent disc herniation,* occurring in more than 5% of the cases, or *adjacent-level pathology. Failed fusion surgery* with a pseudarthrosis may also lead to incapacitating back pain.

DIAGNOSIS

Several diagnostic tools are available for the patient presenting with back pain (12,13). History taking and physical examination are central to this diagnostic process. In general, the patient wants to begin with the recent history, but it helps to learn about the first episode of back or leg pain, perhaps many years before. We need to know if there was a sudden onset or an injury, whether litigation was involved, and so on (29).

History: Evolution of the Pain

Trying to determine the cause of leg pain after surgery, it is useful to classify the leg pain by the time course of its appearance. If the leg pain after surgery is the same as before surgery, the surgery may have been inadequate with residual structural pathology (nociceptive pain) or nerve injury present (neuropathic pain).

Leg pain worse after surgery or not present before surgery may be caused by nerve injury during surgery or new pathology introduced during surgery. If the leg pain disappeared after surgery but reappeared after a period, recurrent pathology is likely.

If there is significant back pain after disc or decompressive surgery, it may be caused by instability or discogenic sources. Significant back pain after a previous fusion operation may be caused by pseudarthrosis or adjacent-level disease.

History: Types of Pain

Leg pain after previous lumbar surgery can be nociceptive (mechanical), neuropathic, psychogenic, or a mixture of these three elements. Pain radiating to the leg may also be referred pain as a result of a low back problem. Nociceptive pain is due to a identifiable structural abnormality activating nociceptors, like pressure on a nerve root. It is usually not constant and increases with activity. In most cases, a structural problem can be demonstrated as the cause of the pain.

When no structural abnormalities can be demonstrated, the pain may be neuropathic. Neuropathic pain is due to neural tissue injury and often associated with sensory abnormalities, such as elevated tactile thresholds (hyperthesia) or abnormal or unfamiliar sensations like burning (dysesthesias), allodynia, or hyperalgesia. The pain is usually felt in an area where there is a sensory abnormality. It usually is constant (day and night) but may increase with activity. Accurate diagnosis of the type of pain is essential because this will have an impact on the type of therapy chosen.

Clinical Examination

Although a clinical examination is more of a subjective assessment, it may provide valuable information (11). The examination begins as the patient is entering the consultation room. Is he or she limping, walking with short steps, or listing to one side? While giving the history, the clinical examination is already under way, and much is revealed by the patient's attitude: depressive, hysterical, obsessional, or malingering. A careful clinical examination is important in the diagnostic work. Painful lumbar flexion may suggest a lumbar disc lesion, instability, or a pseudarthrosis. An extension catch, a jerky resistance halfway through the process of standing up from the stooped position, is a sign of instability. Painful extension can be caused by apophyseal joint lesions or by spondylolisis (27). Careful neurological examination of the lower limb may help to find out which nerve root is affected and to find out if the pain is neuropathic or nociceptive.

Technical Examinations

Standing X-rays with flexion and extension views may show instability and misalignment. Conventional X-rays can sometimes show a pseudarthrosis: if a lytic zone occurs around the fixing material, if there is abnormal movement on the flexion-extension images, or if resorption of the graft occurs.

A CT may show recurrent disc herniation, central or foraminal stenosis, and may detect a pseudarthrosis, especially in the presence of metal implants. The MRI scan is becoming the examination of choice in patients with spinal problems. It shows disc degeneration, annular tears, and central, lateral, and foraminal disc herniations. It allows evaluation of the spinal canal and the diagnosis of central and lateral spinal stenosis (16). Isotope scans may also be helpful in detecting a pseudarthrosis or an infection. Discograms, injection studies, and nerve conduction studies also may prove helpful in selected cases (15).

Psychological Evaluation

Psychological examination of the patient may also be appropriate, particularly when making decisions about treatment, because various psychological factors have been associated with poor outcome (14).

Treatment of the FBSS

Following the diagnostic work-up, the patient will usually fall in one of these diagnostic groups: primarily nociceptive leg pain, primarily neuropathic leg pain, or primarily back pain.

Primarily Nociceptive Leg Pain

The treatment is usually staged. For many patients a combination of analgesics and nonsteroidal antiinflammatory drugs (NSAIDs) may be adequate to manage the pain. If there is residual spinal stenosis, an epidural infiltration at the stenotic level may be indicated. If there is foraminal stenosis, a CT-guided foraminal infiltration with local anesthetic and steroids around the nerve root can relieve the pain and is also a helpful diagnostic tool. If the infiltration has no effect on the pain, probably the foraminal stenosis is not the cause of the pain or the pain may be neuropathic. Further surgery will probably not be effective (26).

Physiotherapy may be used both as symptomatic treatment and as rehabilitation to improve conditioning, reeducate muscles of the back and abdomen, and promote good postural practices (22). If the leg pain is resistant to conservative therapy and if there is a clear cause of the pain, repeat surgery can be considered. In a number of cases, like a recurrent disc herniation, a lateral disc herniation, a subarticular stenosis, and so on, a microsurgical decompression may be sufficient. In other cases, like a foraminal stenosis due to disc collapse or central spinal stenosis due to a degenerative anterolisthesis, the decompression may have to be combined with a fusion. If possible, normal anatomical proportions should be restored using intervertebral cages and internal fixation and stabilization (25).

If repeat surgery is unsuccessful, neuromodulation can be considered, although it is less successful for nociceptive pain. If a neuromodulation trial proves unsuccessful, systemic medication including opioids can be used.

Primarily Neuropathic Leg Pain

Medication management can be successful for patients with neuropathic leg pain after surgery. The most useful medications are anticonvulsants like carbamazepine and gabapentin, tricyclic antidepressants, and opioid analgesics. Infiltrations and repeat surgery have been proven less effective in the treatment of neuropathic leg pain.

If conservative treatment with medications does not improve the condition, spinal cord stimulation can be indicated. Multidisciplinary assessment of the patient and careful screening is important. If the patient proves to be a suitable candidate, a trial stimulation will be used, with final implantation if the trial is successful. The tip of the electrodes is usually placed between T8 and T12. In most patients, the use of single-lead stimulation is adequate, but sometimes a second lead may be required to produce enough paraesthesia cover and corresponding pain relief.

Primarily Low Back Pain

The low back pain may originate from the previously operated level or from an adjacent level. Adjacent-level pain can be discogenic pain, apophyseal joint pain, or sacroiliac joint pain. The anatomical source of the pain can be demonstrated by MRI, technetium scan, but often diagnostic injection of the painful disc or apophyseal joints are necessary to locate the source.

Pain originating from the previously operated level may be due to degenerative disease, instability, failed fusion, or idiopathic (no clear cause). Degenerative disease or instability at the previously operated level is most common after discectomy or decompressive surgery.

Again, the treatment is usually staged. Pain medication, antiinflammatory drugs, injection therapy, and physiotherapy may be adequate to manage the pain. If, however, these remedies are not effective in the long term, other therapies must be sought (24).

In patients with discogenic or apophyseal pain, the symptoms may be so resistant that surgical treatment is considered. The best indications are patients with degenerative changes at one or at the most two levels, with a positive discography and modic changes on MRI images. Interbody fusion currently provides the best results, but total disc replacement in selected cases is gaining popularity, although long-term results with this procedure are not available.

In the event of persisting pain resulting from instability (degenerative antero- or laterolisthesis), an interbody or posterolateral fusion combined with internal fixation may provide good relief of the pain. In failed fusion surgery, with a pseudarthrosis, a repeat fusion attempt may be indicated, often with a combined anterior and posterior approach (360-degree fusion), but the results are often disappointing.

If repeat surgery is not indicated or fails to provide pain relief, a trial of spinal cord stimulation can be considered, although it is still experimental in the treatment of low back pain. Some studies show favorable results. Another option is systemic opioids or intrathecal morphine.

SUMMARY

Chronic low back and leg pain, particularly in patients who have undergone unsuccessful surgery, represents a great therapeutic challenge. Nevertheless, good therapeutic outcomes can be achieved in many patients.

In the treatment of the FBSS, accurate diagnosis of the type of pain is essential. Careful history taking and a physical and psychological examination will allow accurate patient selection for appropriate therapy.

Repeat surgery is often not successful and only indicated if there is a clear anatomical problem with nociceptive pain. Neuromodulatory therapy may produce beneficial effects and is the treatment of choice for neuropathic pain of a nonstructural nature.

REFERENCES

1. Svensson HO, Andersson GBJ. The relationship of low-back pain, work history, work environment, and stress: a retrospective cross-sectional study of 38 to 64 year old women. Spine 1989;14:517-22.
2. Frymoyer JW, Cats-Baril WL. An overview of the incidence and costs of low back pain. Orthop Clin N Am 1991;22:263-71.
3. Papageorgiou AC, Croft PR, Forry S, et al. Estimating the prevalence of low back pain in the general population: evidence from the South Manchester back pain survey. Spine 1995;20:1889-94.
4. Cassidy DJ. The Saskatchewan Health and Back Pain Survey: the prevalence of low back pain and related disability in Saskatchewan. Spine 1998;23:1860-7.

5. Hakelius A. Prognosis in sciatica: a clinical follow-up of surgical and non-surgical treatment. Acta Orthop Scand 1970;129 (Suppl):1-76.

6. Weber H. Lumbar disc herniation: a controlled prospective study with ten years of observation. Spine 1983;8:131-40.

7. Segal R, Stacey BR, Rudy TE, et al. Spinal cord stimulation revisited. Neurol Res 1998;20:391-6.

8. North RB, Ewend MG, Lawton MT, et al. Failed back surgery syndrome: 5-year follow-up after spinal cord stimulator implantation. Neurosurgery 1991;28:692-9.

9. Waddell G, Kummel EG, Lotto WN, et al. Failed lumbar disc surgery and repeat surgery following industrial injuries. J Bone Joint Surg Am 1979;61:201-7.

10. North RB, Campbell JN, James CS, et al. Failed back surgery syndrome: five-year follow up in 102 patients undergoing reoperation. Neurosurgery 1991;28:685-91.

10a. Portenoy R. Mechanisms of clinical pain. Neural Clin 1989;7:205-29.

11. Porter RW. Management of back pain. London: Churchill Livingstone, 1986.

12. Borenstein D. Epidemiology, etiology, diagnostic evaluation, and treatment of low back pain. Curr Opin Rheumatol 1998;10:104-9.

13. Bigos SJ, Müller G. Primary care approach to acute and chronic back problems: definitions and care. In: Loeser JD, ed., Bonica's management of pain (3rd ed.). London: Lippincott, Williams and Wilkins, 2000: 1509-28.

14. Block AR. Psychological screening of spine surgery candidates: risk factors for poor outcome. In: Loeser JD, ed., Bonica's management of pain (3rd ed.). London: Lippincott, Williams and Wilkins, 2000: 1549-57.

15. Gresham JL, Miller R. Evaluation of lumbar spine by discography. Clin Orthop 1969;67:29-41.

16. Boden SD, Davis DO, Dina TS, et al. Abnormal magnetic-resonance scans of the lumbar spine in asymptomatic subjects. A prospective investigation. J Bone Joint Surg Am 1990;72:403-81.

17. Kumar K, Toth C, Nath RK, Lang P. Epidural spinal cord stimulation for treatment of chronic pain—some predictors of success: a 15-year experience. Surg Neurol 1998;50:110-21.

18. Spengler DM, Freeman C, Westbrook R, et al. Low-back pain following multiple lumbar spine procedures: failure of initial selection? Spine 1980;5:356-60.

19. Zucherman J, Schofferman J. Pathology of failed back surgery syndrome. In: White AH, ed., Failed back surgery syndrome. Philadelphia: Hanley & Belfus, 1986: 1-12.

20. Fager CA, Freidberg SR. Analysis of failures and poor results of lumbar spine surgery. Spine 1980;5:87-94.

21. Long DM, Filtzer DL, BenDebba M, et al. Clinical features of the failed-back syndrome. J Neurosurg 1988;69: 61-71.

22. Seeger D. Physiotherapy in low back pain—indications and limits. Schmerz 2001;15:461-7.

23. Burton CV, Kirkaldy-Willis WH, Yong-Hing K, et al. Causes of failure of surgery on the lumbar spine. Clin Orthop 1981;157:191-9.

24. Nachemson A, Zdeblick TA, O'Brien JP. Lumbar disc disease with discogenic pain. What surgical treatment is most effective? Spine 1996;21:1835-8.

25. Brantigan JW, Steffee AD. A carbon fiber implant to aid interbody lumbar fusion. Two-year clinical results in the first 26 patients. Spine 1993;18:2106-17.

26. Wise JJ, Andersson BJ. Role of surgery in the treatment of low back pain and sciatica. In: Loeser JD, ed., Bonica's management of pain (3rd ed.). London: Lippincott, Williams and Wilkins, 2000: 1528-39.

27. Armstrong JR. The causes of unsatisfactory results from the operative treatment of lumbar disc lesions. J Bone Joint Surg 1951;33B:31-5.

28. Burton CV, Kirkaldy-Willis WH, Yong-Hing K, et al. Causes of failure of surgery on the lumbar spine. Clin Orthop 1981;157:191-9.

29. Long DM. Failed back syndrome: etiology, assessment, and treatment. In: Burchiel KJ, ed., Surgical management of pain. New York: Thieme, 2002: 354-64.

30. Fritsch EW, Heisel J, Rupp S. The failed back surgery syndrome: reasons, intraoperative findings, and long-term results: a report of 182 operative treatments. Spine 1996;21:626-33.

24

Mechanical Supplementation by Dynamic Fixation in Degenerative Intervertebral Lumbar Segments: The Wallis System

Jacques Sénégas

BACKGROUND

Necessity being the mother of invention, distal joint repair and replacement began much earlier than analogous work on spinal segments. Indeed, the unique organization of the intervertebral articulations in a kinetic chain provides the capacity to compensate relatively well for the loss of a single mobile segment caused by operative fusion. This explains the continued extensive use of spinal arthrodesis to date. Nonetheless, prompted by progress in the surgical management of distal joint disorders, we began studying and developing nonrigid stabilization of lumbar segments in 1984.

After conducting preliminary biomechanical cadaver studies between 1984 and 1986, we opted for a tension-band system with no bony fixation because of the incompatibility of bony purchase (such as that provided by pedicle screws) with a dynamic stabilization device. The pioneer system we developed and first implanted in 1986 included a titanium interspinous spacer and a cord of woven polyester. Following an observational study in 1988 (1,2), we carried out a prospective controlled study from 1988 to 1993 (3,4). We permitted only cautious, limited diffusion of this device while waiting for assessment of long-term results.

These studies and subsequent limited diffusion showed promising results and an absence of serious complications. We then developed a second-generation device called the Wallis system, which was fundamentally updated and improved. The former metallic interspinous spacer was replaced by a redesigned spacer made of polyetheretherketone (PEEK), a more resilient material, and the cord was replaced by flat bands of woven polyester.

BASIC CONCEPTS

Three aspects are fundamental to understanding the Wallis implant and the mechanical normalization it provides:

1. *Degenerative disc disease is basically a mechanical disorder.* Acute or progressive disc lesions create instability of the motion segment. This instability is best characterized by a loss of stiffness, which contributes to further deterioration and leads to a vicious cycle exacerbated by a concentration of stress on the posterior portion of the disc.

As in any mobile, dynamic system submitted to a force, intervertebral segments undergo acceleration inversely proportional to the moment of inertia. The stiffness of the segment dampens this movement. This braking action preserves a margin of security and contributes to the protection of the disc and intervertebral ligaments. Stiffness, or rigidity, is a mechanical parameter defined in terms of load for a given displacement. It corresponds to the derivative of the load/deformity curve.

Ebara et al. (5) and Mimura et al. (6) demonstrated that segmental laxity or loss of rigidity is constant in degenerative disc disease. This is observed throughout the course of the degenerative process. Early on, before loss of disc height, bending studies reveal a wider range of motion (ROM) corresponding to increased laxity. Even in advanced lesions in which intervertebral mobility is reduced because of disc narrowing, the system still exhibits loss of stiffness. This decrease in rigidity corresponds to an increase in the neutral zone of disc loading over displacement.

The stretching of the connective tissues uniting two vertebrae leads to a force resisting the displacement. The dissipation of kinetic energy in the form of heat is mediated by the viscoelastic properties of these connective tissues. This passive damping would, in fact, be quite insufficient to protect the disc if it were not constantly supplemented by the much more effective active damping provided by the reflex contraction of the powerful paravertebral muscles. Although the dynamic equilibrium of the intervertebral articular system depends on a combination of muscle activity and tension of the passive elements of union, the active system constantly protects the passive elements, which consequently remain within the limits of their elasticity under healthy physiological conditions.

2. *Degenerative disc disease is basically a mechanical disorder occurring in a biological environment.* The disc and intervertebral ligaments can be overloaded and fail when loading is excessive or the active system of damping is deficient. Sustained excessive stresses on the connective tissues of the disc and ligaments prevent normal healing because the cells can only persist and fulfill their functions under a restricted range of mechanical stresses. Under the mechanical conditions just outlined, the intervertebral disc cells that synthesize the extracellular matrix exhibit normal activity. Lotz and Chin (7) have shown that disc cells function normally only within a precise range of mechanical loading. Too much or too little loading leads to direct cell destruction and programmed cell death (apoptosis).

Discs consist almost entirely of connective tissue, with a disappearance of notochord remnants by 20 years of age (8). As in all connective tissues, notably the annulus, cell activity can repair damage if lesions are limited or if the lesional process takes place over time in a manner analogous to stress fractures. In fact, an indisputable healing process can be observed in the intervertebral disc, with a fibroelastic reaction and neovascularization, at least during early degenerative change. However, just as in pseudarthrosis of long bones and in meniscal lesions, when deleterious conditions persist, the healing process can be overwhelmed.

Based on these mechanical and biological aspects of degenerative disc disease, different working hypotheses were involved in the concept of nonrigid stabilization and development of the Wallis system. One was that by increasing the stiffness of the damaged intervertebral segment and by limiting the amplitude of mobility, one provides mechanical normalization, which should slow the progression of degenerative lesions. Moreover, provided that disc height is sufficiently preserved, creation of the proper range of loading stresses on the disc by the interspinous process implant should foster the healing process of the disc tissue. Finally, although many years of follow-up will be necessary for confirmation, it is anticipated that dynamic stabilization will slow the domino effect of accelerated degenerative change in the segments adjacent to the treated level, especially in comparison to treatment by fusion. This brings us to the third aspect fundamental to the Wallis system.

3. Discectomy for herniation of a transitional disc with sacralization of L5
4. Degenerative disc disease at a level adjacent to a fusion or prosthesis
5. Isolated disc resorption, notably with concomitant type-1 modic changes, associated with low back pain
6. Symptomatic narrow canal treated using partial laminectomy consisting of resection of the superior aspect of the laminae (a technique we refer to as the "recalibration" procedure).

The Wallis system should only be used in patients who do not have substantial loss of disc height, that is, only for discs corresponding to stages 2, 3, and 4 of the MRI disc classification proposed by Pfirrmann et al. (12) in which stage 1 is a healthy aspect and stage 5 corresponds to a black disc with severe loss of disc height. Note also that the implant is not intended for the L5-S1 segment because the spinous process of S1 is inadequate for this purpose.

DISCUSSION

Regarding our personal series, the indications for Wallis and fusion were different as reflected by the differences in the inner, preoperative shapes, but the comparison provides a rough frame of reference for those who are not familiar with these diagrams. It was evident from the outset that this new system of dynamic stabilization does not have the inherent drawbacks of fusion or disc replacement: With Wallis, there is less intraoperative bleeding because it is less invasive, operative duration is shorter because the system is simpler, and the procedure is completely reversible. To this should be added the anticipated difference regarding adjacent levels compared to fusion but theoretically not compared to disc replacement. This follow-up evidence has convinced us that to date, the efficacy of Wallis is at least as good as that of fusion. We now have a tentatively validated operative alternative for many young patients with degenerative disc disease for whom fusion, or even disc prosthesis, might seem too radical.

In view of the good long-term results of the first-generation device, there is no reason to believe the good intermediate-term results of the Wallis will not persist. For patients and surgeons, however, it is a fail-safe solution because even if relief fails to persist, the procedure is completely reversible. The patient would be able to start over again with all the original options. Consequently, this method should rapidly assume a specific role along with total disc prostheses in the new stepwise surgical strategy for initial forms of degenerative intervertebral lumbar disc disease.

Regarding the three previously mentioned working hypotheses behind the development of Wallis, the clinical evidence favors the first two. Stabilizing the degenerative segments and limiting amplitudes of mobility with Wallis is associated with clinical findings consistent with a halt in the degenerative process. Levels of pain and functionality have significantly improved over preoperative values. Furthermore, many patients with modic 1 changes exhibit either normal bone or modic 2 changes on follow-up MRIs.

It is still too early to determine whether the anticipated healing of this connective tissue is actually occurring. There is MRI evidence of disc rehydration at follow-up. Many initially black discs are coming back with a normal white signal. Examples are shown in Figures 24.3 and 24.4.

As indicated, it will take years to ascertain whether Wallis has a protective effect on the adjacent discs (third working hypothesis). A fourth, accessory working hypothesis concerned the decision to use a tension binding system rather than screw fixation, to permit this dynamic stabilization to last by avoiding screw toggle and to make it less invasive and more reversible. The two types warrant a comparative study, but for ethical reasons, this would seem likely only in centers in which surgeons expect equivalent advantages and drawbacks from both.

REFERENCES

1. Sénégas J. La ligamentoplastie intervertébrale, alternative à l'arthrodèse dans le traitement des instabilitiés dégénératives. Acta Ortop Belg 1991;57 (Suppl 1):221-6.
2. Sénégas J, Etchevers JP, Baulny D, Grenier F. Widening of the lumbar vertebral canal as an alternative to laminectomy, in the treatment of lumbar stenosis. Fr J Orthop Surg 1988;2:93-9.
3. Sénégas J, Vital JM, Guérin J, Bernard P, M'Barek M, Loreiro M, Bouvet R. Stabilisation lombaire souple. In: GIEDA—Instabilités vertébrales lombaires. Expansion Scientifique Française 1995; Paris:122-32.
4. Sénégas J. Mechanical supplementation by non-rigid fixation in degenerative intervertebral lumbar segments: the Wallis system. Eur Spine J 2002 Oct11; Suppl 2:S164-9.
5. Ebara S, Harada T, Hosono N, et al. Intraoperative measurement of lumbar spinal instability. Spine 1992;17 (3S):44-50.
6. Mimura M, Panjabi M, Oxland TR, et al. Disc degeneration affects the multidirectional flexibility of the lumbar spine. Spine 1994;19:1371-80.
7. Lotz JC, Chin JR. Intervertebral disc cell death is dependent on the magnitude and duration of spinal loading. Spine 2002;25:1477-83.
8. Oegema TR Jr. The role of disc cell heterogeneity in determining disc biochemistry: a speculation. Biochem Soc Trans 2002; Nov30(Pt 6):839-44.
9. Ganey TM, Meisel HJ. A potential role for cell-based therapeutics in the treatment of intervertebral disc herniation. Eur Spine J 2002 Oct11; Suppl 2:S206-14.
10. Hildebrand KA, Jia F, Woo SL. Response of donor and recipient cells after transplantation of cells to the ligament and tendon. Microsc Res Tech 2002 Jul 1;58(1):34-8.
11. Minns RJ, Walsh WK. Preliminary design and experimental studies of a novel soft implant for correcting sagittal plane instability in the lumbar spine. Spine 1997;22:1819-25; discussion 1826-7.
12. Pfirrmann CWA, Metzdorf A, Zanetti M, Hodler J, Boos N. Magnetic resonance classification of lumbar intervertebral disc degeneration. Spine 2001;26:4873-8.

25

Failed Back Surgery Syndrome Is the Syndrome of the Failed Back Surgeon!

Alf L. Nachemson

INTRODUCTION

Even though only a small percentage of patients with low back pain become chronic, they constitute a large burden for themselves and societies in all industrialized countries. The natural history of low back pain has usually been reported in a favorable manner (1–4), that is, rapid recovery within a few weeks, a view lately modified (5). Now it also seems that the economic benefits in the welfare states contribute to the increasing problem of low back disability (6,7).

The prevalence of low back pain at any age from 10 to 85 years of age hovers around 40%. Of these, only 25% ever see a physician, and although 90% will recover and go back to work within 6 weeks, the sheer number of those not recovered after 6 months constitute a large burden for societies as well as spinal surgeons (7). In the vast majority of chronic sufferers, we are unable to pinpoint a definite cause (8).

When patients consult surgeons, we often try to help these patients with some type of invasive procedures, in the last 20 years mostly a spine fusion. Recent U.S. figures show a 100% increase in such procedures in the last 10 years from 150,000 to 300,000 operations per year, approaching the number of total hip replacements and knee arthroplasties (9,10). The literature shows that reoperations for these fused patients within the next 5 years will amount to around 20% to 30%, that is, constituting the failed back surgery syndrome (FBSS) (11–22). Thus FBSS is categorized as those not improving following surgery, remaining severely disabled for a long time, and those who have recurrence of disabling symptoms.

The indications for back surgery in patients with sciatica due to a disc hernia is fairly well established with good evidence for effectiveness (23), but unfortunately for those with chronic back pain alone, this is not the case. In addition we now have scientific evidence that our past efforts have been rather futile. We have been fooling ourselves, our patients, and our societies. At some orthopedic surgical meetings in the United States, Great Britain, and Sweden in 1998, the audience was asked, after having been given a patient's history of chronic back pain with degenerative changes in the lower discs, whether general orthopedic surgeons would refer such a patient to a spine surgeon, and 40% said they would. Then they were asked if they would have a fusion themselves with the same history, and only 7% answered affirmatively.

In this chapter I delineate the five main failures for the dismal results mirrored by the number of conferences held and books published on the "failed spine surgery syndrome." In this context we unfortunately stand out among surgical specialists.

FIRST FAILURE: DISREGARD FOR FAILURE OF MOST DIAGNOSTIC METHODS TO PINPOINT THE PAIN SOURCE

We use various diagnostic labels without scientific evidence (8,24,25). To demonstrate utility, the validation of a diagnostic test requires the determination of sensitivity and specificity against a meaningful gold standard, which in our case should be a treatment method with proven positive effect. Tests such as ordinary radiography (26–29), magnetic resonance imaging (30,31), discography (32–37), or detection of a high-intensity zone with gadolinium enhancement (35) have no proven utility. As stated by Weinstein et al. 2003 in an editorial in *Spine* (38), all these tests have only increased our ability to view disc anatomy but not helped predict which patients with low back pain will benefit from interventions. In addition there is poor inter- and intraobserver agreement for many findings like facet joint arthritis, spinal canal narrowing, degenerative spondylolisthesis (8,40) and bulging (31) discs on MRI (25,39).

There is also controversy on motion segment instability, the measurements and symptoms of which are not defined (41–43). In addition, the very accurate roentgen stereophotographic assessment (44,45) has even failed to show increased mobility or difference between symptomatic and nonsymptomatic patients with spondylolisthesis grade I and II. There could be more examples of diagnostic uncertainties, but suffice to say that spine surgeons often perform large interventions on patients with nonproven diagnostic labels like "disc degeneration," "disappearing disc," "black discs," "instability," (4,46,47), and so on. Clearly such behavior is abnormal. We simply lack a meaningful gold standard for the diagnostic tests (38). Even invasive diagnostic tests like nerve root blocks or temporary external fixation tests have failed to show utility (48–52). A recent study in *Spine* (53) also showed a clear relation between the number of CT and MRI examinations and the relative incidence of spinal surgery, giving further support to the uncertainties of these diagnostic tests.

SECOND FAILURE: DISREGARD FOR THE LACK OF SCIENTIFIC SUPPORT FOR ANY SURGICAL APPROACH FOR CLBP (EXCLUDING SPECIFIC DISEASES)

From 1994 to 2002, I co-coordinated the Cochrane Collaboration Back Group where different authors reviewed the evidence for various treatments of low back pain (54,55). Gibson and Waddell published in 1999 (23) a review of surgery for lumbar disc prolapse and one on degenerative lumbar spondylosis; chronic low back pain (CLBP) due to disc aging or degeneration. At that time there was moderate evidence for disc hernia removal as an effective treatment of sciatica while no randomized trial existed on surgery for chronic low back pain due to "degenerative disc disease."

At the end of 2003, however, four new randomized trials were presented, some even with up to 5-year follow-up; the first two came from Sweden, one on back pain due to mild/moderate spondylolisthesis (13,14) and the larger study on fusion for chronic low back pain in a multicenter randomized trial with a minimum 2-year follow-up of nearly 300 patients (12). In this larger "Swedish Back" study, the conservative arm in the different hospitals varied and was the same that the patients had received before randomization. The results judged by an unbiased observer were significantly better in those fused, irrespective of which of the three surgical methods were used: ordinary posterolateral fusion without screws, fusion with plates and screws, or a "360-degree" fusion (56). The pain on a visual analogue scale (VAS), which improved quite a lot in the surgical group at the 1-year follow-up, seemed to diminish at the 2-year follow-up. Preliminary results at the 5-year minimum follow-up now seem to indicate that all the groups, including those conservatively treated, have the same result (57).

Exactly the same has been now reported by Ekman et al. (58). In these two Swedish randomized control trials (RCTs), no difference in results in the two or three surgical groups was encountered (14,56,59). Where metal implants were used, there were significantly higher rates of complications and reoperations in both studies. In addition, in a recent new inquiry by the Swedish Back Group, reported at the EuroSpine meeting in Prague and published in *European Spine Journal* (2003), 50% of men with anterior fusion had some disturbance in the genital sphere: ejaculation disturbances 41%, sensory disturbances 47%, and retrograde ejaculation 13% (60).

In a Norwegian study published in *Spine* (2003) (61), Brox et al. showed no difference between fusion with screws and plates and a cognitive behavioral treatment program at the 1-year follow-up. Already within 1 year there were 18% complications in the fusion group. Preliminary results from the larger (360 patients) Oxford study led by Fairbanks in Great Britain at the 2-year follow-up seemed to show the same thing (62). Thus we now know that, in general, based on scientific evidence, there is very limited success of spine fusion that fades over time, and in addition there is a significant amount of complications in particular when using screws and plates (14,18,22,56,63,64). In contrast, a Cochrane review on conservative treatment of CLBP consisting of multidisciplinary activation programs has been shown to be effective with reduction of pain and increasing function (65–67) with no serious complications.

Surgery for the clinical diagnosis of spinal stenosis is increasing in the world because of our aging populations (63). Nieggemeyer et al. (68) looked at 30 studies published between 1975 and 1995 describing that decompression alone seems to give better results and fewer complications in this elderly group of patients. Again, in this review, adding instruments to fusion resulted in more complications (69). As in the Atlas study (70), the better results fade with time and Malmivaara et al. (71) in a recent RCT could not find any difference between surgical and conservative treated patients with spinal stenosis in the short (6-month) term. Another not yet published study by Zuckerman et al. (72) showed at 1 year significant improvement with a very simple surgical gadget between spinous processes. Until further scientific evidence is at hand, most surgeons agree that for an elderly patient with severe clinical and radiological spinal stenosis at one or two levels a conservative, limited surgical approach is indicated.

Intradiscal electrothermal treatment (IDET), another invasive method used to treating chronic low back pain was reported by the inventors (73) to give excellent results, but now in randomized trials the efficacy has been questioned (74,75) as have other "denervation" procedures (76,77). Note that in order to be clinically meaningful, the reduction in pain and the improvement in Oswestry functional scale should amount to about 30% (78–80).

THIRD FAILURE: INSTRUMENT COMPANIES AND/OR WELL-SPOKEN COLLEAGUES ADVOCATE NEW EXPENSIVE IMPLANTS

The spine implant industry has been mentioned in the lay economic press as the one showing the biggest growth potential segment of the orthopedic industry and was said also to be the most profitable. This has happened because of the introduction without proper scientific support of the clinical advantages of more than 150 systems of screws and plates for internal fixation, various types of cages, and now an astounding number of disc prostheses (46,81).

We now know that for a one- to two-level fusion for CLBP, these systems offer no advantages in pain reduction even though they appear to have a higher fusion rate, which, however, in no studies has been demonstrated to give improved clinical results. More than 130 patents of disc prostheses implants exist in the literature (81). The preliminary results of randomized controlled trials (82,83) presented from the United States where the FDA nowadays demands such a study before the introduction of a new spinal device has not demonstrated improvement over fusion procedures! A review published by the National Institute for Clinical Excellence (84), on the literature up to October 2003, based on retrospective studies mostly in Europe, found overall clinical results to be satisfactory in at least 60% of cases in three studies that reported outcome. Reoperation rates varied between 3% and 24%, rates of implant-related problems from 1% to 4%, and return to work varied from 0% to 70% but was rarely reported. The final conclusion was that the benefit of prosthetic discs in patients over 45 years of age remains unresolved. The preliminary results from the randomized studies in the United States underscore this statement. If a disc prosthesis is no better than spinal fusion that we now know is of little benefit, then why do a large riskier procedure when equal (61) or perhaps better conservative (66,67) methods exist? There is thus poor scientific support for the intensive marketing of the many implants; screws, plates, cages, and prostheses now seen at all meetings where exhibits exist and the flow of advertisement to orthopedic surgeons all over the world. It is thus not surprising to find the number of operations for CLBP using implants increasing (9,10). The influence of strong marketing is thus noted also among spinal surgeons.

There are now several randomized controlled as well as prospective trials comparing one- or two-level fusions for low back pain, spondylolisthesis, or spinal stenosis with or without internal fixation, finding no difference in the clinical outcome, functional return to work, but significantly rather more complications when implants are used (14,20,56,69, 85–91). We are clearly witnessing a triumph of marketing over scientific evidence!

FOURTH FAILURE: LACK OF CRITICAL READING OF PUBLISHED PAPERS ON SURGERY FOR LOW BACK PAIN, PARTICULARLY REPEAT SURGERY

There exist strict rules for clinical follow-up series (8,92,93), depicted in Table 25.1. Few studies in this area adhere to these criteria. In addition it has been estimated that only 20% of readers of scientific articles really read the methods section (94).

Nowadays the gold standard for evidence of treatment effectiveness of medical conditions consists of randomized controlled trials (94), but these also have to fulfill most criteria seen in Table 25.2—some difficult in a surgical trial, although successful attempts exist (95).

TABLE 25.1. *Guide for follow-up studies*

1. Clear description of patients and of intervention
2. Valid intake and outcome measures
3. Adequate sample size
4. Nonbiased personal follow-up
5. Adequate length of follow-up (>2 years)
6. Sufficient percentage follow-up (>90%)

TABLE 25.2. *Criteria list for the methodological quality assessment (modified from van Tulder et al. [55])*

A. Was the method of randomization adequate?
B. Was the treatment allocation concealed?
C. Were the groups similar at baseline regarding the most important prognostic indicators?
D. Was the patient blinded to the intervention?
E. Was the care provider blinded to the intervention?
F. Was the outcome assessor blinded to the intervention?
G. Were cointerventions avoided or similar?
H. Was the compliance acceptable in all groups?
I. Was the dropout rate described and acceptable?
J. Was the timing of the outcome assessment in all groups similar?
K. Did the analysis include an intention-to-treat-analysis?

FIFTH FAILURE: DISREGARD OF THE PROVEN PREDICTIVE VALUE OF THE PSYCHOSOCIAL FACTORS, IN PARTICULAR FOR REPEAT SURGERY

There is ample evidence in the literature that certain psychosocial factors limit the success of any treatment method, including fusion operations in chronic low back pain patients (19,96,97–103). Even the otherwise successful removal of a disc hernia gives poorer results in patients with certain psychosocial factors (19). The introduction of yellow flags (96,104,105) and illness behavior, Waddell tests (98.99), and the University of Alabama Pain Behavior Rating Scale (100,106,107) all are useful tests to predict success or failure from any conservative or surgical procedure on the back for any nonspecific back pain patient. In particular this is also true for repeat surgery patients (19,64, 108,109,110). It is known that surgeons often misinterpret suffering and ineffective coping in patients with chronic low back pain.

Recent studies in these patients also have elucidated an increased amount in substance P and nerve root growth factor (NGF) (both pronociceptive substances) in the cerebrospinal fluid of patients with nonspecific CLBP (111). In addition, an earlier Spanish study showed a diminution of endorphins in the same type of patients (112). In a recent study by Giesecke et al. (113,114), we have demonstrated increased pain sensitivity and abnormal activation in the brain by functional MRI in several cortical areas of these patients. Psychosocial factors also predict results after disc hernia surgery (115–118).

It has been calculated that repeat surgery is common in the United States (119), whereas in Europe it hovers around 6%. There also seems to be some relation to the number of reoperations to number of primary operations (108).

SUMMARY

We live in an era of evidence-based medicine (54,65,94,120,121), which should lead us spinal surgeons to an evidence-based practice where we use the available scientific reviews together with our clinical expertise and the patients' specific history and physical and psychological findings as guides. From this overview it should be clear that for the most common diagnostic "labels" for chronic low back pain, such as degenerative disc disease, moderate spondylolisthesis in adults, and spinal stenosis, the efficacy of spine fusion remains unclear and the moderately positive early effects not lasting.

In order to avoid FBSS, CLBP without a definite proven cause should not be operated on and a reoperation extremely rarely performed. There might be a few exceptional cases with clearly demonstrable instability of >6 mm in flexion-extension X-rays after previous laminectomies or fractures, a few cases with spinal stenosis and severe leg pain with very short walking distances in patients without psychosocial deterrents for recovery. In addition, the removal of a definite new disc hernia after a minimum 1-year pain-free interval seems to have support (118). The use of artificial discs must await long-term scientifically reliable studies (84). The preliminary trials suggest equivalent results to spinal fusion, which generally is not effective. As we stated in a recent article in the *New England Journal of Medicine* (122), "The emphasis of research efforts should shift from examining how to fuse or replace to examining who really should have an operation".

REFERENCES

1. Nachemson A. Ont i Ryggen. Back pain—causes, diagnosis, treatment. SBU Statens Beredning for Utvordering av medicinsk metodik, Stockholm 1991.
2. Nachemson AL. Newest knowledge of low back pain. a critical look. Clin Orthop 1992;279:8-20.
3. Hillman M, Wright A, Rajaratnam G, Tennant A, Chamberlain MA. Prevalence of low back pain in the community: implications for service provision in Bradford, UK. J Epidemiol Community Health 1996 Jun; 50(3):347-52.
4. Andersson GBJ. The epidemiology of spinal disorders. In: Frymoyer JW (ed.), The adult spine: principles and practice (2nd ed.). New York: Raven Press, 1997;1:93-141.
5. von Korff M, Saunders K. The course of back pain in primary care. Spine 1996;21:2833-7.
6. Nachemson, AL. Chronic pain—the end of the welfare state? Quality of Life Research, 1994;3;S1:11-7.
7. Nachemson A. Epidemiology and the economics of LBP. In: Herkowitz HN, Dvorak J, Bell G, Nordin M, Grob D (eds.), The lumbar spine (3rd ed). Philadelphia: Lippincott Williams and Wilkins, 2003.
8. Nachemson A, Jonsson E. Neck and back pain: the scientific evidence of causes, diagnosis and treatment. Philadelphia: Lippincott, Williams and Wilkins, 2000.
9. Agency for Healthcare Research and Quality. Healthcare Cost and Utilization Project, HCUPnet. www.ahcpr.gov/data/hcup/hcupnet.htm. Accessed June 30, 2003.
10. Mendenhall Associates, Inc. 2002 Spinal Industry Update. Orthopedic Network News 2002;13(4):7-8.
11. Malter AD, McNeney B, Loeser JD, Deyo RA. 5-year reoperation rates after different types of lumbar spine surgery. Spine 1998;23(7):814-28.
12. Fritzell P, Hagg O, Wessberg P, Nordwall A. 2001 Volvo Award Winner in Clinical Studies: Lumbar fusion versus nonsurgical treatment for chronic low back pain: a multicenter randomized controlled trial from the Swedish Lumbar Spine Study Group. Spine 2001;26:2521-32.
13. Moller H, Hedlund R. Surgery versus conservative management in adult isthmic spondylolisthesis—a prospective randomized study: Part I. Spine 2000;25:1711-5.
14. Moller H, Hedlund R. Instrumented and noninstrumented posterolateral fusion in adult spondylolisthesis—a prospective randomized study: Part 2. Spine 2000;25:1716-21.
15. Ciol M, Deyo R, Kreuter W, Bigos S. Characteristics in Medicare beneficiaries associated with reoperation after lumbar spine surgery. Spine 1994;19(12):1329-34.
16. Wilkinson H. The failed back syndrome. etiology and therapy. Philadelphia: Harper & Row, 1991.
17. Gill K, Frymoyer J. Management of treatment failures after decompressive surgery: surgical alternatives and results: In: Frymoyer J (ed.), The adult spine: principles and practice (2nd ed.). Philadelphia: Lippincott-Raven, 1997;2111-33.
18. Turner JA, Ersek M, Herron L, Haselkorn J, Kent D, Ciol MA, Deyo RA. Patient outcomes after lumbar spinal fusions. JAMA 1992;268:907-11. Review.
19. Waddell G, Kummell EG, Lotto WN, Graham JD, Hall H, McCulloch JA. Failed lumbar disc surgery and repeat surgery following industrial injuries. J Bone Joint Surg 1979;61-A:201-7.
20. Bjarke Christensen F, Stender Hansen E, Laursen M, Thomsen K, Bunger CE. Long-term functional outcome of pedicle screw instrumentation as a support for posterolateral spinal fusion: randomized clinical study with a 5-year follow-up. Spine 2002;27:1269-77.
21. Deyo RA, Cherkin DC, Loeser JD, Bigos SJ, Ciol MA. Morbidity and mortality in association with operations on the lumbar spine. The influence of age, diagnosis and procedure. J Bone Joint Surg Am 1992;74(4):536-43.
22. Deyo RA, Ciol MA, Cherkin DC, Loeser JD, Bigos SJ. Lumbar spinal fusion. A cohort study of complications, reoperations, and resource use in the Medicare population. Spine 1993;18:1463-70.
23. Gibson JNA, Grant IC, Waddell G. The Cochrane review of surgery for lumbar disc prolapse and degenerative lumbar spondylolsis. Spine 1999;24:1820-32.
24. Abenhaim L, Rossignol M, Gobeille D, Bonvalot Y, Fines P, Scott S. The prognostic consequences in the making of the initial medical diagnosis of work-related back injuries. Spine 1995;20(7):791-5.
25. Roland M, van Tulder M. Should radiologists change the way they report plain radiography of the spine. Viewpoint. The Lancet 1998;352:229-30.

26. Bigos S, Hansson T, Castillo R, Beecher P, Wortley M. The value of preemployment roentgenographs for predicting acute back injury claims and chronic back pain disability. Clin Orthop 1992;283:124-9.
27. van den Hoogen H. Spinal x-ray findings and non-specific low back pain a systematic review of observational studies. In: van Tulder M, Koes B, Bouter L (eds.), Low back pain in primary care. Amsterdam: EMGO Institute, 1996.
28. van den Hoogen HMM, Koes BW, van Eijk JTM, Bouter LM. On the accuracy of history, physical examination, and erythrocyte sedimentation rate in diagnosing low-back pain in general practice. A criteria-based review of the literature. Spine 1995;20(3):318-27.
29. van Tulder MW, Assendelft WJ, Koes BW, Bouter LM. Spinal radiographic findings and nonspecific low back pain. A systematic review of observational studies. Spine 1997;22(4):427-34.
30. Boden SD, Davis DO, Dina TS, Patronas NJ, Wiesel SW. Abnormal magnetic-resonance scans of the lumbar spine in asymptomatic subjects. A prospective investigation. J Bone Joint Surg Am 1990;72(3):403-8.
31. Boos N, Rieder R, Schade V, Spratt KF, Semmer N, Aebi M. The diagnostic accuracy of magnetic resonance imaging, work perception, and psychosocial factors in identifying symptomatic disc herniations. Spine 1995;20(24):2613-25.
32. Carragee EJ, Tanner CM, Yang B, Brito JL, Truong T. False-positive findings on lumbar discography. Reliability of subjective concordance assessment during provocative disc injection. Spine 1999;24:2542-7.
33. Carragee EJ. Is lumbar discography a determinate of discogenic low back pain: provocative discography reconsidered. Curr Rev Pain 2000;4:301-8. Review.
34. Carragee EJ, Tanner CM, Norbash A, Khurana S, Hayward C, Welsh J, Date E, Truong T, Rossi M, Hagle C. The rates of false positive lumbar discography in select patients without low back complaints. Paper given at the 65th annual meeting of the American Academy of Orthopaedic Surgeons, New Orleans, LA, March 1998.
35. Carragee EJ, Paragioudakis SJ, Khurana S. 2000 Volvo Award Winner in Clinical Studies: Lumbar high-intensity zone and discography in subjects without low back problems. Spine 2000;25:298-92.
36. Carragee EJ, Alamin TE. Discography, a review. Spine J 2001;1(5):364-72.
37. Carragee EJ, Alamin TF, Miller J, Grafe M. Provocative discography in volunteer subjects with mild persistent low back pain. Spine J 2002;2(1):25-34.
38. Weinstein JN, Boden SD, An H. Emerging technology in spine: should we rethink the past or move forward in spite of the past? Spine 2003;28:S1.
39. Brant-Zawadzki MN, Jensen MC, Obuchowski N, Ross JS, Modic MT. Interobserver and intraobserver variability in interpretation of lumbar disc abnormalities: a comparison of two nomenclatures. Spine 1995;20(11):1257-64.
40. Espeland A, Korsbrekke K, Albrektsen G, Larsen JL. Observer variation in plain radiography of the lumbosacral spine. Br J Radiol 1998;71:366-75.
41. Nachemson AL. Scientific diagnosis or unproved label for back pain patients. In: Szpalski M, Gunzburg R, Pope MH (eds.), Lumbar segmental instability. Philadelphia: Lippincott Raven, 1999.
42. Panjabi MH. The stabilizing system of the spine. Part I. Function, dysfunction, adaptation, and enhancement. J Spinal Dis 1992;5(4):383-9.
43. Panjabi MH. The stabilizing system of the spine. Part II. Neutral zone and instability hypothesis. J Spinal Dis 1992;5(4):390-7.
44. Axelsson P. On lumbar spine stabilization. Thesis, Lund University, Sweden, 1996.
45. Danielsson B, Frennered K, Selvik G, Irstam L. Roentgenologic assessment of spondylolisthesis. II. An evaluation of progression. Acta Radiol 1989;30:65-8.
46. Nachemson AL. Instrumented fusion of the lumbar spine for degenerative disorders: a critical look. In: Szpalski M, Gunzburg R, Spengler DM, Nachemson A (eds.), Instrumented fusion of the degenerative lumbar spine. State of the art, questions, and controversies. Philadelphia: Lippincott-Raven, 1996;307-17.
47. Nachemson AL. Challenge of the artificial disc. In: Weinstein JN (ed.), Clinical efficacy and outcome in the diagnosis and treatment of low back pain. New York: Raven Press, 1992;271-8.
48. North RB, Campbell JN, James CS, Conover-Walker MK, Wang H, Piantadosi S, Rybock JD, Long DM. Failed back surgery syndrome, 5-year follow-up in 102 patients undergoing repeated operation. Neurosurgery 1991;28(5):685-91.
49. North RB, Kidd DH, Zahurak M, Piantadosi S. Specificity of diagnostic nerve blocks: a prospective, randomized study of sciatica due to lumbarsacral spine disease. Pain 1996;65(1):77-85.
50. Faraj AA, Akasha K, Mulholland RC. Temporary external fixation for low back pain: is it worth doing? Eur Spine J 1997;6:187-90.
51. Esses SI, Botsford DJ, Kostuik JP. The role of external spinal skeletal fixation in the assessment of low-back disorders. Spine 1989;14:594-601.
52. Soini JR, Seitsalo SK. The external fixation test of the lumbar spine. 30 complications in 25 patients of 100 consecutive patients. Acta Orthop Scand 1993:64:147-9.
53. Lurie JD, Birkmeyer NJ, Weinstein JN. Rates of advanced spinal imaging and spine surgery. Spine 2003;28:616-20.
54. Bombardier C, Esmail R, Nachemson AL, and the Back Review Group Editorial Board. The Cochrane Collaboration Back Review Group for Spinal Disorders. Spine 1997;22(8):837-40.
55. Van Tulder M, Furlan A, Bombardier C, Bouter L, and the Editorial Board of the Cochrane Collaboration Back Review Group. Updated method guidelines for systematic reviews in the Cochrane Collaboration Back Review Group. Spine 2003;28:1290-9.

56. Fritzell P, Hagg O, Nordwall A. Complications in lumbar fusion surgery for chronic low back pain: comparison of three surgical techniques used in a prospective randomized study. A report from the Swedish Lumbar Spine Study Group. Eur Spine J 2003;12:178-89.
57. Nordwall A, Hagg O. Personal communication, Göteborg, Sweden, 2003.
58. Ekman P, Hedlund R, Möller H. Fusion in adult isthmic spondylolisthesis. A long term follow-up of a prospective randomized study. Presented at the annual meeting of the Nordic Spine Deformity Society, Stockholm, August 23, 2003.
59. Fritzell P, Hagg O, Wessberg P, Nordwall A. Chronic low back pain and fusion: a comparison of three surgical techniques: a prospective multicenter randomized study from the Swedish lumbar spine study group. Spine 2002;27:1131-41.
60. Hagg O, Fritzell P, Nordwall A, and the Swedish Lumbar Spine Study Group. Sexual function after surgery for chronic low back pain. Eur Spine J 2003;12:S17-8.
61. Brox JI, Sörensen R, Friis A, Nygaard O, Indahl A et al. Randomized clinical trial of lumbar instrumented fusion and cognitive intervention and exercises in patients with chronic low back pain and disc degeneration. Spine 2003;28:1913-21.
62. Fairbanks J. Personal communication, Oxford, England, 2003.
63. Turner JA, Ersek M, Herron L, Deyo R. Surgery for lumbar spinal stenosis: attempted meta-analysis of the literature. Spine 1992;17(1):1-8.
64. Greenough CG. Outcome assessment of lumbar spinal fusion. In: Szpalski M, Gunzberg R, Spengler DM, Nachemson A (eds.), Instrumented fusion of the degenerative spine: state of the art, questions, and controversies. New York: Lippincott-Raven, 1996;45-54.
65. van Tulder MW, Koes BW, Bouter LM. Conservative treatment of acute and chronic nonspecific low back pain. A systematic review of randomized controlled trials of the most common interventions. Spine 1997;22(18): 2128-56.
66. Guzman J, Esmail R, Karjalainen K, Malmivaara A, Irwin E, Bombardier C. Multidisciplinary rehabilitation for chronic low back pain: systematic review. BMJ 2001;322(7301):1511-6.
67. Schonstein E, Kenny D, Keating J, Koes B, Herbert RD. physical conditioning programs for workers with back and neck pain: a Cochrane Systematic Review. Spine 2003;28:E391.
68. Niggemeyer O, Strauss JM, Schlitz KP. Comparison of surgical procedures for degenerative lumbar spinal stenosis: a meta-analysis of the literature from 1975 to 1995. Eur Spine J 1997;6:423-9.
69. Grob D, Humke T, Dvorak J. Degenerative lumbar spinal stenosis: decompression with and without arthrodesis. J Bone Joint Surg 1995;77-A:1036-41.
70. Atlas SJ, Keller RB, Robson D, Deyo RA, Singer DE. Surgical and no surgical management of lumbar spinal stenosis: four-year outcomes from the Maine Lumbar Spine Study. Spine 2000;25:556-62.
71. Malmivaara A, Heliovaara M, Sainio P, Kinnunen M et al. Operative treatment for moderately severe lumbar spinal stenosis. a randomized controlled trial. Abstract, International Society for the Study of the Lumbar Spine (ISSLS) 30th annual meeting, May 13-17, 2003, Vancouver, Canada.
72. Zucherman J, Hsu K, Hartjen C, Mehalic T, Implicito D. Treatment of lumbar spinal stenosis with an interspinous spacer. SpineLine Sept/Oct. 2003;31-2.
73. Saal JA, Saal JS. Intradiscal electrothermal treatment for chronic discogenic low back pain. Spine 2002;27: 966-74.
74. Freeman BJC, Fraser RD, Cain CMJ, Hall DJ. A randomized, double-blind, controlled efficacy study: intradiscal electrothermal therapy (IDET) versus placebo for the treatment of chronic discogenic low back pain. Eur Spine J 2003;12:S1-23.
75. Pauza K, Howell S, Dreyfuss P, Dawson K, Peloza J, Bogduk N. New data demonstrates IDET efficacy. Presented at the 30th annual meeting of the International Society for the Study of the Lumbar Spine (ISSLS), May 13-17, 2003, Vancouver, Canada.
76. Geurtz JW, van Wijk RM, Wynne HJ, Hammink E, Nuskens E, et al. Radiofrequency lesioning of dorsal root ganglia for chronic lumbosacral radicular pain: a randomised, double-blind, controlled trial. Lancet 2003;36 (9351):21-6.
77. Ercelen O, Bulutcu E, Oktenoglu T, Sasani M, Bozkus H, Cetin Saryoglu A, Ozer F. Radiofrequency lesioning using two different time modalities for the treatment of lumbar discogenic pain: a randomized trial. Spine 2003;28:1922-27.
78. Rowbotham MC. What is a "clinically meaningful" reduction in pain? Editorial Pain 2001;94:131-2.
79. Bombardier C. Outcome assessments in the evaluation of treatment of spinal disorders: summary and general recommendations. Spine 2000;25:3100-3. Review.
80. Bombardier C, Havden J, Beaton DE. Minimal clinically important difference. Low back pain: outcome measures. J Rheumatol 2001;28:431-8.
81. Szpalski M, Gunzburg R, Mayer M. Spine arthroplasty: a historical review. Eur Spine J 2002;Oct 11 Suppl 2:S65-84. E-pub Aug. 13, 2002.
82. Delamarter RB, Fribourg DM, Kanim LEA, Bae H. ProDisc artificial total lumbar disc replacement: introduction and early results from the United States clinical trial. Spine 2003;28(20S):S167-75.
83. McAfee PC, Fedder IL, Saiedy S, Shucosky EM. Experimental design of total disk replacement—experience with a prospective randomized study of the SB Charité. Spine 2003;28(20S):S153-62.
84. National Institute for Clinical Excellence. Interventional Procedure Consultation Document, Prosthetic Intervertebral disc replacement, October 2003. London National Institute for Clinical Excellence. http://www.nice.org.uk.

85. Bono C, Lee C. Critical analysis of trends in fusion for degenerative disc disease over the last 20 years: influence of technique on fusion rate and clinical outcome. Presented at the annual meeting of the International Society for the Study of the Lumbar Spine, May 13-17, 2003, Vancouver, Canada.
86. DeBerard MS, Master KS, Colledge AL, Schleursemer RL, Schlegel JD. Outcomes of posterolateral lumbar fusion in Utah patients receiving workers compensation: a retrospective cohort study. Spine 2001;26: 738-47.
87. Christensen FB, Hansen ES, Eiskjaer SP, Hoy K, Helmig P, et al. Circumferential lumbar spinal fusion with Brantigan cage versus posterolateral fusion with titanium Cotrel-Dubousset instrumentation: a prospective, randomized clinical study of 146 patients. Spine 2002;27:2674-83.
88. Fischgrund JS, Mackay M, Herkowitz HN, Brower R, Montgomery DM, Kurz LT. 1997 Volvo Award Winner in clinical studies. Degenerative lumbar spondylolisthesis with spinal stenosis: a prospective randomized study comparing decompressive laminectomy and arthrodesis with and without spinal instrumentation. Spine 1997; 22:2807-12.
89. France JC, Yaszemski MJ, Lauerman WC, Cain JE, Glover JM, Lawson KJ, Coe JD, Topper SM. A randomized prospective study of posterolateral lumbar fusion. Outcomes with and without pedicle screw instrumentation. Spine 1999;24:553-60.
90. Katz JN, Lipson SJ, Lew RA, Grobler LJ, Weinstein JN, Brick GW, Fossel AH, Liang MH. Lumbar laminectomy alone or with instrumented or noninstrumented arthrodesis in degenerative lumbar spinal stenosis. Patient selection, costs, and surgical outcomes. Spine 1997;22:1123-31.
91. Thomsen K, Christensen FB, Eiskjaer SP, Hansen ES, Fruensgaard S, Bunger CE. 1997 Volvo Award winner in clinical studies. The effect of pedicle screw instrumentation on functional outcome and fusion rates in posterolateral lumbar spinal fusion: a prospective, randomized clinical study. Spine 1997;22:2813-22.
92. Block R. Methodology of clinical back pain trials. Spine 1987;12(5):430-2.
93. Nachemson AL, LaRocca H. Editorial. Spine 1987;12(5):427-9.
94. Sackett DL, Scott Richardson W, Rosenberg W, Haynes RB. Evidence-based medicine. How to practice and teach EBM. New York: Churchill Livingstone, 1997.
95. Moseley JB, O'Malley K, Petersen NJ, Menke TJ, Brody BA, et al. A controlled trial of arthroscopic surgery for osteoarthritis of the knee. N Engl J Med 2002;347(2):81-8.
96. Kendall NAS, Linton SJ, Main CJ. Guide to assessing psychosocial yellow flags in acute low back pain: risk factors for long-term disability and work loss. Accident Rehabilitation & Compensation Insurance Corporation of New Zealand and the National Health Committee, Wellington, NZ, 1997.
97. Waddell G, Main CJ, Morris EW, DiPaola M, Gray ICM. Chronic low back pain, psychologic distress, and illness behavior. Spine 1984;9:209-13.
98. Waddell G, McCulloch JA, Kummel E, Venner RM. Nonorganic physical signs in low back pain. Spine 1980;5:117-23.
99. Waddell G, Newton M, Henderson I, Somerville D, Main CJ. A fear-avoidance beliefs questionnaire (FABQ) and the role of fear-avoidance beliefs in chronic low back pain and disability. Pain 1993;52:157-68.
100. Keefe FJ, Block AR. Development of an observation method for assessing pain behavior in chronic low back pain patients. Behav Ther 1982;13:363-75.
101. Hagg O. Measurement and prediction of outcome. Application in fusion surgery for chronic low back pain. The Swedish Lumbar Spine Study. Thesis, Sahlgrenska Academy at Göteborg University, Göteborg, Sweden, 2002.
102. Greenough CG, Peterson MD, Hadlow S, Fraser RD. Instrumented posterolateral lumbar fusion. Results and comparison with anterior interbody fusion. Spine 1998;23(4):479-86.
103. Greenough CG, Fraser RD. The effects of compensation on recovery from low-back injury. Spine 1989;14:947-55.
104. Fordyce WE. Back pain in the workplace: management of disability in nonspecific conditions: a report of the Task Force on Pain in the workplace of the International Association for the Study of Pain. IASP Press, Seattle, WA, 1995.
105. Fordyce WE. Behavioral methods for chronic pain and illness. St. Louis: CV Mosby, 1966.
106. Fouyas IP, Statham PFX, Sandercock PAG. Cochrane review on the role of surgery in cervical spondylotic radiculomyelopathy. Spine 2002;27:736-47.
107. Ohlund C, Lindstrom I, Areskoug B, Eek C, Peterson LE, Nachemson A. Pain behavior in industrial subacute low back pain. I. Reliability: concurrent and predictive validity of pain behavior assessments. Pain 1994;58:201-9.
108. Ohlund C, Lindstrom I, Eek C, Areskoug B, Nachemson A. The causality field (extrinsic and intrinsic factors) in industrial subacute low back pain patients. Scand J Med Sci Sports 1996;6:98-111.
109. Osterman H, Sund R, Seitsalo S, Kesmimaki I. Risk of multiple reoperation after lumbar discectomy: a population-based study. Spine 2003;28:621-7.
110. Greenough CG, Taylor LJ, Fraser RD. Anterior lumbar fusion: a comparison of noncompensation patients with compensation patients. Clin Orthop 1994;300:30-7.
111. Main CJ, Waddell G. Spine update behavioral responses to examination. A reappraisal of the interpretation of nonorganic signs. Spine 1998;23:2367-71.
112. Clauw DJ, Williams D, Lauerman W, Dahlman M, Aslami A, Nachemson AL, et al. Pain sensitivity as a correlate of clinical status in individuals with chronic low back pain. Spine 1999;24:2035-41.
113. Puig MM, Laorden ML, Miralles FS, Olaso MJ. Endorphin levels in cerebrospinal fluid of patients with postoperative and chronic pain. Anesthesiology 1982;57:1-4.

114. Giesecke T, Gracely RH, Grant MAB, Nachemson AL, Petzke F, et al. Evidence of augmented central pain processing in idiopathic chronic low back pain. Arthritis Rheum (in press).
115. Giesecke T, Gracely RH, Grant MAB, Nachemson AL, Williams DA, Clauw DJ. Evidence of augmented central pain processing in idiopathic chronic low back pain. Eur Spine J 2003;12:S1-12.
116. Graver V, Ljunggren AE, Malt UF, Loeb M, Haaland M, et al. Can psychological traits predict the outcome of lumbar disc surgery when anamnestic and psychological risk factors are controlled for? Results of a prospective cohort study. J Psychosom Res 1995;39:465-76.
117. Hasenbring M, Ulrich HW, Hartmann M, Soyka D. The efficacy of a risk factor-based cognitive behavioral intervention and electromyographic biofeedback in patients with acute sciatic pain. An attempt to prevent chronicity. Spine 1999;24:2525-35.
118. Junge A, Frohlich M, Ahrens S, Hasenbring M, Sandler A, et al. Predictors of bad and good outcome of lumbar spine surgery. A prospective clinical study with 2 years' follow up. Spine 1996;21:1056-64; discussion 1064-5.
119. Schade V, Semmer N, Main CJ, Hora J, Boos N. The impact of clinical, morphological, psychosocial and work-related factors on the outcome of lumbar discectomy. Pain 1999;80:239-49.
120. Cherkin DC, Deyo RA, Loeser JD, Bush T, Waddell G. An international comparison of back surgery rates. Spine 1994;19(11):1201-6.
121. Jadad AR, Cook DJ, Jones A, Klassen TP, Tugwell P, Moher M, Moher D. Methodology and reports of systematic reviews and meta-analyses: a comparison of Cochrane reviews with articles published in paper-based journals. JAMA 1998;280(3):278-80.
122. Dickersin K, Manheimer E. The Cochrane Collaboration: evaluation of health care and services using systematic reviews of the results of randomized controlled trials. Clin Obstet Gynecol 1998;41:315-31.
123. Deyo RA. Nachemson A, Mirza SK. Spinal fusion surgery: the case for restraint. (in press) N Engl J Med, 2003.

26

The Failed System

Gordon Waddell

Spinal surgeons rightly focus on surgery, but that is only 1% to 2% of all patients with back problems. Meetings focus on surgical failures and the technical issues involved, which is not surprising as "no operation in any field of surgery leaves in its wake more human wreckage than surgery on the lumbar spine" (5). That is certainly important, but it may be even more important to think about what happens to the 99% of patients who do not have surgery. The question I want to consider is how surgical thinking has influenced the whole Western approach to back pain.

THE HISTORY OF HEALTH CARE FOR BACK PAIN

The history of health care for back pain (1,14) is closely linked to the emergence of the specialty of orthopedics. Three key ideas from the early to mid 19th century came to dominate the modern management of spinal conditions:

- Back pain is an injury (prior to that time back pain was considered one of the common aches and pains of life)
- Back pain comes from the spine and involves the nervous system (previously it was a muscular or "rheumatic" condition)
- Therapeutic rest (previously some patients might go to "the sick bed," but that was seen as a consequence of illness and not a treatment)

Early orthopedics was mainly about childhood deformities, and orthopedics first took an interest in sciatica because of sciatic scoliosis. In the second half of the 19th century, interest in spinal deformities spread to sciatica and back pain and began to focus on the spine. Previously, back pain and sciatica were regarded as separate conditions, but from that time they were linked in the spine. Ever since, there has been confusion and a lack of clear distinction between the concepts of back pain and sciatica.

The discovery of X-rays opened up a whole new perspective. For the first time it was possible to visualize the spine during life. Soon, every incidental radiographical finding became an explanation for back pain and sciatica—for example, lumbosacral anomalies, facet joint degeneration, and sacroiliac disease. So the 1920s and early 1930s saw a spate of operations to correct these anomalies by sacroiliac fusion, lumbosacral fusion, transversectomy, and facetectomy. (Which may now seem ridiculous, but how will future generations look on our current operations on MRIs?)

Hugh Owen Thomas (1834–1891), the father of English orthopedics, introduced the concept of therapeutic rest, which must be "enforced, uninterrupted and prolonged" and could be achieved by bracing, by bed rest, or later by surgical fusion. Rest became one of the main orthopedic principles for the treatment of fractures, tuberculosis, and joint infection, which was quite reasonable in the days before antibiotics and modern surgery.

TABLE 26.1. *Popular U.S. myths about health care for back problems (after Deyo)*

- Everyone with back pain should have an x-ray of their spine.
- X-rays, CT, and MRI scans can identify the cause of the pain.
- If you have a slipped disk, you need surgery.
- High-tech medicine should be able to fix the problem.

When orthopedics took over the management of sciatica and then back pain, and really did not know how to treat them, it applied its standard principle of rest. From 1900 to the 1990s, orthopedic textbooks advised treatment of acute back pain with bed rest or in a plaster jacket for weeks on end. Modern evidence shows this was not only ineffective, it actually delayed recovery (6). Previously, people with back pain had continued their daily lives and normal activities. Medicine now transformed back pain into a serious disease, the sufferer became a patient, and management actually prescribed disability.

The discovery of "the ruptured disc" (9) brought together these ideas and made them into a marketable package: back pain is an injury, an injury to the spine that involves the nervous system, and a mechanical problem that should be treated according to orthopedic principles. If all else fails, it can be fixed by surgery. For the next 50 years the disc dominated medical thinking about back pain: "the dynasty of the disc." There was rapid growth in disc surgery, closely related to the growth of orthopedics and neurosurgery. Disc surgery has survived the test of time because 80% to 90% of carefully selected patients get good relief from sciatica. But the rapid growth of disc surgery soon exposed its limitations, and it was gradually acknowledged that disc prolapse accounts for less than 5% of all back problems.

Not to be daunted, orthopedic surgeons extended the concept of "disc lesions." If sciatica is caused by disc prolapse, then perhaps back pain might be caused by "disc degeneration," so the answer is spinal fusion. This reestablished the role of surgery and the influence of spinal surgeons in the management of back pain. In the last decade, the introduction of MRI with its myriad incidental, age-related findings and totally seductive images has provided an exponential boost to this thinking (10). The introduction of high-tech medicine and commercial interests has only compounded the problem.

There is a separate debate about the efficacy of spinal surgery, but however important that may be, it only applies to a small minority of patients. Much more important for the present argument, this whole approach has gravely distorted health care for the 99% of people with back trouble who do not have a surgical condition. It leads to back pain being seen as a mechanical or structural problem, so patients expect to be fixed: just like taking their car to a mechanic, it is the doctor's or the therapist's job to fix their back. By the time patients discover there is no magic cure for back pain, they are trapped. They are no longer healthy people with back pain but have become patients with a serious back injury or irreversible degeneration, and totally unrealistic expectations (Table 26.1). Not only is this whole system harmful to many patients, it has diverted resources from research and management of the real problem of back pain.

MODERN EVIDENCE-BASED TREATMENT FOR BACK PAIN

There is now a solid evidence base for the better management of acute and subacute low back pain (4,10). This has led to a complete reversal of management, from the traditional negative strategy of rest to a more positive strategy of advising and supporting patients to remain active and continue their ordinary daily activities as normally as possible.

TABLE 26.2. *Clinical guidelines for acute low back pain*

- Exclude serious disease.
- Provide reassurance.
- Provide simple symptomatic measures.
- Avoid overinvestigation, labeling, and medicalization.
- Continue ordinary activities as normally as possible.
- Advise early return to work.
- 4–6 weeks: Recommend intensive reactivation and rehabilitation.

There are now clinical guidelines in most developed countries, with common messages (Table 26.2) (7,11).

After diagnostic triage, management of nonspecific low back pain is very basic, the main priorities being to provide symptomatic relief, help patients get on with their lives, and avoid turning an everyday bodily symptom into a medical disaster. It is not high-tech medicine or rocket science, but it is the basics that are hardest to get right. Back pain is a primary care problem that is most appropriately managed in primary care, and there is now evidence this can improve clinical outcomes (8,12). This has been extended into occupational health guidelines (3,13). If the basics are right, the rest follows automatically: if the basics are wrong, it becomes very difficult to correct. If patients with back pain are not getting back to their normal activities and work by about 4 to 6 weeks, then what they need is rehabilitation and occupational health, not referral for surgical investigations and opinions.

There is now evidence of a radical shift in public understanding and perceptions about back pain (2,17). There is a shift in primary care management (15–17). There is some evidence that social security and workers' compensation trends for back pain may be reversing, at least in some settings in some countries (15).

CURRENT HEALTH CARE FOR BACK PAIN

Health care for back pain is still in transition, and the debate among conflicting interests is still not resolved. Primary care management of back pain is changing (even if that still has a long way to go), but specialist management is still dominated by the surgical specialties, and that still influences professional and patient teaching, understanding, management, referrals, and expectations. There is still a serious lack of research and resources for effective rehabilitation and occupational health.

It may then be argued that it is not surgery for back pain that fails: it is the surgical approach to back pain. So-called surgical failures are really failures of our whole health care system for back pain. The solution depends on sorting out what spinal surgery can and, equally important, can not do.

Surgical investigations and interventions are effective for surgically treatable conditions such as serious spinal pathology (e.g., fracture, tumor, or infection) or for nerve root problems that fail to resolve with conservative treatment and natural history. Most specialist services are designed for these biomedical conditions, for which they generally provide a reasonable service. However, more than 90% of patients have nonspecific low back pain, which is really not a surgical condition.

Chronic low back pain and disability is a biopsychosocial problem that requires a biopsychosocial solution. A purely biomedical intervention is insufficient in itself, and management must address all of the bio–psycho–social issues. Patients with nonspecific low back pain (LBP) require:

- Accurate and up-to-date information and advice about back pain and how they should deal with it
- Simple, safe, symptomatic relief
- Support and encouragement to get on with their lives
- Those who fail to recover sufficient to (return to) work need additional support to control their symptoms and increase their activity levels
- Occupational health and rehabilitation services

Current health care services, based largely on medical specialty interests, completely fail to address these needs. That is why treatment is so ineffective (as shown by evidence-based medicine and by epidemiological and social security trends over the past 30 years) and why so many of these patients and primary care practitioners are so dissatisfied with specialist care. These services are inappropriate for the large majority of patients with nonspecific low back pain.

Even worse, many specialist consultations are positively harmful on every one of the counts just listed. Spinal surgeons can do far more harm (or good) by the explanations and advice they give to patients they do not operate on than they can by surgery itself. The word is more powerful than the scalpel. Spinal surgeons need to devote much more care and attention to what they say to patients and how they say it.

Even more fundamentally, the current approach (dominated by mechanical and orthopedic concepts) distorts how patients and most health care professionals think about and manage back pain. Instead of addressing the real biological and psychosocial issues, we search blindly and unsuccessfully for a structural "lesion" that can be "fixed." There is a lack of research to develop effective physical treatments for what is basically a physiological musculoskeletal dysfunction. There is a lack of (effective) occupational health and rehabilitation. Expensive specialist and hospital investigations and treatments also consume the largest portion of the health care dollars spent on back pain. There is much ineffective and wasteful use of health care resources for back pain, and that money could be spent more effectively in other ways.

SUMMARY

- The problem of failed spinal surgery and our failed health care system for back problems will only be solved when spinal surgeons recognize and acknowledge the difference between surgically treatable spinal disorders and nonspecific back pain.
- Surgery is not the answer for back pain, and patients with back pain are much safer to stay well away from spinal surgeons. The sooner we admit that the better.
- We must develop more appropriate (nonsurgical) services specifically designed to meet the needs of patients with ordinary backache, but that is another story for another day.

REFERENCES

1. Allan DB, Waddell G. An historical perspective on low back pain and disability. Acta Orthop Scand 1989; 60(suppl 234):1-23.
2. Buchinder R, Jolley D, Wyatt M. Population based intervention to change back pain beliefs and disability: three part evaluation. Brit Med J 2001; 322:1516-20.
3. Carter JT, Birrell LN (eds.). Occupational health guidelines for the management of low back pain. London: Faculty of Occupational Medicine, 2000. www.facoccmed.ac.uk.

4. Cochrane reviews on back pain. The Cochrane Library. Oxford: Update Software. www.cochrane.iwh.on.ca.

5. De Palma AF, Rothman RH. The intervertebral disc. Philadelphia: WB Saunders, 1970.

6. Hagen KB, Hilde G, Jamtvedt G, Winnem M. Bed rest for acute low back pain and sciatica (Cochrane Review). In: The Cochrane Library, Issue 4, 2000. Oxford: Update Software. Also in Spine 2000; 25:2932-9.

7. Koes BW, van Tulder MW, Ostelo R, Burton AK, Waddell G. Clinical guidelines for the management of low back pain in primary care: an international comparison. Spine 2001; 26:2504-13.

8. McGuirk B, King W, Govind J, Lowry J, Bogduk N. The safety, efficacy and cost-effectiveness of evidence-based guidelines for the management of acute low back pain in primary care. Spine 2001; 26:2615-22.

9. Mixter WJ, Barr JS. Rupture of the intervertebral disc with involvement of the spinal canal. N Engl J Med 1934; 211:210-15.

10. Nachemson A, Jonsson E. (eds.). Neck and back pain: the scientific evidence of causes, diagnosis and treatment. Philadelphia: Lippincott, Williams and Wilkins, 2000.

11. RCGP. Clinical guidelines for the management of acute low back pain. London: Royal College of General Practitioners, 1999. www.rcgp.org.uk.

12. Rossignol M, Abenhaim L, Seguin P, et al. Co-ordination of primary health care for back pain: a randomized controlled trial. Spine 2000; 25:251-9.

13. Staal JB, Hlobil H, van Tulder MW, et al. Occupational health guidelines for the management of low back pain: an international comparison. Occup Environ Med 2003; 60:618–26.

14. Waddell G. The back pain revolution. Edinburgh: Churchill Livingstone, 1998. (Note: New edition early 2004.)

15. Waddell G. Recent developments in low back pain: UK 1994-2001. IASP Refresher Course. World Congress on Pain, San Diego. IASP Press, Seattle, August 2002.

16. Waddell G, Aylward M, Sawney P. Low back pain, disability and social security benefits: an international literature and analysis. London: Royal Society of Medicine Press, 2002.

17. Working Backs Scotland. Edinburgh: Health Education Board of Scotland, 2003. www.workingbacksscotland.com.

27

Costs and Effects of Radiofrequency Techniques Integrated in a Multidisciplinary Approach to Low Back Pain

Jan Van Zundert

INTRODUCTION

The management of chronic low back pain represents a major challenge because of its aspecific and complex character. The available treatment options can be subdivided into three major categories: conservative (pharmacological and physical treatment), interventional, and surgical management techniques. Interventional and surgical techniques are only contemplated when pharmacological treatment supplemented with physical exercise failed to provide adequate relief or induced too many side effects. In an area of evidence-based medicine (EBM), the available level of evidence should guide our therapeutic choices. It needs to be said that newer treatment options are often expensive, and their uncontrolled use poses extra constraints on health care budgets. Pharmacoeconomic evaluations are now mandatory for new drugs; those studies are often an integrated part of the product development strategy.

The evaluation of the efficacy, safety, and cost effectiveness of interventional pain management in randomized controlled trials (RCTs) faces several difficulties, however. One of the most important burdens is the fact that the comparator in a double-blind study is a sham intervention, which can, ethically speaking, hardly be offered to patients suffering unbearable pain. Measuring the economic impact of a given interventional treatment option should include a comparison with the currently used golden standard and requires long-term follow-up of parallel groups, an artificial situation that does not reflect daily clinical practice and is often subject to a selection bias. Some of those interventional techniques have been used extensively to the benefit of numerous patients. Treatment outcomes have been documented in case reports, retrospective analysis of patient records and prospective studies, and even in RCTs. Although EBM is a wonderful tool, helping physicians to make the right treatment decision, and pharmacoeconomic studies provide health care funding institutions with a sound basis for judging the cost effectiveness, a broader approach for evaluating the value of interventional treatment options is recommended.

AN ALGORITHM FOR THE MANAGEMENT OF LOW BACK PAIN

The multidisciplinary approach of chronic pain was advocated as an alternative to the traditional fragmented approach (1). In the majority of patients suffering chronic low back pain, no definite etiology can be identified and treatment of the underlying disease is impossible (2). Pain is now accepted as a disease on its own, requiring a multidisciplinary

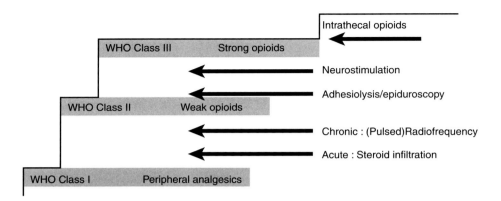

Ongoing Multi-Disciplinary approach:
• Adjuvant analgesics
• Psychologic counselling
• Physical therapy
• Evaluation of causal diagnosis/treatment

FIG. 27.1. Schematic representation of the stepwise approach of chronic low back pain, suggesting progressive use of more invasive therapies within a multidisciplinary setting.

evaluation and elaboration of a treatment scheme whereby the physical, psychological, and cognitive behavior treatment constitute an integral part of the global patient's management. The stepwise approach is represented in Figure 27.1. On a theoretical basis, patients should receive progressively increasingly invasive treatment options until optimal pain control is achieved. In practice, however, attempts are made to identify the causative structure, and treatment will be chosen based on the causative structure and the specificity of the technique.

RADIOFREQUENCY TREATMENT FOR LOW BACK PAIN

Radiofrequency (RF) treatment is considered a minimal invasive percutaneous technique whereby a high-frequency current passes through a carefully positioned insulated needle. The circuit is closed with a ground plate applied to one of the patient's extremities. The friction of the molecules at the electrode tip induces a temperature increase in the surrounding nervous tissue. The mode of action of RF treatment is not completely elucidated yet. Several observations indicate that the heat induction is not the primary mechanism involved. The correct positioning of the needle is controlled by (a) fluoroscopy for correct anatomical location, (b) physiological differentiation of sensorial and motoric stimulation levels, and (c) impedance control. Mechanical low back pain may be attributable to the zygapophyseal joints, the intravertebral disc, and the sacroiliac joint (3).

Radiofrequency percutaneous facet denervation (RF-PFD) has been described in retrospective, prospective, and randomized controlled trials. The RCTs reported by Gallagher et al. and van Kleef et al. (4,5) show a good pain relief lasting up to 6 and 12 months, respectively. The third study from Leclaire et al. (6) did not conclude that RF-PFD is efficacious in the treatment of chronic low back pain. A closer analysis of the patients' selection criteria highlights that in the first two reports the imperative diagnostic blocks with local anesthetic are performed at the level of the medial branches of the distal portions of the spinal posterior rami nerves, whereas in the third study local anesthetic is injected into the facet joint, which may lead to a high level of false-positive results. This suspicion is supported by the fact that 92% of the screened patients were included in the study, although the prevalence of facet pain is only estimated at 10% to 20% (3). These findings clearly indicate that the degree of success of this technique depends a great deal on the accuracy of the diagnosis and subdiagnosis of the causative structure.

Discogenic pain constitutes the most important part of mechanical chronic low back pain. Fine unmyelinated and small myelinated nerve fibers can be demonstrated in the intervertebral disc.

The radiofrequency treatment using SMK electrodes only yielded positive results in the first pilot study (7). These could not be confirmed in the RCT from the same group (8) and even increasing the duration of the treatment from 120s to 360s did not provide accurate pain reduction (9). Flexible catheters are proposed for introduction in the nucleus of the disc. This approach has been documented in a prospective outcome study to provide improvement in 71% of the patients 16 months after the intervention (10). In a placebo-controlled trial, intradiscal electrothermal therapy suggests a positive effect in a well-selected patient population (11).

Sacroiliac (SI) joint pain may result from sacroiliitis (Bechterew's disease), infections, spondylarthropathy, pyogenic or crystal arthropathy, fracture of the sacrum and pelvis, and diastasis (12). Primary pain emanating from the SI joint in the absence of demonstrable pathology is thought to be of mechanical origin and termed a sacroiliac syndrome. RF treatment of the SI joint has been documented in a first pilot study illustrating more than 50% pain reduction in approximately half the patients (13). In a retrospective audit, Yin et al. (14) noted successful outcome in 64% of the patients who underwent sensory stimulation-guided sacral lateral branch RF neurotomy after dual analgesic sacroiliac joint deep interosseous ligament analgesic testing.

Radicular pain irradiating in the leg is called sciatica and has to be differentiated from the earlier described mechanical pain. RF treatment adjacent to the dorsal root ganglion (DRG) in patients suffering radicular pain has been described in prospective and retrospective studies, indicating beneficial outcome in 38% to 76% of the patients (15–17). The RCT conducted by Geurts could not demonstrate an advantage of RF-DRG over sham treatment with local anesthetic (18).

VALUE OF THE EVIDENCE OF RF TREATMENT IN CLINICAL DECISION MAKING

The constant search for the best choice in treatment options, together with the request from policy makers to provide proof of efficacy and safety as well as economic advantages, has stimulated the search for the best evidence allowing clinicians to select the most appropriate treatment option. The practice of EBM consists of integrating the personal clinical expertise and the best available external evidence from systematic research (19). The systematic review on the efficacy of RF treatment from Geurts et al. (20) found "insufficient evidence supporting the effectiveness of most RF treatments for spinal pain" because the trials were underpowered or of poor design. Curiously, although chronic pain is a major public health problem, it is widely undertreated, and part of this phenomenon can be attributed to lack of convincing evidence, particularly for invasive procedures (21).

Generating reliable data on interventional pain management procedures is complicated by (a) the fact that these procedures are only considered for patients suffering pain refractory to conventional treatment and offering a placebo or sham intervention can be considered as unethical, (b) the sham intervention can activate the same receptors as the active procedure, thus questioning the value of the placebo control, and (c) the time required to recruit a sufficiently large patient population according to stringent selection criteria required for reaching statistical significant conclusions. The last point was illustrated in the RCT evaluating the efficacy of RF-DRG for the management of radicular lumbar pain (18).

During the last 4 to 6.5 years, 1,001 patients with chronic low back pain were screened, and only 80 completed the trial. The largest number of patients excluded for this trial had back pain equal to or worse than leg pain, which is common in daily practice (21). If the current enthusiasm for EBM were to result in no clinical intervention being offered (or reimbursed) until and unless it has a strong evidentiary basis, this would be unfortunate (23), leaving the vast majority of patients we see every day without further treatment. Leaders in evidence-based pain medicine have emphasized that EBM offers "tools not rules" (23). For these reasons we strongly advocate considering a disease within a broader perspective and offering multidisciplinary management after multidisciplinary patient evaluation and consultation.

COST-EFFECTIVENESS EVALUATION OF MULTIDISCIPLINARY MANAGEMENT OF CHRONIC (LOW) BACK PAIN

Several types of economic evaluations provide an idea of how the cost of a given treatment compare. We list cost-minimization analysis (CMA), cost-benefit analysis (CBA), cost-effectiveness analysis (CEA), or cost-utility analysis (CUA) (24). Ideally economic evaluation should be incorporated in the protocol for the RCTs. Those evaluations provide a solid base for judging on the benefit offered by a novel pharmacological treatment because the new treatment can be compared in a blinded way to the "best alternative." This comparison is very difficult, however, when dealing with interventional pain management techniques because (a) the sham intervention requires the same equipment as the real intervention and consequently is as expensive, (b) comparison with the "best alternative" means comparing interventional treatment with pharmacological and physical treatment where blinding is impossible, and (c) the complexity of the pathology requires a stepwise approach within a multidisciplinary setting. Medical technology assessment (MTA) may be a better alternative to the evaluation methods just described (25). In MTA, careful and systematic evaluation and linkage of the numerous facets of a health care issue are important to determine its full impact and assess the state of the art and the rational use of health care services, in order to finally support and guide medical decision making (26). The conceptual framework to structure the different aspects was introduced by Tugwell (27), including etiology, quantification of the burden of illness, assessment of therapeutic effectiveness, and economic evaluation of therapies (Fig. 27.2).

With this philosophy in mind, we studied the question "Are the higher costs involved with the multidisciplinary management of low back pain as compared to the fragmented approach justified by a reduction of the costs for society?"

Incidence and Prevalence of Low Back Pain in Belgium

In a prevalence survey (28), a representative sample of the Belgian population was questioned regarding the occurrence of low back pain during the past 6 months, indicating that 6% of the population suffers chronic low back pain and extrapolated 176,400 patients, or

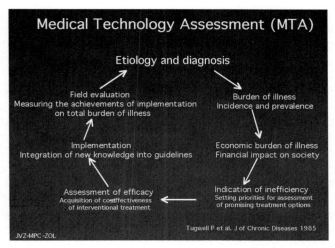

FIG. 27.2. Iterative loop of medical technology assessment. (Reproduced with permission from Tugwell P et al., J Chron Dis 1985.)

17.6 patients per 1,000 inhabitants. These data concur with the epidemiological data from other countries described in the literature. It has been demonstrated that this group uses 75% of the total health care budget for the management of low back pain (29,30).

Economic Costs of Low Back Pain in Belgium

Employers are legally obliged to continue to pay the salary of employees on sick leave. Data from IDEWE (Externe Dienst voor Preventie en Bescherming op het Werk) (31) indicate that 29% of the total number of days sick leave are attributable to low back pain. Although no costs for replacement of the sick employee could be calculated, the total costs for employers and RIZIV amount yearly to €992.6 million. In Belgium yearly, 5.7 million days of absenteeism are paid because of low back pain. The information regarding the loss of income for the patient costs for assistance and supportive tools and the costs of care by family and relatives is not available and could not be taken into consideration.

Treatment Costs of Low Back Pain

Pharmacological treatment consists of non-narcotic analgesics, nonsteroidal antiinflammatory drugs (NSAIDs), and narcotics. IMS data allowed tracking the number of prescriptions issued for low back pain within the different therapeutical classes. The NSAIDs are the most frequently used drugs in this indication with over 1.2 million prescriptions yearly. We estimated that during a doctor's visit, two products were prescribed, adding a budget of €14.5 million to the €20.1 million for the drugs. The total budget of €34.7 million for the pharmacological treatment of low back pain is underestimated because the use of coanalgesics (antidepressants and antiepileptics) for the management of neuropathic pain could not be traced. Even so, the use of over-the-counter painkillers for low back pain is not listed as such in the available data sources.

Physical therapy and revalidation is considered to be the second step in the conservative management of low back pain. In 1999 there were 3 million physiotherapeutic consultations and 41 million consultations done by kinesiotherapists. A point prevalence study (personal communication with KUL Stappaerts, 1999) indicated that 80% of the consultations of kinesiotherapists are done for the locomotor apparatus in analogy with other treatment options. We attributed 70% of the consultations done for pain emanating from the spine to the lower spine. The total cost is estimated at €114.5 million.

Transcutaneous electrical nerve stimulation (TENS) consists of the application of electrodes on the painful area of the skin connected to a pulse generator, a portable device driven by batteries. The physician prescribes the treatment, but a paramedic does the application, testing, and programming. The patient can buy the device after a positive test period. A survey conducted in the Ziekenhuis Oost-Limburg (S. Maninfior, 2000) indicated that 55% of the TENS apparatus are used for the management of low back pain, which means that of the 2,000 machines sold yearly in Belgium, 1,100 are used for low back pain. The test usually requires three consultations. The price of the generator is €297; the electrodes costs €124 annually. The global cost for TENS treatment amounts to €514,769.

The objective of epidural steroid administration is to reduce the inflammation by injecting the drug as close as possible to the causative structure in the epidural space. The intervention is mostly done in a day-care hospital. A survey indicated that in Belgium 50,000 epidural steroid injections are performed yearly and each treatment consists of 2.4 infiltrations (32). Considering that 70% of the interventions are done for the management of low back pain, we estimate that 14,583 patients receive a treatment cycle with epidural steroids. Each treatment cycle starts with an intake consultation, and the patient is seen once after finishing the treatment. The costs of this treatment option can be split into honoraria, day-care hospital fixed budget, medication, and consultation amounting to a total of €4.6 million.

Radiofrequency treatment was used for the treatment of 2,040 patients in 1999. The code does not allow splitting between the different techniques and approaches of other target nerves, obliging us to use the 70%/30% distribution for low back pain. The costs for this management consist of specialists' honoraria, medication, fixed budget for the day-care hospital or hospitalization cost and the medical consultations, and the cost for the diagnostic proof blocks. In Belgium, radiofrequency treatment costs €394,434.

It needs to be said that performing radiofrequency treatment requires an investment in equipment, the generator, and the thermocouple electrodes. The global yearly investment for Belgium based on the sales figures from the producers is estimated to be €178,483. Those investments are currently completely carried by the hospital. The reimbursement of those investments should be obtained from the contribution of the day care and the specialists' honoraria. The low level of the honoraria does not cover those expenses.

Surgery is indicated for decompression of disc herniation in case the patient shows neurological deficit and for patients with degenerative disease of the lumbar spine associated with instability, spinal stenosis, and degenerative spondyloslisthesis. There are two types of spinal surgery, with and without arthrodesis. Arthrodesis uses implants for fusion of two or more vertebrae.

Surgery without arthrodesis was performed 12,899 times in 1999. The total duration of hospital stay was 138,587 days, and each surgical intervention required four medical consultations. The total cost for surgery of the lumbar spine without arthrodesis amounts to €39.3 million.

Surgery with arthrodesis was performed 3,198 times. Besides the costs of hospitalization and consultation, the cost for the implants for a total budget of €8.3 million needs to be considered. The health care budget attributed to surgery with arthrodesis is €21.1 million.

Note: In the global surgery budget for the management of low back pain, the medications used during surgery and the patient contribution is not included.

Epidural neurostimulation is based on the gate theory (33) whereby electrodes are applied to the dorsal column and connected to an implanted pulsed generator. Permanent implantation is preceded by a proof period. The best results are obtained in the management of pain restricted to well-delineated regions. Epidural neurostimulation is reimbursed in Belgium for the management of the failed back surgery syndrome (FBSS).

The cost components of a treatment with epidural neurostimulation are evaluation, epidural implantation of the electrodes for the proof stimulation, the proof period, the permanent implantation, hospitalization, the costs of implanted electrodes that do not result in a permanent implantation (negative electrodes), the price of the stimulator, doctors' and psychiatrists' consultation, and the patient contribution. In Belgium there were 233 neurostimulator implantations for FBSS in 1999, and one third of the cases were replacements. The total cost was €2.1 million.

The intrathecal administration of medication using an implanted pump has the advantage that the opioids bind directly to the opioid receptors of the dorsal column, thus requiring lower doses for pain relief. In case of chronic pain management, an implanted intrathecal catheter connected to an implanted infusion pump provides the intrathecal administration. Permanent implantation is also preceded by a proof period with an external pump. During this proof period, the mode of delivery and the combination and dose of medication is adjusted to achieve optimal pain control. In 1999, 137 pumps were implanted in Belgium and we assume 60% were used for the management of FBSS; thus 82 pumps were implanted for the management of low back pain. As with the neurostimulator, the patient pays a personal contribution for the material. The total cost for the management of low back pain with implantable pumps is €573,309. It must be mentioned that patients return regularly to the pain center for refilling of the pump. Cost of the medication and the consultation could not be evaluated because of the variability in drug cocktails and dose.

Cognitive behavioral treatment is considered effective in the management of certain types of patients suffering low back pain. The frequency of use and the cost of this treatment option could not be evaluated because there is no official registration for this treatment option.

The global cost for the management of low back pain in Belgium is illustrated in Table 27.1. Those figures underestimate the real cost because of the following facts:

- The personal contribution of the patient could not be completely traced.
- The budget spent on alternative treatments is not listed.
- The costs of psychological treatment could not be evaluated.

TABLE 27.1. *Overview of the cost of treatment of low back pain in Belgium in 1999*

	Total cost € × 10^3	% Cost
Total conservative treatments	149,759	80.08
Medication	34,717	18.56
Revalidation	114,528	61.24
TENS	515	0.28
Total conservative treatments	149,759	80.08
Total interventional treatments	7,707	4.12
Total surgery	29,539	15.80
Total	**187,005**	

TABLE 27.2. *Overview of the cost of invasive pain management in Belgium in 1999 (inclusive of TENS)*

	Number of patients	Total Cost $€ \times 10^3$	% Cost	Cost per patient $€$
TENS	1,100	515	1.36	468
Epidural steroid injections	14,583	4,605	12.20	316
Radiofrequency treatments	1,428	394	1.04	276
Epidural neuromodulation	233	2,134	5.65	9,160
Intrathecal drug administration	82	573	1.52	6,992
Surgery without arthrodesis	12,899	8,448	22.73	655
Surgery with arthrodesis	3,198	21,091	55.85	6,595
Total	**33,523**	**187,005**		

- The description of the different (interventional) pain management techniques is not accurate in the official registry.
- The management of chronic low back pain following accidents on the workplace is not accounted for in the official statistics.

The interventional treatment options account for approximately 20% of the total budget spent on the management of low back pain, and 85% is attributed to surgery. The distribution of the costs for interventional pain management is illustrated in Table 27.2.

Close analysis of these data points to the fragmented use of the different treatment options. Algorithms for the management of chronic pain clearly prefer the use of the least invasive and least expensive procedures first. Only when those treatment options fail are the more invasive and more expensive treatments envisioned. The more invasive procedures should be used in a multidimensional environment with sufficient attention to psychosocial counseling and revalidation.

During the last decade, more attention has been paid to the multidisciplinary management of low back pain. According to Waddel (34),

An historic review shows that there is no change in the pathology or prevalence of low back pain in the United States and the United Kingdom, although neither delivers the kind of care recommended by recent evidence based guidelines. Medical care for low back pain in the United States is specialist-oriented, of high technology, and of high cost, but 40% of American patients seek chiropractic care for low back pain instead. Despite the different health care systems, treatment availability, and costs, there seems to be little difference in clinical outcomes or the social impact of low back pain in the two countries. There is growing dissatisfaction with health care for low back pain on both sides of the Atlantic. Future health care for patients with nonspecific low back pain should be designed to meet their specific needs.

This describes precisely the role of the multidisciplinary pain centers. Waddel's remarks, comparing pain management with two completely different health care systems, led to comparing the costs for managing low back pain in Belgium with those from The Netherlands. The authorities demonstrated a high interest in chronic pain, advocating and funding the development of multidisciplinary pain centers. The use of interventional pain management techniques is reimbursed in well-defined protocols. Those initiatives led to a structured and coordinated approach of chronic pain within a multidimensional environment. The comparison of the frequency of use of the different techniques between the two countries is illustrated in Table 27.3.

TABLE 27.3. *Comparison of the number of treatments for low back pain in Belgium (Belg) and in The Netherlands (NL)*

	Total no. Belg	Total no. NL	No. per 1,000 inhabitants Belg	No. per 1,000 inhabitants NL	Ratio Belg: NL
Medication	1,883,000	1,784,527	188,30	118.97	1.6:1
TENS	1,100	5,000	0,11	0.33	**1:3**
Epidural steroids	35,000	17,640	3,50	0.48	3.3:1
Radiofrequency	1,428	6,011	0,14	0.40	**1.2:8**
Epidural neurostimulation	233	89	0,02	0.01	3.9:1
Intrathecal drug administration	82	32	0,01	0.00	3.8:1
Surgery without arthrodesis	12,899	3,528	1,29	0.24	5.5:1
Surgery with arthrodesis	3,198	1,851	0,32	0.12	2.6:1

We notice that the use of medication is 33% lower in The Netherlands than in Belgium. The exact figures regarding physical therapy and kinesiotherapy could not be obtained. In view of a stepwise approach whereby conservative treatment options should be used to the point that no additional benefit can be expected, there is only reimbursement for nine kinesiotherapeutic sessions for the management of low back pain.

Among the interventional treatment modalities, TENS and radiofrequency are used three times more often in The Netherlands. It needs to be mentioned that in The Netherlands TENS is reimbursed, which is not the case in Belgium, and radiofrequency treatment is not correctly financed in Belgium. The epidural steroid administration is more frequently used in Belgium than in The Netherlands. In The Netherlands the major part of epidural steroid administrations is done with the transforaminal approach under fluoroscopic guidance (nerve root infiltration).

The biggest difference is seen in the frequency of surgical interventions. Per 1,000 inhabitants, the number of surgical interventions without arthrodesis is 19% of the number in Belgium and the surgical interventions with arthrodesis in The Netherlands is 37% of the number in Belgium. This has a direct consequence on the use of neuromodulation techniques, which are mainly indicated for the management of low back pain attributable to failed back surgery syndrome. The more frequent use of those interventional techniques is responsible for a €21.9 million higher cost in Belgium. The costs for the therapeutic options that could be calculated for both countries are €72.5 million for Belgium, which is theoretically €36.2 million more expensive than in The Netherlands.

SUMMARY

Chronic low back pain is a complex, multidimensional problem requiring a multidisciplinary evaluation and management. The newer interventional treatment modalities offer new perspectives for patients suffering pain refractory to conventional treatment. Frequently proposed treatment algorithms point toward a progressive and integrated use of the least invasive interventions before moving on to more invasive techniques. The cost analysis clearly indicates that minimal invasive techniques, such as radiofrequency treatment, are less expensive, and their appropriate use may prevent the need for more invasive and more expensive techniques.

ACKNOWLEDGMENTS

The author wants to express his gratitude to Professor K. Kesteloot (Katholieke Universiteit Leuven) for the support and guidance with his dissertation "Cost and Effects of a Multidisciplinary Approach of (Chronic) Low Back Pain." He also thanks Nicole Van den Hecke for the administrative support and coordination of this manuscript and the original dissertation.

REFERENCES

1. Flor H, Fydrich T, Turk DC. Efficacy of multidisciplinary pain treatment centers: a meta-analytic review. Pain 1992;49:221-30.
2. Spitzer W. Report on Quebeck Task force on low back pain. Spine 1987;12:S1-S59.
3. Schwarzer AC, Wang SC, O'Driscoll D, Harrington T, Bogduk N, Laurent R. The ability of computed tomography to identify a painful zygapophyseal joint in patients with chronic low back pain. Spine 1995;20: 907-12.
4. Gallagher J, Vadi PLP, Wesley JR. Radiofrequency facet joint denervation in the treatment of low back pain—a prospective controlled double-blind study in assess to efficacy. Pain Clinic 1994;7:193-8.
5. van Kleef M, Barendse GA, Kessels F, Voets HM, Weber WE, de Lange S. Randomized trial of radiofrequency lumbar facet denervation for chronic low back pain. Spine 1999;24: 1937-42.
6. Leclaire R, Fortin L, Lambert R, Bergeron YM, Rossignol M. Radiofrequency facet denervation in the treatment of low back pain: a placebo-controlled clinical trial to assess efficacy. Spine 2001;26:1411-6.
7. van Kleef M, Barendse G, Wilmink JT, Lousberg R, Bulstra SK, Weber WE, Sluijter ME. Percutaneous intradiscal radio-frequency thermocoagulation in chronic non-specific low back pain. Pain Clinic 1996;9:259-68.
8. Barendse G, Berg SGv, Kessels F, Weber WE, van Kleef M. Randomized controlled trial of percutaneous intradiscal radiofrequency thermocoagulation for chronic discogenic back pain: lack of effect form a 90-second 70°C lesion. Spine 2001;26:287-92.
9. Ercelen O, Bulutcu E, Oktenoglu T, Sasani M, Bozkus H, Cetin Saryoglu A, Ozer F. Radiofrequency lesioning using two different time modalities for the treatment of lumbar discogenic pain: a randomized trial. Spine 2003;28:1922-7.
10. Saal JA, Saal JS. Intradiscal electrothermal treatment for chronic discogenic low back pain: a prospective outcome study with minimum 1-year follow-up. Spine 2000;25:2622-7.
11. Pauza KJ, Howell S, Dreyfuss P, Peloza JH, Dawson K, Bogduk N. A randomized, placebo-controlled trial of intradiscal electrothermal therapy for the treatment of discogenic low back pain. Spine J 2004;4:27-35.
12. Ferrante FM, King LF, Roche SA, Kim PS, Aranda M, Delaney LR, Mardini IA, Mannes AJ. Radiofrequency sacroiliac joint denervation for sacroiliac syndrome. Reg Anesth Pain Med 2001;26:137-42.
13. Cohen SP, Abdi S. Lateral branch blocks as a treatment for sacroiliac joint pain: a pilot study. Reg Anesth Pain Med 2003;28:113-9.
14. Yin W, Willard F, Carreiro J, Dreyfuss P. Sensory stimulation-guided sacroiliac joint radiofrequency neurotomy: technique based on neuroanatomy of the dorsal sacral plexus. Spine 2003;28:2419-25.
15. Sluijter ME, Metha M (eds.). Treatment of chronic back and neck pain by percutaneous thermal lesions, in persistent pain, modern methods of treatment. London: Academic Press, 1981.
16. Nash TP. Percutaneous radiofrequency lesioning of dorsal root ganglia for intractable pain. Pain 1986;24:67-73.
17. van Wijk RM, Geurts JW, Wynne HJ. Long-lasting analgesic effect of radiofrequency treatment of the lumbosacral dorsal root ganglion. J Neurosurg 2001;94:227-31.
18. Geurts JWM, van Wijk RM, Wynne HJ, Hammink E, Buskens E, Lousberg R, Knape JT, Groen GJ. Radiofrequency lesioning of dorsal root ganglia for chronic lumbosacral radicular pain. A randomised, double blind, controlled trial. Lancet 2003;361:21-6.
19. Sackett DL, Richardson WS, Rosenberg W. Evidence-based medicine: what it is and what it isn't. BMJ 1997;312:71-2.
20. Geurts J, van Wijk RM, Stolker R, Groen GJ. Efficacy of radiofrequency procedures for the treatment of spinal pain: a systematic review of randomized clinical trials. Reg Anesth Pain Med 2001;26:394-400.
21. Carr DB, Goudas LC. Burning questions, randomized controlled trials, and the pain doctor's dilemma. Reg Anesth Pain Med 2003;28:360-1.
22. Petrovic P, Kalso E, Peterson KM, Ingvar M. Placebo and opioid analgesia—imaging a shared neuronal network. Science 2002;295:1737-40.
23. Carr DB, Goudas LC. Evidence-based pain medicine: the good, the bad, and the ugly. Reg Anesth Pain Med 2001;26:389-93.
24. Drummond MF (ed.). Methods for the economic evaluation of health care programmes (2nd ed.). Oxford, UK: Oxford University Press, 1997.
25. Goossens MEJB (ed.). Economic evaluation of cognitive behavioral rehabilitation for chronic musculoskeletal pain. Doctoral thesis, Amsterdam University, Amsterdam,1999.
26. Lawrence VA, Tugwell P, Gafni A, Kosuwon W, Spitzer WO. Acute low back pain and economics of therapy: the iterative loop approach. J Clin Epidemiol 1992;45:301-11.
27. Tugwell P, Bennett K, Sackett DL, Haynes RB. The measurement iterative loop: a framework for the critical appraisal of need, benefits and costs of health care interventions. J Chron Dis 1985;38:339-51.
28. Masquelier E, le Polain B, Vissers K, Crombez G, De Laat A. Rugpijn in België: een epidemiologische enquête. Newsletter Belgian Pain Society 2002;11.

29. Nachemson AL. Lagerugpijn—het einde van de vezorginsstaat. Toespraak bij opening van Pijn Kennis Centrum. Maastricht: Academisch Ziekenhuis, 1994.
30. Spitzer W. Scientific approach to the assessment and management of activity-related spinal disorders. Report of the Quebec Task Force on Spinal Disorders. Spine 1987;Suppl:12-7.
31. Moens G. Externe Dienst voor Preventie en Bescherming op het Werk. Brussels: IDWE, 2001.
32. Van Zundert J, Van Buyten JP. Current use of epidural corticosteroids in Belgium: results of a recent survey. Pain Digest 1999;9:228-9.
33. Wall PD. The gate control theory of pain mechanisms. A re-examination and re-statement. Brain 1978;101:1-18.
34. Waddell G. Low back pain: a twentieth century health care enigma. Spine 1996;21:2820-5.

28

Central Registration of Complications: Spine Tango—A European Spine Registry

Christoph P. Röder, Amer Ibrahim EL-Kerdi, Dieter Grob, and Max Aebi

New joint replacement registries are widely implemented across national and international organizations. The need for a continuous long-term postmarket surveillance of implants as well as surgical failures has been recognized and has become increasingly important to ensure the quality assurance of treatments and prosthetic components. Registry data with large case numbers represents an acceptable alternative to controlled randomized clinical trials, which are often difficult to conduct in orthopedic surgery. The variety of implants and procedures in spinal surgery not only represents the same need for long-term monitoring of procedures and postsurgical product performance as in the joint replacement subspecialties, but it also makes the establishment of a comprehensive spine registry for all major pathologies and interventions a must.

In cooperation with the Institute for Evaluative Research in Orthopaedic Surgery (MEM-CED) of the University of Bern, Switzerland, the Spine Society of Europe (SSE) launched Spine Tango in the fall of 2003: the first modular and multilevel European online registry for spinal surgery. Within Spine Tango, the major challenge in registry design and structure is the definition of and agreement on a core set of questions as a common European data set. Additional questions for national or individual interest can also be dynamically added to the core data set. Moreover, an automated implant tracking system was set up that allows highly precise product documentation without additional workload for clinical staff members.

INTRODUCTION

All over the world, efforts are made to set up registries on regional, state, or even national levels, and consequently the number of articles in the literature reflects the establishment and activity of all these new and young institutions (1,3,7,11,12). The Swedish hip registry is considered one of the oldest and best functioning registries. It has already proven valuable in eliminating poorly performing materials and implants and was key in changing treatment practices on an evidence-based background (4). Imitating the Swedish model, registries have been, or are now set up, in Germany (7), Canada (1), New Zealand (12), Norway (3), Finland, England, as well as in many Eastern European countries. With their focus enlarged beyond major joint replacements, such as total hip and knee arthroplasty, new registries are set up for joint replacement procedures that are less frequently performed like shoulder and elbow arthroplasties (11).

All authors stress the fact that their registry questionnaires should be considered a minimal data set in order to avoid overworking the surgeon and thus lowering response rates (3,7,12). In addition, many registries try to construct their questionnaires in such a way that data collection is rendered a team effort among operating room staff, surgeons, secretaries, and residents.

Spine surgery represents a challenge for all registry endeavors. The variety of levels, pathologies, accesses, and surgical techniques renders as failures all attempts to invent a short yet comprehensive questionnaire. Therefore, institutions that have developed questionnaires or registries have focused on certain main aspects of spinal surgery. The North American Spine Society has developed mainly patient-based questionnaires for cervical and lumbar spinal problems in addition to scoliosis (2,9). The Swedish spine registry was even named The Swedish National Register for Lumbar Spine Surgery, indicating that the focus was on lumbar pathologies and interventions only (14). As compared to older registration and documentation initiatives in other orthopedic subspecialties (6), the outcomes movement has led to a dramatic shift toward patient-based documentation (5,15). Hence the burden of answering large and detailed questionnaires was taken away from the busy clinician and put into the hand of the patient, who has been empowered with more responsibility to participate in decision making and quality assessment. What makes up a modern surgeon-based documentation system was described by one of the authors of the Swedish spine registry with three words: "simplicity, simplicity, simplicity" (personal communication).

SPINE TANGO—THE EUROPEAN INITIATIVE

Under the auspices of the SSE, a project was launched to design and implement a documentation system for spinal surgery in 2000. This effort was introduced as the "Spine Tango" and conducted in collaboration with the Institute for Evaluative Research in Orthopaedic Surgery, University of Bern, which enjoys a profound expertise in documentation and data collection because it has been hosting arguably the oldest and most detailed hip arthroplasty registry in the world, set up by Professor M. E. Müller. While its first records date back to 1968, there are currently over 48,000 primary interventions, 12,000 revisions, and roughly 71,000 follow-up controls archived in the database. Data collection took place on a voluntary basis and was standardized according to the International Documentation and Evaluation System (IDES) (10). Data was collected in over 40 hospitals in various European countries, which included Austria, Belgium, Switzerland, Germany, Great Britain, France, Italy, and The Netherlands.

The Spine Tango is the first spine registry initiative to face the challenge of developing a comprehensive questionnaire covering all major spine pathologies and interventions, as well as spanning all anatomical levels. To accomplish this task, a technically demanding computer application was an obvious prerequisite. The need for such an application coincided with the prototype release of a centralized data management technology platform developed by the MEM-CED. The decision to employ electronic technologies to enhance centralized data collection seemed obvious to the Spine Tango team, given the cumbersome and inaccurate paper-based methods utilized to date. Paper-based forms are traditionally filled in by clinical users, sent to the central data collection office, and then entered into a database using various customized local software solutions, which are sometimes optionally interfaced to optical character or mark readers. The enormous human and financial resources needed to read paper-based data, and especially to correct and complete invalid datasheets, were the driving force behind changing these outdated methods by migrating data entry technologically back to the peripheral user. All the while, new documentation features and interfaces are introduced to further alleviate the burden of registering data.

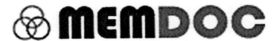

FIG. 28.1. The MEMDOC portal (www.memdoc.org).

MEDICAL IT INNOVATIONS

The MEM-CED novel documentation system is slowly being recognized as a powerful generic centralized data management application. Along with its numerous simplified tools for collecting medical, implant, radiological, and patient data, a real information technology innovation was developed. Embedded in an orthopedic technology platform called MEMDOC (Fig. 28.1), the academic online registry application currently offers a wide array of questionnaires and online tools for data collection and administration. In addition to the Spine Tango, it offers the orthopedic community the EFORT and IDES registries for total hip arthroplasty, the IDES total knee arthroplasty registry, as well as several ongoing multicenter studies for restricted user communities, which deal with spine trauma, children's fractures, brain trauma, motion-preserving spine stabilization, and other spinal implants.

Data can be collected and extracted using several complementary solutions (Fig. 28.2). The most direct method of data entry is using the online interface, but a second alternative offline solution employs handheld barcode readers. A third possibility of data collection is based on a MEMDOC proprietary online interface to traditional paper-based data registration using an optical mark reader. Regardless by which preferred method data is registered, all data is finally routed back to the online-accessible central database where the user can verify, edit, and submit data. Online validation rules guarantee that only medically and logically valid and complete data sets are submitted. Otherwise, the data set is rejected and users are warned to perform corrections. This ensures the quality and integrity of data stored in the database. Once data is submitted, it cannot be altered anymore. Various online features are in place for online data analysis to recuperate time spent for documentation. Forms can be printed out in a question-and-answer format, and soon the documented information will be available within an editable text body so the collected data can be used to create user-customizable reports and letters. Additionally, direct online-accessible real-time queries of personal user statistics and comparison with

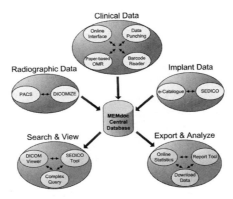

FIG. 28.2. Overview of documentation IT solution.

the data pool for benchmarking are possible. Moreover, data can be downloaded to the user's own computers for further customized statistical analysis. An online tool to upload up to six digital X-rays per documented case is also available.

Due to the nature of the doctor/patient relationship and the sensitivity of health care data, exchanging and collecting information on the Web brings with it many concerns regarding privacy and confidentiality. As such, the official security policy of the MEM-CED and the MEMDOC portal is to take every measure possible to guarantee the security and integrity of entrusted data. This is accomplished by using only ISO-compliant systems with a physically secure and segregated network setup protected by firewalls and antivirus filtering. In addition, all transfer of data is done via 128-bit encrypted channels conforming to the highest levels of security similar to those utilized in e-business solutions.

DOCMOD—THE ANSWER TO LEGAL AND PSYCHOLOGICAL ISSUES

Medical data sets crossing or getting stored outside national boundaries cause discomfort to both representatives of medical and judicial communities. Moreover, in some instances, participating physicians dislike sending their data to a central server that is neither located within their national borders nor belongs to an institution to which they are directly affiliated, even if they are legally permitted to do so. Recognizing the need for a solution to these essentially psychological and legal restraints to central data management, the MEM-CED has initiated the development of a modular documentation system called DocMod.

In addition to providing a more convincing legal framework, if any are mandated by national governments, this solution offers medical societies and hospital centers the opportunity to overtake a larger amount of administrative control and accountability over their users as well as data. This formulation involves the local hosting of a small encapsulated Web server application (Fig. 28.3) powered with a unique interface to the central database. In essence, all users and clinics opting for entrance to the centrally hosted registry or study can only gain access via the DocMod peripheral system. Although purely anonymous user and patient data sets are submitted to the MEM-CED central database,

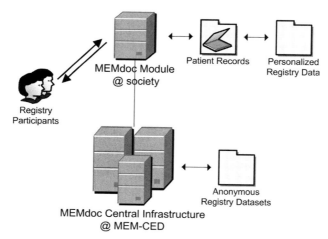

FIG. 28.3. Setup and communication of DocMod with the central infrastructure hosted at the MEM-CED.

the module maintains the hosting of all personalized user and patient information as well as receiving a complete copy of all submitted data.

A EUROPEAN REGISTRY—UNITY IN DIVERSITY

The biggest obstacle in establishing a European registry is the heterogeneity of interests and ideas regarding content and techniques of documentation. There is no doubt that the Internet represents the ideal and cheapest solution possible to network all players and to gather data sets in a central database. In addition, no costly hardware and software purchases are necessary to run or maintain the installation because system upgrades and maintenance are only conducted at the central control unit. Nevertheless, the amalgamation of different sets of questions into a single questionnaire to satisfy various European, national, and regional, or even individual needs, while still ensuring the possibility to only extract the data of interest to the respective user, remains the insurmountable obstacle of any documentation system.

In developing an online tool for a European mission, the MEM-CED has engineered an IT solution that measures up to the expected complexity of several levels of content within one and the same questionnaire. After a core data set for a European register has been adopted, each participating nation can define additional questions it would like to incorporate into its national documentation system. Participating surgeons can consequently still choose their national registry questionnaire but also fulfill European standards. Moreover, they are provided with an online tool to generate questions for their individual in-house interests. This is accomplished by introducing a new scheme of real-time retrospective and prospective documentation. In such a system, each study questionnaire is divided into subforms that best emulate the data collection work flow in hospitals (Fig. 28.4). The overwhelming advantage of such a model is that subforms can potentially be filled out by different users independently of each other, all the while validation rules built within the generic system ensure that data is logically and medically validated before submission.

Because data sharing is defined on the department level, all surgeons within this department can make use of the individually created sets of added-on questions, whereas users outside of the department or the hospital cannot see nor use these extensions. To increase flexibility and application tidiness, the various sets of additionally created questions are provided in te form of a menu of optional packages that can be actively selected and linked to the European and national questions, hence enabling the concept of multilevel documentation. The European core data is anonymously pooled at the central data collection unit, and benchmarks are created. Hospitals are given the opportunity to compare

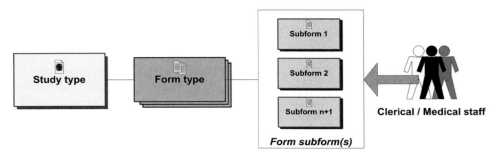

FIG. 28.4. Breakdown of study forms into sizable subforms.

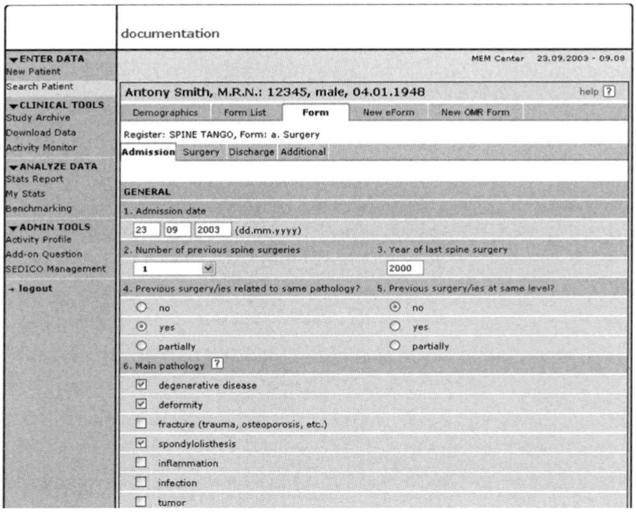

FIG. 28.5. Spine Tango admission subform.

their core parameters with the European or national averages by performing online live queries to the database. The national data sets belong to the society under whose auspices the registry was established. Only the surgeon who entered the data is able to retrieve the complete set of parameters including patient-based information.

Far more difficult then constructing this complicated IT architecture is the definition of a core data set for the various orthopedic subspecialties. Regarding a core questionnaire for the Spine Tango, an initiative was taken in cooperation with the Spine Department at the Schulthess Clinic, Zurich, Switzerland, to work out a set of questions suitable for a European spine registry. For reasons of data validation, possibilities of real-time documentation, and sharing of documentation workload, the core questions are subdivided into five subforms: admission, main pathology, surgery, surgical measures, and discharge (Fig. 28.5). Under the additional menu, several optional modules are also available: social, clinical assessment cervicothoracic, clinical assessment lumbar, imaging, functional tests and invasive imaging, and the Oswestry score. Moreover, a second intervention surgery and surgical measures subform for combined access or two-step intervention can be activated for a precise documentation of cases with two accesses or even two interventions within one hospital stay. The intention is to provide users who have an interest to document information beyond the core data set with standard add-on modules.

IMPLANT DOCUMENTATION—HIGH TECH
FOR PRECISION AND TIME SAVING

One of the main reasons for setting up joint replacement and implant registries is the fact that many implants enter the market with only laboratory testing. However, the real testing arenas for implants are the patients themselves, where all factors affecting implant performance like design, choice of materials, manufacturing issues, patient characteristics, and surgical techniques come into play (8). A minimum follow-up of 10 years is normally required to judge a joint replacement realistically as successful (13). However, many institutions that are in possession of such data can often not compare it with other authors because of the technological and content limitation of the different utilized methods of data collection and analysis.

Implants are also an essential part of modern spinal surgery, and the increased use of artificial materials over the past years makes postmarket surveillance of products as necessary as in the joint replacement sector. To finally overcome the compatibility problems of documentation techniques, parameters of interest, and consequently to follow new or questionable product and implant designs over extended postoperative periods, the MEM-CED has integrated a unique implant-tracking tool to complement the documentation system.

A major European implant producer has introduced a barcode-based implant tracking system for its own ordering and stocking purposes. The so-called SEDICO (secure data integration concept) system is marketed in an open partner concept because other large implant producers are already participating and increasingly using the new technology. All materials with article and lot numbers in barcode format are registered with a barcode scanner when they are unwrapped by the operating room (OR) staff and delivered to the surgeon. Via telephone modem, the article and lot numbers are sent to the producers for restocking. Hospitals, which are part of the fast-growing SEDICO user community and document with the MEMDOC online system, can rely on the automated background linking of article and lot numbers of implants to their documented cases.

Hence a unique and proprietary interface is in place ensuring that a copy of all implant data sets is sent independently to the registry database and made available online within minutes. As a result, not only a single product can be evaluated precisely, but also an early warning system for poorly performing implants is established because all other implants belonging to a respective production run can be recalled using the lot numbers. Users who do not want to or cannot install the SEDICO system are offered updated online product catalogs of all participating implant suppliers within the documentation system. With the search tools in place, an implant can be selected and also linked to the respective case. However, lot numbers are not registered with this implant-tracking search option.

REFERENCES

1. Bourne RB. The planning and implementation of the Canadian Joint Replacement Registry. Bull Hosp Jt Dis 1999;58(3):128-32.
2. Daltroy LH, Cats-Baril WL, Katz JN, Fossel AH, Liang MH. The North American spine society lumbar spine outcome assessment instrument: reliability and validity tests. Spine 1996;21(6):741-9.
3. Havelin LI. The Norwegian Joint Registry. Bull Hosp Jt Dis 1999;58(3):139-47.
4. Herberts P, Malchau H. How outcome studies have changed total hip arthroplasty practices in Sweden. Clin Orthop 1997;344:44-60.
5. Johanson NA. Outcomes assessment. In: JJ Callaghan, AG Rosenberg, HE Rubash (eds.), The adult hip. Philadelphia: Lippincott-Raven, 1998;853-63.
6. Johnston RC, Fitzgerald RH, Harris WH, Poss R, Muller ME, Sledge CB. Clinical and radiographic evaluation of total hip replacement. A standard system of terminology for reporting results. J Bone Joint Surg Am 1990;72(2):161-8.
7. Lang I, Willert HG. [Experiences with the German Endoprosthesis Register]. Z Arztl Fortbild Qualitatssich 2001;95(3):203-8.
8. Maloney WJ. National joint replacement registries: has the time come? J Bone Joint Surg Am 2001;83-A(10):1582-5.
9. NASS. N. A. S. S.: www.spine.org.
10. Paterson D. The International Documentation and Evaluation System (IDES). Orthopedics 1993;16(1):11-14.
11. Rahme H, Jacobsen MB, Salomonsson B. The Swedish Elbow Arthroplasty Register and the Swedish Shoulder Arthroplasty Register: two new Swedish arthroplasty registers. Acta Orthop Scand 2001;72(2): 107-12.
12. Rothwell AG. Development of the New Zealand Joint Register. Bull Hosp Jt Dis 1999;58(3):148-60.
13. Sochart DH, Long AJ, Porter ML. Joint responsibility: the need for a national arthroplasty register. BMJ 1996;313(7049):66-7.
14. Stromqvist B, Jonsson B, Fritzell P, Hagg O, Larsson BE, Lind B. The Swedish National Register for lumbar spine surgery: Swedish Society for Spinal Surgery. Acta Orthop Scand 2001;72(2):99-106.
15. Weinstein JN, Deyo RA. Clinical research: issues in data collection. Spine 2000;25(24):3104-9.

Subject Index